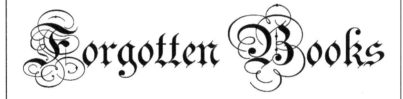

ISBN 978-1-5277-9738-3
PIBN 10899759

1 MONTH OF
FREE
READING

at

www.ForgottenBooks.com

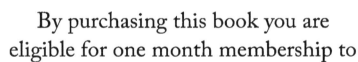

By purchasing this book you are eligible for one month membership to ForgottenBooks.com, giving you unlimited access to our entire collection of over 1,000,000 titles via our web site and mobile apps.

To claim your free month visit:

www.forgottenbooks.com/free899759

English
Français
Deutsche
Italiano
Español
Português

www.forgottenbooks.com

Mythology Photography **Fiction**
Fishing Christianity **Art** Cooking
Essays Buddhism Freemasonry
Medicine **Biology** Music **Ancient**
Egypt Evolution Carpentry Physics
Dance Geology **Mathematics** Fitness
Shakespeare **Folklore** Yoga Marketing
Confidence Immortality Biographies
Poetry **Psychology** Witchcraft
Electronics Chemistry History **Law**
Accounting **Philosophy** Anthropology
Alchemy Drama Quantum Mechanics
Atheism Sexual Health **Ancient History**
Entrepreneurship Languages Sport
Paleontology Needlework Islam
Metaphysics Investment Archaeology
Parenting Statistics Criminology
Motivational

V.

KARL PEARSON, F.R.S. *Price 5s. net.*

VI.

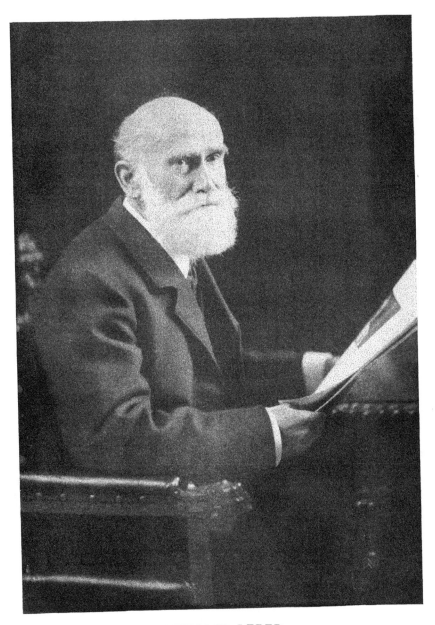

THEODOR LEBER

(1840—1917)

" Ueber hereditäre und congenital-angelegte Sehnervenleiden," 1871.

HEREDITARY OPTIC ATROPHY
(LEBER'S DISEASE)

Introductory. This condition is one of the less rare of the hereditary diseases if rarity can be measured by the number of pedigrees of the disease available; indeed no other condition provides us with a larger proportion of extensive, fully worked-out pedigrees from which to deduce the hereditary features of the disease. Material regarding hereditary optic atrophy has been slowly accumulating since 1871 when Leber published his now famous paper entitled "Ueber hereditäre und congenital-angelegte Sehnervenleiden[1]," which brought about the full recognition of the clinical features constituting the disease and its hereditary etiology. The impetus provided by this paper to the study of hereditary optic atrophy is undoubted, and has been so widely acknowledged as to lead to the frequent reference to the condition as "Leber's disease" in all countries of the world; the description of the disease there given is so complete from the point of view of its clinical features that little knowledge has since been added to that aspect of the subject, and this is surely a great testimony considering how few cases had been previously described. Leber must have relied almost entirely upon his own close observations made on nine cases only in four families, together with reports of six allied cases, and on von Graefe's account of examples of the disease in three brothers published in 1858[2]; a number of other reported possible cases are reviewed by him in his historical survey of the subject, but they are all, as he states, so incompletely described that they can be placed with no certainty in any category. To give an example of the inadequacy of these earlier accounts I will quote from Beer[3], who provided the earliest and the most interesting of them in 1817. He wrote:

Ofters als den grauen Staar findet man die Amaurose wahrhaft erblich; so zwar dass die meisten Glieder einer Familie durch mehr als eine Generation in einer bestimmten Lebensperiode am schwarzen Staar erblinden.

Anmerkung—Ich kenne mehr als eine Familie bei welcher dieses wirklich der Fall ist und vorzügliche Aufmerksamkeit verdient eine derselben, deren weibliche Glieder schon in der dritten Generation vollkommen und unaufhaltsam amaurotisch werden, sobald die Menstruation aufhört, doch blieben bisher alle diejenigen davon verschont, welche Kinder getragen und geboren hatten. Aber auch bei den männlichen Gliedern dieser unglücklichen Familie, welche sowie die weiblichen durchaus sehr dunkelbraune Augen haben, zeigt sich ohne Ausnahme offenbar ein Opportunität zur amaurotischen Gesichtsschwäche, obwohl bisher keines derselben wirklich erblindet ist.

The nature of the doubts regarding this commonly quoted reference will become clear on examination of the pedigrees given below and the facts deduced from them.

The uncertainty of the earlier accounts for purposes of identification is commonly attributed to the absence of an ophthalmoscopic examination; I would dissent from this view, for it is clear that in the large majority of cases the diagnosis based on a complete clinical history alone should be undoubted and should never be confused with

---

[1] *Bibl.* No. 8.   [2] *Bibl.* No. 3.   [3] *Bibl.* No. 1.

other hereditary conditions, though isolated cases, in which the family history of the disease is negative or is not available, may well be taken to refer to some other type of amblyopia perhaps temporary in character. The mode of onset of the disease, the nature of the visual defect, the stationary character which it assumes after a brief period, the absence of other symptoms, the knowledge of multiple cases in the family and the probably unaffected parentage, can leave little doubt of the nature of the malady, whereas the associated ophthalmoscopic appearances are by no means confined to this disease, and vary so markedly as to be regarded in any individual case as confirmatory rather than primarily diagnostic in character.

The lack of additional knowledge since 1871, which might have been expected to follow a wide and general experience of the disease, is a testimony to Leber's thoroughness: much however has since been learned regarding the hereditary character and such other features of the condition as may be gleaned from an examination of the statistics of a long series of recorded cases.

The impetus provided by Leber's paper certainly came at a fortunate time, and the seed sown by him was, maybe, rendered fruitful by the preparation of the ground at this period, when a small but enthusiastic group of people were becoming aware of the need for the collection of material, and the massing of facts concerning heredity, with a view to their statistical treatment. Few published pedigrees of hereditary optic atrophy followed immediately upon the appearance of Leber's paper; shortly however there was evidence of a rapid growth in the number of pedigrees which became available, not only of this disease but of many others, so that for six hereditary conditions[1] of which the Galton Laboratory has complete collections of pedigrees I find the following total numbers published in ten-year periods respectively:

1840–49	1850–59	1860–69	1870–79	1880–89	1890–99	1900–09
25	59	62	160	185	172	359

It is evident that after 1870 the problem of heredity was coming to the fore and the need for facts and pedigrees as a means of investigating the operation of its laws was before the minds of many men. The interest was becoming widespread, but Francis Galton was surely the pioneer who most effectively showed the way to all who sought exact knowledge concerning the potency of parentage, and rendered Leber's work doubly valuable at this time when a clear exposition of the main features of the disease, by which its recognition could be made, became all important.

I find nothing of interest to add to Leber's accounts of the few earlier published doubtful cases. One can only to-day be surprised that there was not a much wider recognition of the disease at a much earlier date; it would appear that the majority of mankind are incapable of grasping the entity of a symptom complex which constitutes a disease until some master mind comes forward and defines the condition in no uncertain terms—thus it is that most of the earlier accounts of hereditary optic

[1] Colour-Blindness, Retinitis Pigmentosa, Hereditary Optic Atrophy, Haemophilia, Congenital Cataract, Hereditary Multiple Exostoses.

atrophy, prior to the work of Leber, are vague and full of omissions which lead to an uncertain picture and render the diagnosis doubtful.

The main features of hereditary optic atrophy to be considered include (a) the sex incidence of the disease; (b) the character of the onset of the disease and the age at which it occurs; (c) the clinical signs and symptoms of the disease; (d) the course and prognosis of hereditary optic atrophy; (e) the association of other disabilities with hereditary optic atrophy; and (f) the hereditary character of the disease and its mode of transmission.

(a) *The Sex Incidence of the Disease.* It has been customary, in the literature of Ophthalmology and Genetics, to class hereditary optic atrophy amongst sex-limited diseases; my material has compelled me to question this classification, and to consider in some detail the whole question of the sex-limitation of conditions usually placed in this category—how truly any of them can be described as sex-limited and whether the limitation is inherent in sex-attributes or can be modified by other physical conditions; or again whether one can point to any features common to all sex-limited hereditary diseases which might point the way to the underlying source of the sex-selection. The facts which lead me to these considerations are as follows: the material upon which I have to work has been collected from published reports of cases, which have provided me with some 240 pedigrees of the disease covering 1182 affected individuals; 32 of these pedigrees, including 164 affected members, represent Japanese families, but the main bulk of the material refers to European peoples.

The first fact which became apparent on examination of the pedigrees was the relatively great number of females amongst the Japanese affected population; on proceeding to find the sex incidence for the two series of cases the following figures were obtained:

	Males	Females	Male Sex Incidence
European Population	863	155	$84\cdot8 \pm 0\cdot8$
Japanese „	97	67	$59\cdot1 \pm 2\cdot6$

Clearly it is not permissible, even by the European standard, to speak of hereditary optic atrophy as a sex-limited disease, and if we refer to it as "relatively sex-limited" how are we to explain the Japanese figures? The Japanese series is taken almost entirely from a paper in *von Graefes Archiv*, published by Kawakami, in 1926[1], which gives a very extensive pedigree worked out by the author himself, and includes a collection of pedigrees published by other Japanese ophthalmologists; the paper is particularly valuable owing to the inaccessibility of Japanese ophthalmological literature to European readers, but so few details are given that it is not possible to attempt any explanation of the source of this very marked difference between the values of the sex incidence for the eastern and western races, nor is it possible to determine whether from the clinical point of view the Japanese cases are really homogeneous with those provided by Europeans. It becomes of urgent interest to obtain further and more complete statistics of hereditary disease as exhibited by the eastern races.

[1] *Bibl.* No. 137.

If then one cannot, with any measure of accuracy, speak of hereditary optic atrophy as a sex-limited disease, it becomes of some interest to enquire what is the position with regard to other diseases usually placed in this category. The following table gives the sex incidence, based on such material as is available to me, for general examples:

Disease	♂	♀	Male Sex Incidence
Haemophilia	—	—	100 °/₀
Congenital Stationary Night-Blindness*	130	1	99·2 °/₀
Congenital Colour-Blindness	880	99	89·9 °/₀
Pseudo-Hypertrophic Muscular Paralysis	47	6	88·7 °/₀
Hereditary Optic Atrophy (in Europeans)	863	155	84·8 °/₀

* Sex-limited type of the disease only.

On examination of the values given in this table it becomes very doubtful as to whether a real inherent significance can be claimed for any one of them, or whether any of them can be definitely accepted as a measure of the sex incidence characteristic of the diseases to which they refer. Thus the value given for haemophilia is based entirely upon Professor Bulloch's views as stated below; the views of so critical an observer, based on an analysis of his wide experience, carry great weight, but on this point they are, as he states, not universally accepted; congenital stationary night-blindness of sex-limited type is an extremely rare disease and one cannot feel sure that the sex incidence of 99·2 based on 131 cases only would not be markedly modified if there were more chance of an affected male marrying a woman of an affected stock; the value given for congenital colour-blindness based on all the material available to me could we know be varied within wide limits by so selecting the material as to include a greater proportion of cases in which affected males married females of affected stock.

The numbers in the case of pseudo-hypertrophic muscular paralysis are too few to provide anything more than a provisional value of the sex incidence, and finally, as we have seen, the sex incidence of hereditary optic atrophy varies markedly as we pass from European to Japanese cases. With this caution I publish the table as illustrating the range of values which the sex incidence may exhibit in collections of material referring to what are known as sex-limited diseases. This series of values could be shown to follow an almost continuous course down to a percentage of 44·6 for the male sex incidence in blue sclerotics, as indicated in the last section of this Nettleship Memorial Volume, and it would appear to be a matter of choice, if viewed from this consideration alone, where the line should be drawn between conditions which may be regarded as only exceptionally manifested in females and those which may be looked upon as liable to affect either sex; a glance at the pedigrees, however, reveals that this is not so, and that the mechanism of heredity for the conditions mentioned above departs in some very fundamental way from the laws in operation for the case of, say, hereditary multiple exostoses, with a male sex incidence of 70 °/₀; the mode of transmission of a disease and the potentiality to transmit on the part of women who do not manifest any defect are the more effective differentiating criteria, and when combined with a knowledge of the sex incidence they leave no doubt regarding the type of inheritance to which a disease conforms.

The sole condition within my experience which appears to be perhaps truly sex-limited is haemophilia, a disease characterised by "an excessive and chronic liability to immoderate haemorrhage." The outstanding authority on this subject, who has most carefully analysed all available material, is Professor Bulloch[1], who writes: "So far as we can find, after studying the contents of some 900 papers on haemophilia, no case has yet been described in a female which bears more than a superficial resemblance to the disease as found in the male." Is there any reason why women should not suffer from haemophilia? Histories of cases suggest that there probably may be, for as Bulloch points out, the inherent defect which underlies the condition in man varies from time to time in its manifestation—the condition is often described as a *periodic* tendency to bleed—moreover a severe bleeding tends to temporarily cure the condition, unless it kills, for after a haemorrhage the bleeder may not behave differently from a normal individual even while wounded. Now all this is very interesting when we consider the question as to why women do not show symptoms of the disease, and it seems by no means improbable that there are basic physiological reasons, inherent in the female sex, which protect it from exhibiting this particular disease, even when really all the potentialities responsible for it in the male are present. It is conceivable also that for physiological reasons it would be impossible for a woman with true haemophilia to survive puberty or to bear children, and that thus stocks in which females show the affection must tend to become extinct. Haemophilia is thus a possibly unique example of a sex-limited hereditary disease which fulfils its title and for which one can maybe glimpse a suggestion that the source of the protection to the female lies in her physiological attributes. No such explanation could be offered in the case of the other conditions which enter any table affecting respectively the light sense, the colour sense, the functional capacity of the optic nerve, or the degeneration of muscular tissue in certain characteristically restricted areas of the body; indeed we may well ask ourselves why other muscular dystrophies which affect characteristically a different set of muscles appear to attack either sex almost indiscriminately as also does another type of night-blindness.

It has long been recognised in a rather vague way that hereditary disease tends to select man rather than woman as an instrument in which to manifest its peculiarities and crippling effects; Darwin extends the scope of this statement in his *Origin of Species* where he writes: "It is a fact of some importance to us that peculiarities appearing in the males of our domestic breeds are often transmitted either exclusively or in a much greater degree to the males alone." The problem, however, of seeking some inherent and inevitable reason for this selection in the attributes of sex becomes one of extraordinary difficulty when we are faced with the position presented by hereditary optic atrophy with its sex incidence differing entirely from one race to another. On examination of the Japanese pedigrees (see Plate LXIII) one can have little doubt of the group of hereditary diseases to which they belong, for the mode of transmission in these cases

[1] *Treasury of Human Inheritance*, Vol. I. pp. 169, 175—181, 194.

closely resembles that exhibited by the European pedigrees, but to refer to the condition as sex-limited in Japan is grossly misleading.

(b) *The Character of the Onset of the Disease and the Age at which it occurs.* If the onset of the disease may be taken to include the active phase of the disease during which its symptoms progress, it is described in individual cases as sudden, as rapid or as characterised by a gradual or by a slow progression of symptoms, and there is no doubt that cases occur which would be aptly placed in each of these categories; on reading the histories of cases, however, it becomes evident that there is no general standard as to what constitutes suddenness or rapidity in the onset of the disease, and that the descriptions of cases in these respects are subject to very large personal equations on the part of patient and physician. It is indeed unlikely that any individual ophthalmologist sees sufficient cases of the disease to enable him to form a standard, from his own experience, on the basis of which to classify cases; when I seek, from an analysis of all available reported cases, to provide him with such a standard, the difficulties of the undertaking seem to be insuperable. I have tried to discover what proportion of cases reach a maximum disability in less than one, two, three months, and so on, but so relatively few histories give any exact period during which progress of symptoms was noted—and the difficulty in doing so is obvious—that I think it wiser to say nothing more definite than that probably a majority of cases reach their maximum disability within two months from the time at which the patient becomes aware of his failing vision, and that it is relatively rare for symptoms to advance after six months. Even this cautious statement may be misleading, for it is by no means unlikely that it is the cases which run a short progressive course and are under the care of the ophthalmologist throughout the period during which the disease advances, which tend to be fully described; hence the mass of cases of which no definite information is given may tend to be those which progress slowly and over a longer period. Again, the recorded onset dates from the moment at which the patient noticed some defect in his vision and this is almost certainly a variable stage in the course of the disease, dependent upon the individuality of the patient, whether he is observant or is slow to note slight changes in his vision, whether he readily takes alarm or is slow to believe that all is not well, and whether the nature of his work or mode of living are such as to inevitably reveal early changes in vision. The particular site of the early pathological process too may very largely determine the stage at which defect becomes recognisable to the patient, and the problem is further complicated by the fact that the onset in the two eyes is frequently not simultaneous and affection of one eye may readily escape notice until the second eye becomes affected.

The onset is thus in hereditary optic atrophy a very indefinite term, the particular significance of which may vary from one case to another, nevertheless it is usually characteristic of the disease and serves at once to differentiate the condition from retinitis pigmentosa. Patients as a rule do not easily describe what they first notice when a function is failing, but I think it is clear that a large number of individuals do experience at first the sensation of a mist or cloud before the eyes which gradually becomes thicker; some definitely realise that they can no longer see clearly what they look at but can get an impression of objects outside the field of direct vision; there is no doubt that in many cases there is a sudden momentary recognition of very gross defect which surely must be explained by some corresponding sudden breakdown of functioning tissue[1]. One reads repeatedly of individuals who "suddenly became blind"; they are as a matter of fact probably not wholly blind but retain a certain amount of peripheral vision; for example: VII. 6 of Fig. 716 noticed on his way to school one morning that his vision suddenly became dim, and that when he reached school he was unable to see to read; II. 3 of Fig. 890 found on attempting to leave his bed one morning that he was nearly blind, he had had a good night's rest and had seen well and been in his usual health the night before; II. 14 of Fig. 717 suddenly noticed when he was out walking that the road "looked as if I could not get any further, as if it ended in the sky"; within a week he had to give up his work and was never able to return to it. It must be agreed that if the onset in hereditary optic atrophy appears to be too indefinite to provide any standardisation, it does provide in individual cases very dramatic and overwhelming experiences absolutely incompatible with retinitis pigmentosa, the onset of which disease is characterised first by night-blindness alone and then by an always slow progressive closing-in of the peripheral fields of vision, leaving central direct vision unimpaired until a late stage of the disease. Thus, whilst the patient with hereditary optic atrophy is usually able to go about alone with safety but cannot read or recognise objects which he looks at—he may for example know that somebody passes him in the street but cannot say whether it is a man or a woman—the patient with retinitis pigmentosa cannot so safely go about alone but can see to read till a late stage of the disease when complete blindness for him ensues.

The age at which the onset in hereditary optic atrophy occurs, or the age at which the patient first noticed some interference in vision[2], is stated in a considerable proportion of the recorded cases, and it has been possible to construct graphs to show the grade of liability to develop the disease at each period of life in males and females; here again, as with regard to the sex incidence of the disease, the Japanese and European series show such marked divergences that it is not possible to regard the combined material as homogeneous, and the Japanese material must be treated separately and tentatively until adequate statistics are available and some explanation of the differences can be found.

The following table gives the mean age of onset for each sex of the two series and its variation as measured by the standard deviation:

	No.	Mean	Standard Deviation
European ♂	(669)	$23.23 \pm .26$	$9.98 \pm .18$
,, ♀	(113)	$25.15 \pm .84$	$13.27 \pm .60$
Japanese ♂	(74)	$21.30 \pm .67$	$8.53 \pm .47$
,, ♀	(48)	$20.50 \pm .76$	$7.82 \pm .54$

[1] Perhaps in some of these cases the "sudden" recognition may be explained by a temporary interference, through dust, say, with the better eye, revealing the bad state of the worn eye.

[2] I have already published a paper on this subject in *Annals of Eugenics*, Vol. III. pp. 269—276, but propose to incorporate some of my conclusions given there in this introduction, for the sake of completeness and for the benefit of readers who have not access to the former publication.

Now these values suggest that whatever factors operate to determine the age of onset in the males of the Japanese race, they operate at the same age for Japanese females, and in both cases at an age earlier than for European races; the numbers for the Japanese race are small but so far as they carry any weight they do perhaps fall into line with the view that eastern races develop earlier than western, and it would appear to be legitimate to combine the statistics from the two sexes as homogeneous material. When, however, we regard the different values for males and females of European races, something further requires explanation in the increased variability of the female. The frequency distributions corresponding to the four series are as follows:

Age at Onset in Years	Europeans		Japanese	
	♂	♀	♂	♀
0—3	15	6	—	—
4—7	19	3	1	—
8—11	26	12	2	2
12—15	50	16	20	14
16—19	119	5	20	11
20—23	194	10	11	10
24—27	94	15	3	6
28—31	70	10	8	1
32—35	28	10	4	1
36—39	10	8	1	1
40—43	13	10	3	1
44—47	7	3	—	—
48—51	14	4	1	1
52—55	3	—	—	—
56—59	5	—	—	—
60—63	1	—	—	—
64—67	1	1	—	—

The graph[1] given on p. 333, based on these values, illustrates the frequency percentage of cases in which the onset occurred within each age group for males and females of the two series; it suggests that the factors determining the onset differ markedly in the male and female of European races and supports the view that the combined male and female data for the Japanese race provide homogeneous material.

We know that a temporary condition closely resembling hereditary optic atrophy in its symptoms may be induced in a susceptible subject as a result of toxic influences, and it is reasonable to suppose that a toxic influence, or indeed any disturbance of normal health, has power to precipitate the onset in the presence of the tendency to the hereditary form of the disease; we might expect therefore that the female curve would show some excess of early cases, as a result of the physiological disturbances associated with the onset of menstruation, or again that the curve between the ages of 20 and 43 years might be influenced by the toxic effects of pregnancy. The numbers which contribute to the female curve are too small to determine whether or no such factors are the source of the difference between the curves for European males and females, moreover on this hypothesis we need to ask why the Japanese female curve

[1] The graph is given in this form instead of as a histogram in order to show the differences between the four series in one diagram.

shows no evidence of similar disturbances but on the contrary follows very closely the male curve for the race. To call attention to another fact shown by the female curve—the climacteric appears to have no significance with regard to the onset of the disease, yet the contrary is very commonly stated. Perhaps if a woman is liable to

HEREDITARY OPTIC ATROPHY. AGE OF ONSET OF THE DISEASE.

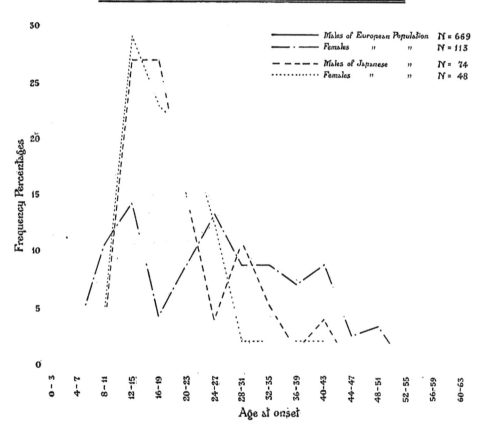

the disease at all she is bound to suffer from periods of lowered resistance or low vitality which would give the tendency an opportunity to manifest itself before the time of the menopause, but whatever the explanation may be I think we may insist that the onset of hereditary optic atrophy must not be added to the list of ills liable to befall woman at this period of her life.

Now the onset of this disease is a profoundly disturbing event for the patient and one would think that he would almost invariably seek for a cause and would connect the occurrence with any associated illness or indisposition if it be present; yet an examination of my records reveals only very few cases in which such an association is suggested; the suggestions moreover are usually entirely inadequate as causative measures; thus one man said the onset followed a cold bath, five cases attributed the onset to the result of a cold, one to worry, one to a fright, one to the result of a fatiguing march and so on. The great majority of cases apparently offer no suggestion and several individuals emphasise their good health at the time and refer to a recent holiday. Thus I think we may accept the fact that the onset of the disease cannot usually be accounted for by any demonstrable ill-health, but the disease appears to be primarily an atrophy, and the fact that the initial stages are frequently associated, as we shall see, with inflammatory signs does suggest that some toxic exciting cause has been in operation in many cases. It is clear, however, that external exciting causes are limited in their action; they can only precipitate the onset of the disease in the presence of an inherent tendency and within a restricted interval from the time at which the condition would be manifested in any case, for the ages of onset in siblings and in uncle and nephew are highly correlated, as is shown below in the section on the inheritance of the disease, and this indicates that the observed character has a definite organic basis; it can perhaps be to some degree modified but cannot be determined by chance individual experiences.

On examining the male curve for Europeans we see that the majority of cases occur within the period which should be of maximum efficiency when all tissues, so far as we can judge from growth curves provided by Professor Ruger and Miss Stoessiger from Galton's data (*Bibl.* No. 145), are at their prime; this fact would appear to be consistent with the view that the condition arises from an inherent defect of vitality; structures grow and develop normally, and then a lack of vital endurance becomes apparent and a breakdown of function follows. The sequence is suggestive of what may be presumed to occur in dementia praecox, and it would be of interest to have for comparison curves descriptive of the age of onset in that disease. Is such a curve to illustrate the age of onset characteristic of abiotrophic disease in general? It has been suggested that retinitis pigmentosa is an abiotrophic disease, the seat of the defect being the percipient layer of the retinal epithelium; such a view is perhaps not generally accepted, but if the above curve is characteristic of the age of onset for abiotrophic disease in general it provides an argument against the acceptance of retinitis pigmentosa in this category of diseases, for its onset is usually at an early age and only rarely occurs as late as 20 years. Perhaps I am precipitate in accepting hereditary optic atrophy as an abiotrophic disease, but no less an authority than Sir William Gowers places it in this category; it is difficult on this assumption to explain the cases of subsequent improvement and even what must be described as cure in some few individuals. The male curve alone is of permanent interest, for evidently some special stimulus has to be in operation before the female can exhibit the disease at all and the numbers in her case are too few to have more than a suggestive interest.

I have tried to fit a curve to the series of observations of age of onset represented by the male European series but have failed to do so; none of the types of curves which so commonly describe series of observations of an anatomical or physiological character fits our frequency distribution with any degree of closeness; the chief difficulty is the great number of cases in which the age of onset is given at 20 years. Perhaps some error has arisen through the tendency to state the age of onset at 20 years when knowledge was uncertain and "about 20" was interpreted as 20, or there may be some more fundamental factor underlying the failure of this material to fall into line with common experience; the frequency distribution does not suggest heterogeneity of material.

I have endeavoured to come to some decision as to whether or no there is ante-dating in the age of onset on passing from one generation to the next. The question arose on finding, from my correlation table for age of onset in uncles and nephews, that the average age of onset in the nephews was three years earlier than the corre-sponding age in uncles. This fact alone does not demonstrate antedating, for the nephew and his generation tend to be the patients who are under observation when the case is reported, and members of this generation have frequently not yet reached the age at which a late onset may occur; moreover, exact knowledge of the age of onset in members of the previous generation who became affected early in life is liable to be forgotten. Completed histories providing information of affected sibships in two successive generations, i.e. those in which no further cases of the defect can reasonably be expected to occur, provide the age of onset in 84 males of the first generation and in 112 males of the second. I have omitted from this investigation all sibships in which females occur, also the offspring of affected mothers, for there is evidence that affection of the mother tends to hasten the onset in her offspring, and that the presence of affected females in a sibship may be taken to indicate some reinforcement of the stimulus leading to the defect which also tends to hasten the onset[1]. Calculated from this carefully selected material the mean age of onset for 84 males of the first generation is 24·91 years and the corresponding value for 112 males of the second generation is 24·14 years; these values are approximately equal within the probable errors, and I think we may conclude that there is no evidence of antedating in the age of onset of hereditary optic atrophy in passing from one generation to the next.

(c) *The Clinical Signs and Symptoms of the Disease.* In most cases the sole symptom complained of by patients suffering from hereditary optic atrophy is diminution of vision; this lowering of visual acuity is always marked and in rare cases blindness is described; the defect is primarily a central one, characterised most commonly by a central scotoma which may be relative or absolute, interfering with direct vision and thus depriving the patient of the power to read or to do any fine work, but enabling him to retain a measure of independence with regard to mobility. The central scotoma can usually be defined and its extent measured, but in a small proportion of cases no scotoma can be demonstrated. The absence of a central scotoma cannot I think neces-sarily be taken to indicate a less severe defect, indeed it may perhaps point to a more widespread affection; the visual acuity in these cases is often very low and in a

---

[1] The mean age of onset for 92 males who have affected sisters is 19·96 years.

considerable proportion of them the onset of the disease had been at a very early age. If the disease is an abiotrophy and is the manifestation of an inherent lack of vital endurance, the ready affection of the most highly specialised tissues is to be looked for and the central scotoma is what one might expect to find, but it is not easy to explain why on such a hypothesis the breakdown should be sudden and should remain so limited in its action, or why the progress of the affection should be stayed and remain stationary after only so short a progression of symptoms.

It is not possible from my material to obtain any idea as to how far the visual acuity is below the normal in regions immediately surrounding the scotomatous area, but a considerable proportion of cases are reported to show a contraction of the peripheral fields of vision. There would appear to be, within the field, a zone of greatest resistance to the disease which so far as one can judge almost invariably retains a certain amount of vision. Such are the facts so far as I can give them but they are difficult to interpret and the relationship, if any, of the peripheral contraction to the central scotoma is very obscure; there is no hint of the peripheral contraction appearing at a later stage of the disease as a normal sequence of events due say to the spread of the disease or impairment of the circulation following the degeneration of retinal vessels.

In a large proportion of cases no information is given regarding the presence or absence of central scotomata and peripheral contraction of the visual fields; the following table, however, shows the percentage of cases in which the occurrence or absence of the two defects has been noted; the percentages are based on cases for which a definite statement is made and must not be taken to refer to all cases of the disease; it may well be that there is a tendency to make no statement when no defect is found and that thus our percentages showing presence of the defect are based on selected material and are too high to apply to the disease in general; any selection there may have been is, however, presumably the same for the two sexes and thus I think we may point to some increased liability on the part of the female to exhibit a peripheral contraction. It is

Percentage of Cases showing Central Scotomata and Peripheral Contraction of the Visual Fields.

Sex	No.	Central Scotoma Present	No.	Peripheral Contraction Present	No.	Central Scotoma and Peripheral Contraction	
						Present	Absent
♂	270	88·1 °/₀	212	42·5 °/₀	179	34·6 °/₀	9·5 °/₀
♀	50	82·0 °/₀	50	62·0 °/₀	42	45·2 °/₀	4·8 °/₀

difficult to account for the peripheral contraction of the fields in hereditary optic atrophy and I find no evidence from the histories that the patient himself is aware of this defect; when one considers the extreme care needful in perimetric examinations, the common variation in the fields determined by this means on different occasions, and the dependence of any particular determination not alone on the observer but also on the state of mind and fatigue of the patient, one should be cautious in suggesting any interpretation of the figures given above. It is not improbable that the peripheral contraction exhibited by these cases is sometimes a secondary affection, only indirectly induced by the optic atrophy, and that perhaps it may then be a manifestation of an accompanying hysterical amblyopia, which would account for the tendency to a greater frequency of the symptom in women. The special stimulus required to induce optic atrophy in women may well involve a strain upon the nervous system which would tend to a functional breakdown of this nature; I do not know whether the peripheral contraction in our cases remains stationary, or whether any observations have been made with regard to its cure or progress; it is well recognised as a symptom of long duration and difficult to cure in hysterical amblyopia[1]. We may remember too that sufferers from hereditary optic atrophy appear to be liable to headaches of the migrainous type and that such headaches are commonly accompanied by a temporary contraction of the peripheral fields; perhaps an explanation of the visual phenomena in migraine might throw some light on the source of the peripheral contraction in hereditary optic atrophy.

The only other symptom generally shown by patients with hereditary optic atrophy is colour-blindness, but tests for this symptom are rarely carried out with any precision; the defect is evidently often a very gross one but, as is natural when the patient is presenting more urgent symptoms, it is customary to pay little attention to it; some interference with the perception of colours is always to be expected in optic atrophy whether the case be hereditary or otherwise. There is no evidence that hereditary optic atrophy tends to occur in the subjects of congenital colour-blindness, and I have no record of any observation in which an acquired disturbance of colour vision was noted prior to the onset of hereditary optic atrophy as indicated by the lowering of visual acuity for form; this may be of significance as an indication of the reality of the *sudden* onsets so often described in this disease; we know that in temporary disabilities of vision, arising from toxic processes or trauma, the colour vision commonly appears to be interfered with earlier than the vision for form and recovers later. The reader may find interest in Benedict's observations on Colour-Blindness in his paper on Atrophy of the Optic Nerve, published in 1864[2].

I would much prefer to write no word concerning the physical signs to be looked for on ophthalmoscopic examination, as characteristic of hereditary optic atrophy, for they vary greatly from one case to another; they are often difficult to explain and their intensity would appear to bear little relationship to the severity of the accompanying symptoms. The main difficulty occurs in the early stages of the disease when a profound disturbance of function is already in operation and the appearance of the fundus may vary from that of complete normality to that indicative of an acute inflammatory reaction—with reddening of the nerve head, blurring of its margins,

---

[1] One ophthalmologist writes that he cannot recollect that any of the fields in his cases suggested hysteria, nor did the few female cases seen by him suggest hysterical individuals. Nettleship refers to the "aggravated hysteria" seen in some stocks carrying Leber's disease (*Bibl.* No. 85, p. cxvii).

[2] *Bibl.* No. 5. See also Part II of this volume on *Colour-Blindness*, pp. 174—180.

dilatation and tortuosity of the vessels and perhaps some small haemorrhages. There may, on the other hand, be signs of atrophy of the nerve at a very early stage following the onset of symptoms; such signs are limited in extent and usually consist of paleness of the temporal side of the disc corresponding to the section of the nerve which provides the macular region, the fibres of which constitute the papillo-macular bundle.

Signs of inflammation are so commonly present in the early stages of the disease as to have led to the view that some exciting cause of a toxic or irritating nature has precipitated the onset of the inherent defect; the history of a few cases might justify this conclusion, but the reading of some hundreds of similar histories gives no hint of the nature of the exciting cause, which certainly cannot usually be attributed to the use of tobacco or alcohol, to sexual excess or to the action of any acute infection, and the idea grows upon one that perhaps the inflammatory signs are really due to a natural effort on the part of surrounding tissues to come to the aid of a failing function, the effort manifesting itself by an increased circulation in the region. Or the circulatory hyperaemia may follow some slight constriction due to the replacement of shrinking nerve fibres by interstitial tissue which is so prominent a feature in the process of optic nerve degeneration. Whatever may be their source, the inflammatory signs are temporary and soon subside, giving place to signs of atrophy which gradually progress and appear from the accounts to advance after the diminution of vision has become stationary; after a period of years it is not infrequent to read of the complete discoloration of the disc, which now has sharply defined margins and narrowing of the arteries, whereas at an earlier stage the sector of the disc corresponding to the papillo-macular fibres alone is pale.

It is a notable fact that once the disc has attained these atrophic signs, it never recovers its normal appearance even though the sight may so markedly improve as to allow of reading and close work. Paleness of the disc is a quite untrustworthy descriptive term; there is no standard as to what constitutes a pale disc and the normal colour evidently varies within considerable limits from one individual to another; a whitish disc is certainly compatible with very good vision and may have no pathological significance; it is not improbable that the colour of the disc varies to some extent through life just as does the colour of the complexion. A disc in which the sector corresponding to the papillo-macular fibres is paler than the rest is certainly under suspicion and a disc that is seen to grow pale progressively is pathological. Thus hereditary optic atrophy eventually always leads to a pale or white disc at any rate affecting part of its area but a pale disc is not always indicative of optic atrophy.

It would be far easier to point to the significance of the signs and symptoms of hereditary optic atrophy if we knew something of the pathology of the disease and its etiology; as a matter of fact, no examination of signs and symptoms is of the slightest use in predicting the prognosis of the disease, or in determining the diagnosis, which must depend almost entirely upon the character of the onset combined with a knowledge of the family history, or on the failure to respond to treatment. There has never to my knowledge been a post-mortem examination of a case of the disease and the primary seat of the affection has not yet been definitely determined. It is certainly a fact that direct vision is first involved and the nerve fibres of the papillo-macular bundle first show the defect; these fibres, however, may still have a normal appearance at a time when direct vision is markedly lowered and we cannot say whether the trouble may not commence by a degeneration of the ganglion cells of the retina in the macular region, or whether, on the other hand, the primary lesion may be in the optic nerve fibres of the papillo-macular bundle outside the eye when they have assumed their axial position in the nerve. It is of considerable significance that one eye alone may be affected, though, in such cases, the second eye perhaps invariably becomes affected after an interval, which may be a few days only or, in rare cases, may extend to several years.

Affections of the optic nerve are often difficult to explain, for example, raised intracranial pressure is perhaps the most common cause of optic neuritis, yet large cerebral tumours may produce no visual disturbance over a long period of time, whereas in other cases quite small growths may lead to the most distressing and rapidly advancing symptoms of the disease; the mechanism of the process is far from clear.

It is not particularly illuminating to be told that the cause of a disease is hereditary and that it is due to an inherent lack of vital endurance leading to the early death of apparently some small section only of a structure; moreover, if this be the position, the cases of improvement and cure are not readily explained.

The failure, relative or absolute, to respond to treatment is the sole factor which can be relied upon to differentiate hereditary optic atrophy from a toxic amblyopia— it is the painful characteristic of all hereditary disease, and herein lies the moral— Hereditary disease can only be cured by its prevention!

(d) *The Course and Prognosis of Hereditary Optic Atrophy.* I have endeavoured to obtain some idea as to whether this disease is likely to shorten life or whether the individuals who become its victims tend to be short-lived people, and whether there is any truth in the statements which have been made regarding the increased early death-rate believed to be possibly an inherent characteristic of stock carrying hereditary optic atrophy; little definite knowledge can be claimed on any of these points but some facts bearing on them can be derived from my material.

It is unfortunate that the age at death of cases who have died is so rarely given; my whole series provides the age at death of only 38 affected individuals; of these, five were over 80 years of age; one man who died at 80 had been affected for 61 years; another man, aged 90, had suffered from the disease for 60 years—clearly then the disease is able to run a very protracted course and is not incompatible with a long life. The following table gives the duration of the disease in 347 cases at the time of the latest record; very few of these people were dead when the record was made; the significance of the table is thus extremely limited, but it does I think justify the suggestion that it is not alone the exceptional individuals who are able to survive long periods of the disease. If there were any marked tendency to a relatively early death associated with the disease I have little doubt that the collection of histories given below would provide some evidence of it

The inheritance of longevity is an established fact; hence stocks which exhibit

Duration of Disease at time of latest Record.

Time since Onset of Disease	No. of Cases
Under 1 year	67
1—10 years	117
11—20 ,,	62
21—30 ,,	48
31—40 ,,	33
41—50 ,,	15
51—60 ,,	4
61 years	1

a heavy mortality in early childhood are to be expected. Now certain pedigrees of hereditary optic atrophy will be seen to show this characteristic, which is not necessarily confined to sibships containing affected members but may be no less conspicuous a feature of sibships unaffected by the disease; notable examples are Figs. 707, 729, 733, 774, and many other pedigrees will be found to show the association. It is possible by a selection of pedigrees showing a markedly heavy early death-rate to obtain 60 sibships members of which suffered from hereditary optic atrophy in which no fewer than 39 °/$_o$ of the children died young. If from the same pedigrees we select unaffected sibships showing a heavy child mortality we find 82 such sibships in which no fewer than 47 °/$_o$ died young. The actual figures on which these percentages are based are as follows:

	No.	Affected	Not Affected	Early Deaths	Percentage of Early Deaths
A. Affected Sibships	60	136	381	202	39·1
B. Unaffected Sibships	82	—	461	215	46·6

Without pledging myself to any view as to whether the association of high child mortality with hereditary optic atrophy in these selected sibships of selected pedigrees is a chance or a significant relationship, I do not think it would be easy, if possible, to obtain figures showing a similar degree of association from an equal number of pedigrees of other non-fatal hereditary diseases. I should like to emphasise the fact that there has been a selection of cases and that other pedigrees or sibships exhibiting hereditary optic atrophy could be selected to illustrate an absence of early deaths. It will be noted that the average size of family in the sibships showing a heavy early death-rate is very large; this is perhaps only an expression of the fact that to have many early deaths in a family there must have been many children to die; we need further to remember that the affected sibships contain also members who have probably not died young since the affection does not commonly become manifest until adult age; thus in selecting sibships showing a heavy early death-rate for inclusion in my table I have probably, unconsciously, made a selection of large families.

The early deaths show no significant sex selection, which might be expected to appear if the cause were at all intimately linked with hereditary optic atrophy; of 173 cases, 101 were males, providing a sex ratio differing little from that for deaths under 5 years in the general population.

Regarding the prognosis of the disease I shall quote freely from my former paper[1]. The histories of my collection do not in many cases provide any means of judging whether improvement has occurred or not, and in almost all cases the information is vague and indefinite; in practice, however, no ophthalmologist feels particularly hopeful regarding the outlook for the patient who comes to him suffering from hereditary optic atrophy. My records include 211 cases in males which appear to have shown no improvement over a period of years, and 86 cases in which improvement has been noted; that is to say, 29 °/₀ of these males showed some measure of improvement; 12 of the 86 improved cases showed complete recovery of vision, 15 showed marked improvement and 59 improved to some less extent. The common story in the case of the patient who does not mend is that of a rapid onset, with progression of symptoms during a short and limited period when the maximum disability is reached; henceforth the condition remains stationary. The percentage of 29 almost certainly indicates too high a rate of improvement from the fact that there is probably a tendency to note improvement when it is found and to make no comment when the condition is found to be unchanged; it however constitutes a maximum value and it may be set against a minimum value of 10 °/₀ based on the supposition that only 86 of my whole series of 837 males showed improvement; the true value undoubtedly lies somewhere between these two and perhaps it is nearer to the upper limit than to the lower. The figures regarding improvement in females are too small to be of any value, but such as they are I find 15 cases improved or recovered and 37 cases in which no improvement occurred but, by an interesting coincidence, the maximum and minimum recovery or improvement rates work out at 29 °/₀ and 10 °/₀ respectively, that is, to precisely the same values as those given above for males.

I have examined my material in considerable detail in the attempt to find evidence of some factor which may be of significance in determining the prognosis of the individual case; the result is disappointing. The points which I thought might have some bearing on the outlook for the individual are: (1) The age of onset of the disease. (2) The family history with regard to improvement. (3) The presence or absence of central scotomata and peripheral contraction of the visual fields. (4) The association of severe headaches and giddiness with the disease. (5) The habits of the patient with regard to smoking and drinking. Such tentative conclusions as I have been able to reach are as follows:

(1) For 75 males who showed improvement the age of onset is given; it was earlier than 16 years in 26·7 °/₀ of cases, whereas in the 200 cases which showed no improvement the age of onset had been earlier than 16 years in only 9·5 °/₀ of cases; thus an early onset would appear to denote a relatively favourable outlook, though no percentages based upon such small numbers can be very convincing.

(2) On reading through the histories of cases one cannot fail to notice that

<hr />

[1] *Bibl.* No. 148.

improvement occurs more readily in some stocks than in others, and that as a matter of fact not only is the liability to the disease inherited but also its prognosis for the individual. I tried to obtain a statistical demonstration of this fact and was able to form the following table.

Progress of Hereditary Optic Atrophy in pairs of Brothers.

First Brother

		Vision Improved	Vision not Improved	Totals
Second Brother	Vision Improved	30	28	58
	Vision not Improved	28	172	200
	Totals	58	200	258

The number of cases in which we are told whether improvement has occurred in more than one brother is small but it suffices to show that the prognosis of the disease is controlled by heredity to precisely the same extent as are a great variety of other measurable characters. The correlation coefficient calculated from this table is ·600 ± ·059·

(3) It is not possible to discover whether any prediction can be based upon the presence of demonstrable scotomata or of peripheral contraction in the fields of vision as the necessary information on which to base any conclusion is given in too few cases.

(4) Very severe headaches, sometimes of the migraine type, are not infrequently found in association with hereditary optic atrophy; there is evidence that the association is not always a chance one for in certain of these cases the headaches make their appearance at the time of the onset of the disease and cease when the condition has become stationary and visual symptoms have ceased to progress; the headaches are not of a uniform character and the pain in different individuals may be localised in the frontal, temporal or occipital regions or the top of the head; sometimes giddiness also is complained of with or without accompanying headaches. Thus records may be found in the histories provided of 71 affected males who suffered from headaches and giddiness (10 of the cases suffered from giddiness only) and of these 12 showed improvement, 36 showed no improvement regarding the optic atrophy and of 23 no information concerning the progress of the case is given. These figures indicate that a maximum number of 25 °/₀ of the affected males, who had associated headaches, showed some improvement; a minimum of 17 °/₀ improved, if we accept the hypothesis that no information may be taken to indicate no improvement. These figures, compared with the maximum and minimum recovery rates of 29 °/₀ and 10 °/₀ respectively for the whole series of cases, indicate that no prognosis can be based on the presence or absence of headaches and giddiness; the numbers are very few and the only safe conclusion to be drawn from them is that very severe accompanying headaches are not incompatible with recovery and do not appear to influence the prognosis unfavourably

in cases of hereditary optic atrophy in males. It should not be inferred that only 71 of the total number of affected males suffered from headaches; in the majority of cases information on this point is either not sought or is not noted by the recorder.

(5) A patient sensitive to nicotine and suffering from tobacco amblyopia may so closely resemble a case of hereditary optic atrophy as to be indistinguishable from it in the early stages of the disease. When long series of cases are available the two conditions are sharply differentiated by the frequency distributions for age of onset the maximum incidence in tobacco amblyopia is rather above the age of 50[1] or when physical health is perhaps failing, whereas in hereditary optic atrophy the maximum incidence corresponds with the period of maximum physical efficiency; the onset in tobacco amblyopia is perhaps more insidious; moreover, Traquair[2] writes that he has always found the scotomata more dense and more defined in Leber's disease than in tobacco amblyopia. Usually the diagnosis becomes evident on watching the progress of the disease as the one condition shows no response to treatment whilst cure may be expected in nicotine poisoning on the absolute cessation of smoking.

It is, therefore, of particular interest to observe how cases of hereditary optic atrophy are affected by tobacco. No patient presenting himself for treatment would fail to be questioned regarding his habits with respect to tobacco and alcohol, but the information obtained, combined with a knowledge of the progress of the case, is so rarely included in the published report, that it is not possible to come to any conclusion as to whether the habits of the patient have a bearing on the prognosis of the case. That the influence of tobacco on the progress of the case is not at once obvious is a surprising and significant fact.

The question of the influence of tobacco smoking on the prognosis of hereditary optic atrophy is rather a complex one; it may well be that the onset of the disease is precipitated by heavy smoking in the susceptible individual and that the cessation of smoking may thus lead to improvement of an associated tobacco amblyopia. The patient whose onset has occurred without any obvious provocation is not in quite the same position with regard to treatment; this may account for some cases in which marked improvement has occurred in patients who have been addicted to heavy smoking; we need to remember, however, that tobacco amblyopia is not hereditary and does not tend to occur in members of the same family, whereas the correlation for improvement in pairs of brothers suffering from hereditary optic atrophy was seen to be $\cdot600 \pm \cdot059$.

My material provides no information regarding the effect of alcohol; any habit which tends to lower vitality and powers of resistance must tend to impede recovery in chronic illness whatever its nature may be.

(e) *The Association of other Disabilities with Hereditary Optic Atrophy.* When the etiology and pathology of a disease are very obscure and little can be found to point the way, there is always the possibility that associated disease may help to an explanation of the primary symptoms. In the case of hereditary optic atrophy anatomical considerations led to the suggestion that possibly some inherited disorder

[1] *Bibl.* No. 147.   [2] *Bibl.* No. 153.

of the pituitary gland was the source of the trouble, and that its over activity and enlargement at the period of adolescence and at the menopause in women might account for the onset of the disease. Now, do we know that there is over activity in the pituitary body at these periods? How is over activity measured? Do we know that there is enlargement of the gland at these periods? We do know that there may be hypertrophy of structure if the secretion of a gland be excessive or if it be inadequate for the needs of the body, but I am very doubtful whether we can say that the pituitary gland enlarges to a measurable extent during adolescence and at the menopause in women; in any case the menopause in women cannot be regarded as of any significance in the matter of her affection with hereditary optic atrophy. We do not know that the subjects of acromegaly or of hypopituitarism exhibit any liability to visual disturbance, unless in acromegaly the gland be sufficiently enlarged to produce pressure symptoms as in tumour formation; furthermore a search through the histories given will reveal no hint of symptoms suggestive of an associated pituitary disorder as the underlying source of the eye affection. Tumours of the pituitary body pressing on the optic chiasma may lead to optic neuritis and temporal hemianopia, but not characteristically to a defect of the papillo-macular bundle and to an accompanying central scotoma. However this may be, the suggestion has received a good deal of consideration; the cases appended provide 60 reports of radiological examination of the skull in affected individuals, with a view to determining whether there is any abnormality in the region of the pituitary fossa. Of these cases 34 showed no abnormality; the remaining 26 showed enlargement of the fossa in 14 cases; in two cases the fossa was said to be small; blurring or prominence of the posterior clinoid processes is reported in a number of cases; irregular outline of the fossa, enlargement of the sphenoidal cells, and shadows due possibly to bony deposits are also described; in five cases from three pedigrees[1] actual measurements of the fossa in millimetres are given but no note is made as to the points from which measurements are taken.

I have no experience of radiology, but it surely is an exceedingly difficult matter to determine by this means, in any but extreme cases, what does and what does not constitute a normal sella turcica. Do we know from measurements on the skull itself what are the normal limits of this fossa relatively to the size of the skull? To the ordinary man it is not particularly convincing to be told that the fossa is enlarged, that the posterior clinoid processes are blurred, or that the sphenoidal cells are large, and one wonders whether the blurring may not sometimes be due to thickening on more superficial parts of the skull, even though stereoscopic apparatus is used. I believe there has been no standardisation on the part of the radiologist regarding the normal limits of this fossa; his reports appear to be based on general impressions determined by his individual experience. General impressions so often prove to be wide of the truth when we put them to the statistical test, that one always needs to use great caution in making deductions from them. I have, however, no doubt that the distinguished ophthalmologist who originated the suggestion had good grounds for doing so in the cases which were before him at the time.

[1] Figs. 704, 737, 779.

A careful search through my material reveals no disease characteristically associated with hereditary optic atrophy; the symptoms of headache and giddiness occur frequently but perhaps not more so than in the general population; anybody who has seen a troublesome liability to migraine cured by a correction for slight errors in refraction will readily agree that its common occurrence in a disease which involves a profound disturbance of vision can be of only slight significance. If the underlying source of the disease be an inherent lack of vitality, it becomes of interest to see whether its incidence in a parent has any effect upon his fertility. Such scanty statistics as I am able to provide referring to this point are given in the following table, but facts deduced from them must be rather tentative and inconclusive.

	Mothers Affected		Fathers Affected	
	No. of Sibships	Average Size of Family	No. of Sibships	Average Size of Family
Sibships without Early Deaths or Miscarriages	28	4·0	110	3·2
Sibships including Early Deaths or Miscarriages	13	8·3	24	5·3
Totals	41	5·4 ± 0·4	134	3·6 ± 0·2

It is true that 3·2 is a rather low average size of family for 110 affected fathers of the class from which most of these families come, but we cannot be sure that there is not some limitation of families on the part of a partially blind father, who is unwilling to increase his responsibilities; moreover, not all the sibships considered are complete. All the affected parents who have contributed to the table were over 40 years of age and thus the families of affected mothers are likely to be nearly all complete, but the families of affected fathers may in a number of cases still be increased.

(f) *The Hereditary Character of the Disease and its Mode of Transmission.* We know that a great variety of general characters—physical, physiological and psychological—are transmitted equally by mother and father to their offspring, whether it be male or female, and that the correlation coefficient which measures the degree of resemblance between parent and child in these cases is about ·50; we know further that the resemblance between pairs of siblings is about the same as that between parent and child. When we are dealing with anomalous conditions, such as hereditary diseases involve, these statements can no longer be assumed to hold, indeed, they manifestly do not hold in the sex-limited diseases which are predominantly manifest in males and are usually transmitted by the unaffected mother to her sons alone, and it becomes of great interest to try and obtain some measure of the extent to which such conditions are controlled by heredity.

Statistical difficulties arise on attempting to measure the intensity of the hereditary factor from parent to child from collections of family histories such as my material provides; I therefore welcomed the opportunity to obtain a measure of the association of certain features of the disease as they occur in pairs of brothers and in other pairs of relations. Such features are the age at onset of the disease and the tendency to improvement of symptoms; the correlations found and the tables from which they were calculated are mostly given in my former paper[1]; I reproduce the correlation coefficients here for purposes of reference, and because of their special interest in demonstrating that a single feature of a relatively sex-limited hereditary disease, in the transmission of which the father takes little part and the mother commonly shows no manifest affection, is controlled by heredity to precisely the same degree as are the general characters which may be present in and transmitted by both parents.

	No.	Correlation Coefficients
Age of Onset in Pairs of Siblings (Japanese)	190	+ ·5073 ± ·0356
,, ,, ,, Pairs of Brothers (European)	812	+ ·5104 ± ·0175
,, ,, ,, Brothers and Sisters (European)	152	+ ·6233 ± ·0335
,, ,, ,, Nephew and Maternal Uncle (European)	393	+ ·2090 ± ·0325
,, ,, ,, Pairs of Male First Cousins (European)	390	+ ·1159 ± ·0337
Improvement of Symptoms—Pairs of Brothers	258	+ ·6002 ± ·0594

There is some tendency to-day to doubt the existence of sex-limited hereditary diseases which follow Lossen's Law in that the mode of transmission is entirely through the female line. It was believed at one time that haemophilia probably always conformed to this law, but it has now been unmistakably demonstrated[2] that the haemophilic male is capable of transmitting the disease if he live long enough to do so. Following this, statements have been made to the effect that hereditary optic atrophy also would be shown to be commonly transmitted through the male if pedigrees were sufficiently extensive to show that his daughters' sons were liable to be affected. Now this assuredly is not the case. A number of the pedigrees sufficient to justify my dogmatism show normal grandsons of affected males but many more pedigrees show affected individuals who were known to have an unaffected maternal grandfather, moreover the nature of this affection is not one which like colour-blindness can be concealed from the knowledge of the affected individual and his relations. I would ask anybody who has the slightest doubt regarding the fact that there is some very fundamental distinction in the mechanism of transmission, between the cases of say colour-blindness and hereditary optic atrophy, to examine the pedigrees of colour-blindness in Part II of this Nettleship volume, and compare them with those of the present memoir. There is no doubt that this disease is transmitted very generally through the female who is commonly unaffected, and that in a large proportion of histories the transmission has probably been confined to the female line; I suspect further that this disease and haemophilia present parallel examples, and that it is not alone the fatality of haemophilia with its liability to early death which leads to its very common transmission through the female line only. The actual figures obtained from my pedigrees are shown on p. 347.

Thus of 573 affected males no fewer than 95 °/₀ owe their affection to the mother, and of 88 females 84 °/₀ obtain affection through the mother. I give the corresponding figures for Japanese cases, for comparative purposes, though the

---

[1] *Bibl.* No. 148.   [2] *Bibl.* No. 143.

Source of Disease in Hereditary Optic Atrophy (Europeans).

	Males		Females	
	No.	Percentage	No.	Percentage
Mother Affected	85	14·8	38	43·2
Mother's Stock Affected	460	80·3	36	40·9
Transmission through Mother	545	95·1 ± 0·6	74	84·1 ± 2·6
Father Affected	23	4·0	12	13·6
Father's Stock Affected	5	0·9	2	2·3
Transmission through Father	28	4·9 ± 0·6	14	15·9 ± 2·6
Totals	573		88	

Source of Disease in Hereditary Optic Atrophy (Japanese).

	Males		Females	
	No.	Percentage	No.	Percentage
Mother Affected	24	34·8	22	57·9
Mother's Stock Affected	36	52·2	13	34·2
Transmission through Mother	60	87·0 ± 2·7	35	92·1 ± 3·0
Father Affected	8	11·6	2	5·3
Father's Stock Affected	1	1·4	1	2·6
Transmission through Father	9	13·0 ± 2·7	3	7·9 ± 3·0
Totals	69		38	

numbers are very small and the percentages they provide should not be regarded seriously until further material is available; they are of special interest, however, as indicating that though the sex incidence in the two series differs so markedly the mode of transmission of the disease in Japanese cases evidently closely resembles that for Europeans. On examining the pedigrees which provide the relatively rare cases of apparent transmission through the father, I find that there is usually no knowledge of the mother's stock and that thus in some of the cases the responsibility probably does not belong to the father; I think it is clear, however, that under special conditions he is undoubtedly able to transmit the disease either directly to his children or indirectly through his daughters to his grandchildren. I find no clue to what these conditions may be, but the fact that in certain stocks the transmission through the father can be seen to readily occur suggests that the power to do so is determined by some linked factor which is inherited with the disease. If from the above tables we omitted a few pedigrees such as Fig. 764 or Fig. 916 the percentages showing transmission through the father would be considerably reduced.

In a former part of this volume (p. 282) I included a table showing a predominantly male sex incidence in a number of hereditary diseases, as they had been actually observed to occur; the table was accompanied by a warning that the figures have only a restricted significance and cannot be assumed to represent the inherent relative liability of each sex to show the disease. With a similar warning I now publish a further table showing the relative apparent responsibility of men and women for the transmission of hereditary disease in a number of cases.

The Transmission of Hereditary Disease.

	Through Mother	Through Father	Percentage through Mother	Male Sex Incidence
Hereditary Optic Atrophy (Europeans)	619	42	93·6	84·8
Retinitis Pigmentosa	214	113	65·4	55·6
Ectopia Lentis	91	56	61·9	53·7
Diabetes	55	35	60·1	66·7
Blue Sclerotics	229	158	59·2	44·6
Night-Blindness*	99	81	55·6	52·3
Congenital Cataract	242	313	43·6	50·1
Multiple Exostoses	157	336	31·8	70·2

* The type in which both sexes are affected.

This table is of interest as showing the heavy actual responsibility of women in this matter, whatever may be the underlying causes operating to produce this state of affairs; the underlying causes are certainly inherent in the case of optic atrophy, in other cases they may be very complex varying from one disease to another and probably reacted upon by economic and social conditions varying from one period to another or from one country to another. I do not know whether one can attribute the exceptional heavily predominating transmission through the father in multiple exostoses to gross deformity preventing child-bearing in affected females; the male sex incidence is very high in this disease and the percentages given should always be considered relatively to the sex incidence. Whilst emphasising the need for caution in the interpretation of this table as a whole, I have no doubt with regard to hereditary optic atrophy that if the sisters of affected males abstained from parentage the disease would be almost exterminated.

The following table gives some analysis of the affected sibships provided by the

	Father Affected Mother Normal	Mother Affected Father Normal		Both Parents Normal Mother's Stock Affected		Both Parents Normal No Knowledge of Mother's Stock	
	A + B (15)† i	A (17)† ii	B (19)† iii	A (171)† iv	B (22)† v	A (41)† vi	B (18)† vii
No. of Affected Sons	18	39	31	325	42	98	34
,, ,, Affected Daughters	10	—	25	—	28	—	28
,, ,, Unaffected Sons	15	6	16	142	13	33	10
,, ,, Unaffected Daughters*	11	24	20	313	37	104	31
Percentage of Sons Affected	[54·5]	[86·7]	[66·0]	69·6 ± 1·4	76·4 ± 3·9	74·8 ± 2·6	77·3 ± 4·3
,, ,, Daughters Affected	[47·6]	—	[55·6]	—	43·1 ± 4·1	—	47·5 ± 4·4
,, ,, Males in Sibships	[61·1]	[65·2]	[51·1]	59·9 ± 1·2	45·8 ± 3·1	55·7 ± 2·2	42·7 ± 3·3
,, ,, Sibship Affected	[51·9]	[56·5]	[60·9]	41·7 ± 1·2	58·3 ± 3·0	41·7 ± 2·2	60·2 ± 3·3

Only affected Sibships are included in this table. A refers to Sibships in which males only are affected.
B refers to Sibships in which affected males and females occur.

* The daughters of this row are such as show no manifest defect, but they may have latent defect and they may in some cases have transmitted the disease.   † = Number of Sibships.

pedigrees; in some columns the numbers are too small to carry much weight, but collectively the table is suggestive and certain deductions can be drawn from it. Thus, nothing definite can be deduced from column i as the numbers are so small, but it provides no support for the view that fathers are unable to influence the transmission of the disease and that when an affected father has affected offspring, they must be attributed to the mother; this column is not directly comparable with the others in so far as the A and B groups are combined, moreover we have records of over a hundred affected fathers whose offspring are entirely normal and therefore do not appear in this table; this very significant fact must be remembered on examining the figures here given. In colour-blindness an affected father very rarely transmits the defect directly to his offspring, but when he marries into an affected stock we look for the relatively exceptional colour-blind females amongst his offspring; my material provides no evidence that a similar parentage is responsible for the occurrence of hereditary optic atrophy in females. Again little can be deduced from columns ii and iii; percentages based on such small numbers are very uncertain quantities but these columns definitely indicate some very fundamental distinction between the mode of transmission in colour-blindness and hereditary optic atrophy in so far as the colour-blind mother has very generally, but not quite always, all her sons colour-blind.

Columns iv and v of the table appear to be homogeneous respectively with columns vi and vii and their numbers might justifiably be combined; they show the extremely high percentage of affected males; when the parentage is such as to lead to manifest affection in the daughters the percentage of affected sons tends to be even further raised. Evidently some special stimulus is in operation when females become affected; its presence can be glimpsed in the high correlation coefficient of ·62 for age of onset between brother and sister and in the low average age of onset (19·96) for brothers who have affected sisters; further there are indications that the correlations between age of onset in pairs of sisters and in male and female first cousins are definitely raised; the tendency to an increased percentage of affected sons in sibships containing affected daughters is thus not an unexpected occurrence. The marked increase in the percentage of the sibship affected when females occur showing manifest defect will be noted, but it must be remembered that some of this increase may perhaps be explained by an increased amount of latent defect in the columns A which has become manifest in columns B and so influences the percentage. The high proportion of males in the sibships in which males alone are affected is not all accounted for by the fact that the nature of the case determines at least one male in the family.

I have sought for some definite indication regarding the nature of the special conditions which lead to the manifestation of hereditary optic atrophy in women but have had no success; I would however call attention to the facts that, as shown in the table given above, of 74 affected females, 38 $°/_{\circ}$ or 43·2 $°/_{\circ}$ had affected mothers, whilst of 545 affected males only 14·8 $°/_{\circ}$ had affected mothers; these facts are suggestive but the sequence leading to the occurrence of this disease in women is far more obscure than in the case of colour-blindness.

Some warm appreciation of the work of Nettleship on Leber's disease is due. In

1909 he collected all the material which was then available on the subject and considered in some detail many of the points which have been here investigated; his paper was of great value to me when I was collecting pedigrees, but the available material has so markedly increased since his work was undertaken that I thought it better to make an entirely independent analysis; it is a pleasure to find how much support the increased data bring to his conclusions. I on the other hand would claim his support in my procedure with regard to the question whether cases of this disease which arise very early in life are truly homogeneous with those which occur at a later age. Nettleship writes:

"Cases of family or hereditary congenital optic atrophy have been described as if forming a group in some way distinct from Leber's disease. I believe that most of these are true Leber's disease setting in very early in life or perhaps sometimes before birth...and I doubt whether we have at present sufficient evidence to justify us in setting up any of these family infantile cases as a distinct group[1]."

Before Nettleship, Hormuth in 1900[2] also collected the then available material concerning hereditary optic atrophy; he reports the clinical details of cases more fully than does Nettleship and has been very helpful to me for purposes of verification and reference.

I am greatly indebted to Mr C. H. Usher and to Professor Karl Pearson for reading the manuscript of this paper and making many valuable suggestions regarding it, also to the Medical Research Council for the continuation of the grant which has enabled me to prepare another portion of this Nettleship Memorial Volume.

NAME INDEX TO THE CHRONOLOGICAL BIBLIOGRAPHY AND TO THE RECORDERS OF PEDIGREES[3].

---

[1] *Bibl.* No. 85, p. cxx.   [2] *Bibl.* No. 64.

[3] Bibliography numbers are always placed before pedigree numbers.

BIBLIOGRAPHY

(An asterisk refers to papers which have not been seen.)

1. BEER, G. J.: *Lehre von den Augenkrankheiten.* Wien, 1817. [Bd. II, S. 443 contains what is perhaps the earliest reference to hereditary optic atrophy.]

2. LUCAS, P.: *Traité philosophique et physiologique de l'Hérédité naturelle.* Paris, 1847. [T. I, pp. 399–401 refers to probable cases of hereditary optic atrophy.] See Fig. 759.

3. VON GRAEFE, A.: Ein ungewöhnlicher Fall von hereditärer Amaurose. *Archiv f. Ophthalmologie.* Bd. IV, Abth. ii, S. 266–268. Berlin, 1858. See Fig. 865.

4. SEDGWICK, W.: Hereditary Amaurosis. *Medical Times and Gazette.* Vol. I for 1862, p. 309. London, 1862. See Fig. 815.

5. BENEDICT, M.: Der Daltonismus bei Sehnervenatrophie. *Archiv j. Ophthalmologie.* Bd. X, Abth. ii, S. 855–910. Berlin, 1864.

6. HUTCHINSON, J.: Report on Cases of Congenital Amaurosis. *Royal London Ophthalmic Hospital Reports.* Vol. V, pp. 347–352. London, 1866. See Fig. 813.

7. HUTCHINSON, J.: Statistical Details of four years' Experience in respect to the form of Amaurosis supposed to be due to Tobacco. *Royal London Ophthalmic Hospital Reports.* Vol. VII, pp. 169–185. London, 1871. See Fig. 863.

8. LEBER, T.: Ueber hereditäre und congenital-angelegte Sehnervenleiden. *Archiv f. Ophthalmologie.* Bd. XVII, Abth. II, S. 249–291. Berlin, 1871. See Figs. 721, 742, 772, 809.

9. DAGUENET, V. and GALEZOWSKI, X.: D'Amaurose congénitale. *Journal d'Ophtalmologie.* T. I, pp. 342–366. Paris, 1872. See Fig. 760.

10. PROUFF, M.: *Sur une Forme d'Atrophie papillaire.* Thèse. Paris, 1873. See Fig. 760.

11. ALEXANDER: Drei Fälle von hereditären Sehnervenleiden. *Klinische Monatsblätter f. Augenheilkunde.* Bd. XII, S. 62–66. Erlangen, 1874. See Fig. 817.

12. PUFAHL, C. L. M.: Ueber hereditäre Amblyopie. *Berliner klinische Wochenschrift.* Bd. XIII, S. 128–130. Berlin, 1876. See Fig. 864.

13. *SCHILLING, H.: *Über Gesichtsfeldamblyopie ohne ophthalmoskopischen Befund.* Dissertation. Berlin, 1876. See Fig. 839.

14. *PUFAHL, C. L. M.: Amblyopia hereditaria. *Beiträge z. praktische Augenheilkunde.* Bd. III, S. 75. Leipzig, 1878. See Fig. 892.

15. Fuchs, E.: Neuritis in Folge hereditärer Anlage. *Klinische Monatsblätter f. Augenheilkunde.* Bd. xvii, S. 332—337. Stuttgart, 1879. See Figs. 761, 811, 825.

16. Higgens, C.: Three Cases of Simple Atrophy of the Optic Nerves occurring in Members of the same Family. *Lancet.* Vol. ii for 1881, p. 869. London, 1881. See Fig. 850.

17. Mooren, A.: *Fünf Lustren ophthalmologischer Wirksamkeit.* Wiesbaden, 1882. [Hereditary optic atrophy is described pp. 249—250.] See Figs. 741, 807, 852, 895.

18. Samelsohn, J.: Zur Anatomie und Nosologie der retrobulbären Neuritis. [Amblyopia centralis.] *Archiv f. Ophthalmologie.* Bd. xxviii, Abth. i, S. 1—110. Berlin, 1882.

19. Schlüter, F.: *Ueber Neuritis Optica.* Dissertation. Berlin, 1882. See Figs. 788, 869, 870.

20. de Keersmaecker: De l'Atrophie axiale du Nerf optique observée chez plusieurs membres d'une même Famille. *Recueil d'Ophtalmologie.* Sér. 3, T. iv, pp. 193—203. Paris, 1883. See Fig. 727.

21. Rampoldi, R.: Amaurosi di Atrofia ottica in quattro Generazioni. *Annali di Ottalmologia.* Anno xii, pp. 269—271. Pavia, 1883. See Fig. 776.

22. Holz, R.: *Drei Fälle von genuiner Atrophia nervorum opticorum simplex progressiva bei Geschwistern.* Dissertation. Greifswald, 1885. See Fig. 889.

23. Norris, W. F.: Hereditary Atrophy of the Optic Nerves. *Transactions, American Ophthalmological Society.* Vol. iii, pp. 355—359, 662—678. Boston, 1885. See Figs. 750, 881.

24. Story, J. B.: Hereditary Amaurosis. *Ophthalmic Review.* Vol. iv, pp. 33—38. London, 1885. See Fig. 851.

25. Gevers, H.: *Zur Symptomatologie der eigentlichen nicht durch Intoxication bedingten retrobulbären Neuritis.* Dissertation. Berlin, 1887. [The case here described is the same as that previously described by Schlüter. See Bibl. 19 and Fig. 788.]

26. Jakobsohn, E.: Casuistische Beiträge zur angeborenen Sehnervenatrophie. *Centralblatt f. praktische Augenheilkunde.* Bd. xi, S. 362—363. Leipzig, 1887. See Fig. 771.

27. Suckling, C. W.: Hereditary Optic Atrophy. *Lancet.* Vol. ii for 1887, p. 1271. London, 1887. See Fig. 904.

28. Browne, E. A.: Optic Atrophy in three Brothers. *Transactions, Ophthalmological Society of U.K.* Vol. viii, pp. 235—239. London, 1888. See Fig. 876.

29. Habershon, S. H.: Hereditary Optic Atrophy. *Transactions, Ophthalmological Society of U.K.* Vol. viii, pp. 190—234. London, 1888. See Figs. 746, 786, 789, 790, 871, 872, 875.

30. Haswell, J. F.: A Case of Hereditary Amblyopia. *British Medical Journal.* Vol. ii for 1888, p. 1279. London, 1888. See Fig. 795.

31. Thomsen: Hereditärer retrobulbärer Neuritis. *Münchener medicinische Wochenschrift.* Bd. xxxv, S. 222. München, 1888. See Fig. 802.

32. Lawford, J. B.: Notes of some out-patient Cases in the Eye Department. *St Thomas's Hospital Reports.* Vol. xvii, pp. 157—170. London, 1889. See Figs. 804, 822.

33. de Wecker, L. and Landolt, E.: *Traité complet d'Ophtalmologie.* T. iv. Paris, 1889. [Hereditary Neuritis is described pp. 478—483, pedigree in footnote p. 485.]

34. Nicolaï, C.: Eenige Gevallen van Atrophia N. optici in ééne Familie. *Nederlandsch Tijdschrift voor Geneeskunde.* Bd. xxvi, S. 118. Amsterdam, 1890. See Fig. 862.

35. Sym, W. G.: A case of Hereditary Amaurosis. *Edinburgh Medical Journal.* Vol. xxxvi, Part ii. pp. 1131—1136. Edinburgh, 1891. See Fig. 803.

36. Despagnet, F.: De la Névrite optique héréditaire. *Recueil d'Ophtalmologie.* Anno xiv. Sér. 3, pp. 387—398. Paris, 1892. See Fig. 882.

37. Somya, J. R.: Ein Beitrag zur Kenntniss der hereditären retrobulbären Neuritis. *Klinische Monatsblätter f. Augenheilkunde.* Bd. xxx, S. 256—261. Stuttgart, 1892. See Fig. 758.

38. Taylor, S. J.: Hereditary Optic Atrophy. *Transactions, Ophthalmological Society of U.K.* Vol. xii, pp. 146—156. London, 1892. See Fig. 749.

39. Daussat, C.: *Étude sur la Névrite optique.* Thèse. Lyon, 1893.

40. Gould, G. M.: Homeochronous Hereditary Optic-nerve Atrophy, extending through six Generations. *Annals of Ophthalmology and Otology.* Vol. ii, pp. 303—307. St Louis, 1893. See Fig. 706.

41. Müller: Genuine Atrophie der Optici bei drei Brüdern. *Klinische Monatsblätter f. Augenheilkunde.* Bd. xxxi, S. 26—27. Stuttgart, 1893. See Fig. 805.

42. Oliver, C. A.: A short note upon so-called "Hereditary Optic Nerve Atrophy" as a contribution to the question of Transmission of Structural Peculiarity. *Proceedings, American Philosophical Society.*

Vol. xxxii, pp. 269—271. Philadelphia, 1894. [Refers to what should be a valuable pedigree but the information given is too slight for reproduction.]

43. BARRETT, J. W.: Two cases of Optic Neuritis occurring in Brothers, each with Central Colour Scotomata. *Australian Medical Journal.* Vol. xvii, pp. 504—505. Melbourne, 1895. See Fig. 900.

44. DODD, O.: Hereditary Retro-bulbar Neuritis. *Annals of Ophthalmology and Otology.* Vol. iv, pp. 300—304. St Louis, 1895. See Fig. 823.

45. LINDE, M.: Neuritische Atrophie des Sehnerven bei Mutter und Kind. *Centralblatt f. praktische Augenheilkunde.* Bd. xix, S. 363—364. Leipzig, 1895. [The case is thought by the recorder to have probably been of syphilitic origin in mother and daughter.]

46. WESTHOFF, C. H. A.: Hereditäre retrobulbäre Neuritis optica. *Centralblatt f. praktische Augenheilkunde.* Bd. xix, S. 168—173. Leipzig, 1895. See Fig. 767.

47. BATTEN, R. D.: A Family suffering from Hereditary Optic Atrophy. *Transactions, Ophthalmological Society of U.K.* Vol. xvi, pp. 125—130. London, 1896. See Fig. 755.

48. KAUFFMANN: Leber's Disease in two Brothers. *Lancet.* Vol. i for 1896, p. 626. London, 1896. See Fig. 848.

49. NOLTE, F.: *Beitrag zu der Lehre von der Erblichkeit von Augenerkrankungen.* Dissertation. Marburg, 1896. [A slight section is given on hereditary optic atrophy pp. 22—26; bibliography pp. 35—36; a brief account is given of the family history described more fully at a later date by Kuhk. See Fig. 751.]

50. OGILVIE, M. B.: Optic Atrophy in three Brothers. *Transactions, Ophthalmological Society of U.K.* Vol. xvi, pp. 111—124. London, 1896. See Fig. 774.

51. VELHAGEN, C.: Ueber hereditäre Sehnervenatrophie. *Deutsche medizinische Wochenschrift.* Bd. xxii, S. 841—842. Leipzig, 1896. See Fig. 821.

52. HIGIER, H.: Zur Klinik der familiären Opticusaffectionen. *Deutsche Zeitschrift f. Nervenheilkunde.* Bd. x, S. 489—505. Leipzig, 1897. See Fig. 787.

53. *LEITNER, W.: [On Hereditary Optic Atrophy.] *Szemészet.* Vol. for 1897. Budapest, 1897. See Figs. 740, 842. [The notes of these cases are taken from Nettleship. Bibl. No. 85, p. clxxvi.]

54. *LOR: Un cas d'atrophie optique familiale. *Cercle méd. de Bruxelles.* November, 1897. [Notes of case taken from *Revue générale d'Ophtalmologie.* T. xvii, p. 132. Paris, 1898.] See Fig. 806.

55. SNELL, S.: Hereditary or Congenital Optic Atrophy and allied Cases. *Transactions, Ophthalmological Society of U.K.* Vol. xvii, pp. 66—81. London, 1897. See Figs. 752, 757, 826, 829, 877.

56. KLOPFER, G.: *Neuritis optica infolge von Heredität und congenitaler Anlage (Leber).* Dissertation. Tübingen, 1898. See Fig. 719.

57. *LEITNER, W.: [On Hereditary Optic Atrophy.] *Szemészet.* Vol. for 1898. Budapest, 1898. See Fig. 739. [The notes of this case are taken from Nettleship. Bibl. No. 85, p. clxxvii.]

58. POSEY, W. C.: Hereditary Optic Nerve Atrophy. A report of three cases, representing members of three successive generations affected by the disease. *Annals of Ophthalmology.* Vol. vii, pp. 357—371. St Louis, 1898. See Fig. 748.

59. BUISSON, G.: Contribution à l'Étude de la Névrite optique rétrobulbaire familiale et Héréditaire. Thèse. Paris, 1899. See Figs. 747, 833.

60. MAGERS, J.: *Ueber hereditäre Sehnervenatrophie und hereditäre Choroiditis.* Dissertation. Jena. 1899. See Fig. 893.

61. STRZEMINSKI: Trois Cas de Névrite optique rétro-bulbaire héréditaire dans une même Famille. *Annales d'Oculistique.* T. cxxi, pp. 99—112. Paris, 1899. See Fig. 832.

62. HANSELL, HOWARD F.: A Case of Double Retrobulbar Optic Neuritis, Hereditary in Origin. *Transactions, American Ophthalmological Society.* Vol. ix, pp. 114—117. Hartford, 1900. See Fig. 890.

63. HAWKES, C. S.: Hereditary Optic Atrophy. *Australasian Medical Gazette.* Vol. xix, pp. 228—229. Sydney, 1900. See Figs. 731, 732.

64. HORMUTH, P.: *Beiträge zur Lehre von den hereditären Sehnervenleiden.* Dissertation. Heidelberg, 1900. See Figs. 777, 782, 849, 853—859, 861, 866, 867, 878, 879.

65. *GALLEMAERTS: Atrophie optique héréditaire. *La Policlinique.* T. x. Bruxelles, 1901. See Fig. 891.

66. MATHIEU, J.: Contribution à l'Étude de la Névrite optique rétrobulbaire héréditaire. Thèse. Paris. 1901. See Fig. 836.

67. HEINSBERGER, P.: Zur Casuistik der retrobulbären Neuritis optica auf hereditärer Grundlage. Dissertation. Giessen, 1902. See Figs. 783, 860.

68. LADDER, H.: Einen Fall von familiärer retrobulbären Neuritis. *Wiener klinische Wochenschrift.* Bd. xv, S. 1264—1265. Wien, 1902. See Fig. 835.

69. VELHAGEN, C.: Atrophia nervi optici hereditaria. *Münchener medicinische Wochenschrift.* Bd. XLIX, S. 941. München, 1902. See Fig. 883.

70. NETTLESHIP, E.: A Case of Family Optic Neuritis (Leber's Disease) in which perfect Recovery of Sight took place. *Transactions, Ophthalmological Society of U.K.* Vol. XXIII, pp. 108—110. London, 1903. See Fig. 818.

71. BICKERTON, R. E.: Hereditary Optic Atrophy in two Brothers. *Transactions, Ophthalmological Society of U.K.* Vol. XXIV, pp. 178—180. London, 1904. See Fig. 908.

72. BRAMWELL, B.: Hereditary Optic Atrophy. *Clinical Studies.* Vol. II, pp. 44—55. Edinburgh, 1904. See Fig. 710.

73. KNAPP, A.: Hereditary Optic Atrophy. *Archives of Ophthalmology.* Vol. XXXIII, pp. 383—385. New York, 1904. See Fig. 827.

74. KOWALEWSKI: Familiäre Opticus-Atrophie. *Centralblatt f. praktische Augenheilkunde.* Bd. XXX, S. 114—115. Leipzig, 1906. See Fig. 808.

75. COSTE, A.: *De l'Atrophie papillaire familiale.* Thèse. Toulouse, 1907. See Fig. 734.

76. GUNN, R. M.: Family Optic Atrophy in Mother and two Children. *Transactions, Ophthalmological Society of U.K.* Vol. XXVII, pp. 221—225. London, 1907. See Fig. 810.

77. LAWSON, A.: Family Optic Atrophy in Mother and Son. *Transactions, Ophthalmological Society of U.K.* Vol. XXVII, pp. 169—170. London, 1907. See Fig. 906.

78. FORTUNATI, A. and MINGAZZINI, G.: Contributo clinico allo Studio della "Neuritis Optica Familiaris (hereditaria)." *Il Policlinico.* Vol. XV, Sez. Medica, pp. 97—116. Roma, 1908. See Figs. 812, 885.

79. HANCOCK, W. I.: Hereditary Optic Atrophy [Leber's Disease]. *Royal London Ophthalmic Hospital Reports.* Vol. XVII, Part ii, pp. 167—177. London, 1908. See Fig. 728.

80. WAGENMANN, A.: Ueber hereditäre Sehnervenentzündung. *Münchener medicinische Wochenschrift.* Bd. XLV, S. 104. München, 1908. See Figs. 773, 831.

81. BACH: Hereditäre familiäre Sehnervenatrophie. *Münchener medicinische Wochenschrift.* Bd. LVI, S. 210. München, 1909. See Fig. 744.

82. BATTEN, R. D.: Two Cases of Hereditary Optic Atrophy in a Family with Recovery in one Case. *Transactions, Ophthalmological Society of U.K.* Vol. XXIX, pp. 144—149. London, 1909. See Fig. 780.

83. BEHR, C.: Die komplizierte, hereditär-familiäre Optikusatrophie des Kindesalters. *Klinische Monatsblätter f. Augenheilkunde.* Bd. XLVII, S. 138—160. Stuttgart, 1909. See Figs. 816, 820, 824.

84. LOEB, C.: Hereditary Blindness and its Prevention. *Annals of Ophthalmology.* Vol. XVIII, pp. 1—47. St Louis, 1909. See Fig. 901.

85. NETTLESHIP, E.: Some Hereditary Diseases of the Eye. *Transactions, Ophthalmological Society of U.K.* Vol. XXIX, pp. lvii—cxcviii. London, 1909. See Figs. 725, 726, 736, 739, 740, 745, 746, 749, 775, 781, 784, 785, 786, 790, 827, 842, 868, 875.

86. RAYMOND, F. and KOENIG, E.: Atrophie héréditaire de la Papille. *Recueil d'Ophtalmologie.* Sér. 3, T. 31, pp. 65—84. Paris, 1909. See Figs. 743, 791, 792, 793.

87. CLEMESHA, J. C.: An Example of Leber's Disease. *American Journal of Ophthalmology.* Vol. XXVII, pp. 139—141. St Louis, 1910. See Fig. 847.

88. CLIMENKO, H.: Retrobulbar Optic Neuritis Familiaris. *Journal of Nervous and Mental Disease.* Vol. XXXVII, p. 303. New York, 1910. See Fig. 898.

89. HAUSHALTER, P.: Un Cas de Névrite optique familiale et héréditaire. *Archives de Médecine des Enfants.* T. XIII, pp. 765—766. Paris, 1910. See Fig. 769.

90. MÜGGE, F.: Hereditäre Neuritis optica. *Deutsche medizinische Wochenschrift.* Bd. XXXVI, S. 2366. Leipzig, 1910. See Figs. 766, 905.

91. RÖNNE, H.: Ueber das Gesichtsfeld bei hereditärer Opticusatrophie (Leber). *Klinische Monatsblätter f. Augenheilkunde.* Bd. XLVIII, Supplement, S. 331—333. Stuttgart, 1910. See Figs. 896, 899.

92. LUTZ, A.: Über einige Stammbäume und die Anwendung der mendelschen Regeln auf die Ophthalmologie. *Archiv f. Ophthalmologie.* Bd. LXXIX, S. 393—427. Leipzig, 1911. See Fig. 796.

93. MÜGGE, F.: Ein Beitrag zur Leberschen familiären Optikusatrophie. *Zeitschrift f. Augenheilkunde.* Bd. XXV, S. 236—253. Berlin, 1911. See Figs. 722, 735.

94. VALUDE, E.: *Observations cliniques d'Atrophie Optique.*—Névrite rétrobulbaire familiale—Atrophie Optique traumatique. *Annales d'Oculistique.* T. CXLVI, pp. 341—345. Paris, 1911. See Fig. 907.

95. BRUNER, W. E.: Hereditary Optic Atrophy with X-Ray Findings. *Transactions, American Ophthalmological Society.* Vol. XIII, pp. 162—174. Philadelphia, 1912. See Figs. 756, 902.

96. GUZMANN, E.: Ueber hereditäre familiäre Sehnervenatrophie. *Wiener klinische Wochenschrift.* Bd. XXVI, S. 139—141. Wien, 1913. See Fig. 835.

97. NETTLESHIP, E. and THOMPSON, A. H.: A Pedigree of Leber's Disease. *Proceedings, Royal Society of Medicine.* Vol. VI, Part 3, Sect. Ophthalmology, pp. 8—15. London, 1913. See Fig. 729.

98. PEARSON, K., NETTLESHIP, E. and USHER, C. H.: *A Monograph on Albinism in Man.* Part IV. London, 1913. See Fig. 779.

99. TAKASHIMA, S.: Sechs Fälle der komplizierten hereditär-familiären Optikus-Atrophie des Kindesalters (Behr). *Klinische Monatsblätter f. Augenheilkunde.* Bd. LI, S. 714—722. Stuttgart, 1913. See Fig. 820.

100. TAYLOR, J. and GORDON HOLMES, M.: Two Families with several Members in each suffering from Optic Atrophy. *Transactions, Ophthalmological Society of U.K.* Vol. XXXIII, pp. 95—115. London, 1913. See Figs. 717, 800.

101. WILBRAND, H. and SAENGER, A.: Die hereditäre Neuritis Optica. *Die Neurologie des Auges.* Bd. V, S. 135—173. Wiesbaden, 1913. See Figs. 762, 763, 814, 819, 909.

102. WORTON, A. S.: Hereditary Optic Neuritis. *Lancet.* Vol. II for 1913, pp. 1112—1114. London, 1913. See Fig. 724.

103. DE GRAAF, J. H. F.: Neuritis Optica hereditaria. *Geneeskundig Tijdschrift voor Nederlandsch-Indië.* Deel LIV, pp. 111—112. Batavia, 1914. See Fig. 778.

104. KUHK, R.: *Beitrag zur Lehre von der retrobulbären Neuritis Optici auf hereditärer Grundlage.* Dissertation. Marburg, 1914. See Fig. 751.

105. VAN LINT, A. and KLEEFELD, G.: Névrite optique familiale; (2 frères, 1 sœur) insuffisance thyroïdienne. *Annales d Oculistique.* T. CLII, pp. 110—122. Paris, 1914. See Fig. 713.

106. POCKLEY, E.: Leber's Disease (Hereditary Optic Atrophy). *Medical Journal of Australia.* Vol. I, pp. 189—191. Sydney, 1915. See Fig. 880.

107. POSEY, W. C.: The Hereditary Form of Retrobulbar Neuritis (or Leber's Disease). *Annals of Ophthalmology.* Vol. XXIV, pp. 423—424. St Louis, 1915. See Figs. 873, 874.

108. FISHER. J. H.: Leber's Disease (Hereditary Optic Atrophy); a Suggestion as to its Cause. *Transactions, Ophthalmological Society of U.K.* Vol. XXXVI, pp. 298—318. London, 1916. See Fig. 844.

109. EVANS, J. JAMESON: Hereditary Optic Atrophy. *Birmingham Medical Review.* Vol. LXXXI, pp. 95—103. Birmingham, 1917. See Figs. 768, 770.

110. FISHER, J. H.: A further Case of Leber's Disease, and two allied Cases associated with Changes in the Sella Turcica. *Transactions, Ophthalmological Society of U.K.* Vol. XXXVII, pp. 251—263. London, 1917. See Fig. 845.

111. HENSEN, H.: Ueber Neuritis Optica hereditaria. *Klinische Monatsblätter f. Augenheilkunde.* Bd. LIX, S. 33—42. Stuttgart, 1917. See Figs. 830, 894.

112. POLLOCK, W. B. I.: Two Cases of Leber s Disease (Hereditary Optic Atrophy) with X-ray Examination of the Sella Turcica. *Transactions, Ophthalmological Society of U.K.* Vol. XXXVII, pp. 247—251. London, 1917. See Fig. 846.

113. VOSSIUS, A.: Über familiäre Opticusatrophie. *Medizinische Klinik.* Bd. XIII, S. 850. Berlin, 1917. See Fig. 801.

114. ZENTMAYER, W.: Hereditary Optic Nerve Atrophy. *American Journal of Ophthalmology.* Ser. 3, Vol. I, pp. 791—792. Chicago, 1918. See Figs. 753, 754.

115. IMAMURA, S. and ICHIKAWA, K.: Atrophie optique familiale. *Revue Neurologique.* T. XXVI, pp. 277—282. Paris, 1919. See Fig. 932.

116. FLEISCHER, B. and JOSENHANS, W.: Ein Beitrag zur Frage der Vererbung der familiären Sehnervenatrophie (Leber'schen Krankheit). *Archiv f. Rassen- u. Gesellschafts-Biologie.* Bd. 13, S. 129—163. Leipzig, 1920. See Fig. 705.

117. DU SEUTRE, J.: Une Famille atteinte de la Maladie de Leber. *Archives d'Ophtalmologie.* T. XXXVII, pp. 545—550. Paris, 1920. See Fig. 828.

118. BARTH, F.: Ein weiterer Beitrag zur Vererbung der familiären Sehnervenatrophie (Leber'schen Krankheit). *Klinische Monatsblätter f. Augenheilkunde.* Bd. LXVI, S. 581—590. Stuttgart, 1921. See Fig. 719.

119. GRISCOM, J. M.: Hereditary Optic Atrophy. *American Journal of Ophthalmology.* Ser. 3, Vol. IV, pp. 347—352. Chicago, 1921. See Fig. 764.

120. MORLET, C.: Hereditary Optic Atrophy as a possible Menace to the Community. *Medical Journal of Australia.* Vol. II for 1921, pp. 499—502. Sydney, 1921. See Fig. 730.

121. ALAJMO, B.: Neurite Ottica retrobulbare ereditaria. *Giornale di Oculistica.* Vol. III, pp. 93—121. Napoli, 1922. See Fig. 709.

122. LAGRANGE, H.: De l'Atrophie optique héréditaire. *Archives d'Ophtalmologie.* T. XXXIX, pp. 530—539. Paris, 1922. See Fig. 765.

123. VOGT, A.: Ueber geschlechtsgebundene Vererbung von Augenleiden. *Schweizerische medizinische Wochenschrift.* Bd. LII, S. 77—83. Basel, 1922. See Fig. 738.

124. DREXEL, K. T.: Inwieweit stimmen der wirklichen Erfahrungen über die Vererbung der familiären, hereditären Sehnervenatrophie (Lebersche Krankheit) überein mit der Theorie der Vererbung der geschlechtsgebundenen Krankheiten? *Archiv f. Augenheilkunde.* Bd. XCIII, S. 49—116. München, 1923.

125. GINZBURG, J. J.: Beitrag zur Kenntnis der Leberschen Krankheit. *Klinische Monatsblätter f. Augenheilkunde.* Bd. LXXI, S. 734—738. Stuttgart, 1923. See Fig. 834.

126. HIRSCH, J.: Ueber familiare hereditäre Sehnervenatrophie. *Klinische Monatsblätter f. Augenheilkunde.* Bd. LXX, S. 710—715. Stuttgart, 1923. See Fig. 707.

127. BAUDOT, R.: Sur un Cas d'Atrophie Optique Héréditaire [Maladie de Leber]. *Revue médicale de l'Est.* T. LII, pp. 296—299. Nancy, 1924. See Fig. 843.

128. *BERESINSKAJA, D.: Ein Fall von familiärer Sehnervenatrophie. *Russ. Ophth. Jour.*, 1924. [Abstract taken from *Klinische Monatsblätter f. Augenheilkunde.* Bd. LXXIV, S. 267. Stuttgart, 1925.] See Fig. 897.

129. BURROUGHS, A. E.: Two Cases of Leber's Disease, or Familial Optic Atrophy with Enlargement of the Pituitary Fossae. *Transactions, Ophthalmological Society of U.K.* Vol. XLIV, pp. 399—403. London, 1924. See Fig. 887.

130. VAN HEUVEN, G. J. and OLTMANS, G.: Over Neuritis Optica Hereditaria. *Nederlandsch Tijdschrift voor Geneeskunde.* Vol. LXVIII, pp. 1958—1965. Haarlem, 1924. See Figs. 712, 714, 733.

131. WAARDENBURG, P. J.: Beitrag zur Vererbung der familiären Sehnervenatrophie [Leberschen Krankheit]. *Klinische Monatsblatter f. Augenheilkunde.* Bd. LXXIII, S. 619—652. Stuttgart, 1924. See Figs. 708, 718, 797.

132. VAN HEUVEN, J. A.: Bijdrage tot de Casuistick der Neuritis Optica Hereditaria. *Nederlandsch Tijdschrift voor Geneeskunde.* Vol. LXIX, Helft i, pp. 1723—1724. Haarlem, 1925. See Fig. 798.

133. LANG: A Case of Hereditary Optic Atrophy is shown at a meeting of the Ophthalmological Society of Vienna. The meeting is reported and family history described in *Klinische Monatsblätter f. Augenheilkunde.* Bd. LXXV, S. 780. Stuttgart, 1925. See Fig. 888.

134. MANSILLA, G.: Neuritis retrobulbar familiar. *El Siglo Médico.* T. LXXVI, pp. 186—187. Madrid, 1925. See Fig. 799.

135. MEYER-RIEMSLOH, B.: Ueber hereditäre Sehnervenatrophie [Lebersche Krankheit]. *Klinische Monatsblätter f. Augenheilkunde.* Bd. LXXIV, S. 340—355. Stuttgart, 1925. See Fig. 716.

136. PINES, I. L. J. and TRON, F.: Hereditäre Neuritis Optica [Lebersche Sehnervenatrophie]. *Zeitschrift f. d. ges. Neurologie u. Psychiatrie.* Bd. XCV, S. 762—776. Berlin, 1925. See Fig. 723.

137. KAWAKAMI, R.: Beiträge zur Vererbung der familiären Sehnervenatrophie. *Archiv f. Ophthalmologie.* Bd. CXVI, S. 568—595. Berlin, 1926. See Figs. 911—941.

138. SCHONENBERGER, F.: Beitrag zur Kenntnis der homochron-hereditären Opticusatrophie. *Archiv der Julius Klaus-Stiftung.* Bd. II, S. 59—70. Zürich, 1926. See Figs 738, 838, 841.

139. ALSBERG: Hereditäre Sehnervenatrophie bei Vater und Sohn. *Klinische Monatsblätter f. Augenheilkunde.* Bd. LXXIX, S. 832. Stuttgart, 1927. See Fig. 903.

140. FAVIER, R.: *Contribution à l'Étude de l'Atrophie optique héréditaire et familiale.* Thèse. Paris, 1927. See Fig. 840.

141. KROPP, L.: Zur Differentialdiagnose der Leber'schen familiären Optikusatrophie. *Zeitschrift f. Augenheilkunde.* Bd. LXII, S. 57—62. Berlin, 1927. See Figs. 711, 715.

142. LUNDSGAARD, K. K. K.: Lebers hereditäre Sehnervenatrophie mit Stammtafel. *Hospitalstidende.* Bd. LXX, S. 32—34. København, 1927. See Fig. 910.

143. NISSÉ, B. S.: The Evidence of Transmission of Haemophilia through the male with a new Haemophilic Pedigree. *Annals of Eugenics.* Vol. II, pp. 25—40. Cambridge, 1927.

144. REEDER, J. E.: Hereditary Optic Atrophy. *American Journal of Ophthalmology.* Vol. X, pp. 429—431. Chicago, 1927. See Fig. 720.

145. RUGER, H. A. and STOESSIGER, B.: On the Growth Curves of Certain Characters in Man Males). *Annals of Eugenics.* Vol. II, pp. 76—110. Cambridge, 1927.

PLATE XLVIII.   DESCRIPTIONS OF PEDIGREE PLATES   357

146. USHER, C. H.: Two Pedigrees of Hereditary Optic Atrophy. *British Journal of Ophthalmology*. Vol. XI, pp. 417—437. London, 1927. See Figs. 704, 737.

147. USHER, C. H. and ELDERTON, E. M.: An Analysis of the Consumption of Tobacco and Alcohol in Cases of Tobacco Amblyopia. *Annals of Eugenics*. Vol. II, pp. 245—289. Cambridge, 1927.

148. BELL, J.: The Age of Onset in Hereditary Optic Atrophy. *Annals of Eugenics*. Vol. III, pp. 269—276. Cambridge, 1928.

149. BRIDE, T. M.: Three Cases of Optic Atrophy. ? Leber's Disease. *Transactions, Ophthalmological Society of U.K.* Vol. XLVIII, p. 422. London, 1928. See Fig. 794.

150. DWORJETZ, M.: Ueber die Berechtigung der Bezeichnung "Atrophia Nervi Optici." *Klinische Monatsblätter f. Augenheilkunde*. Bd. LXXX, S. 30—36. Stuttgart, 1928.

151. HOGG, G. H.: Hereditary Optic Atrophy. *Medical Journal of Australia*. Vol. I for 1928, pp. 372—374. Sydney, 1928. See Figs. 837, 886.

152. MANN, I. C.: Retinitis Pigmentosa and Leber's Hereditary Optic Atrophy occurring in Cousins. *Annals of Eugenics*. Vol. III, pp. 77—83. Cambridge, 1928. See Fig. 884.

153. TRAQUAIR, H. M.: Tobacco Amblyopia. *Lancet*. Vol. II for 1928, pp. 1173—1177. London, 1928.

DESCRIPTIONS OF PEDIGREE PLATES

PLATE XLVIII. Fig. 704. *Usher's Case B.* Fourteen males and two females with hereditary optic atrophy in a very fully worked-out pedigree which extends to six generations; most of the individuals of generations V and VI are below the age at which the onset of the disease usually occurs. Ten cases in generation III occur in the offspring of five unaffected sisters of whom II. 7 had four sons, all affected, and four unaffected daughters, three of them however having each an affected son. II. 8 had nine children of whom only one son and two daughters lived to adult age; the son was affected, neither daughter had affected offspring; III. 15 and 22 died in childhood, III. 21 died aged 16, III. 23 died in infancy. II. 10 had fourteen children of whom two sons and seven daughters grew up and of these one son and two daughters were affected; four children died in infancy or were stillborn, III. 31 died aged 12 from "water in head," III. 28 was phthisical and unable to work for twelve years; none of the married daughters of this sibship had affected offspring. II. 13 had a son who was affected and six daughters who were unaffected but of the four who were married three had each an affected son. II. 17 had two sons (of whom one died in infancy, one was affected), and two unaffected daughters who had not transmitted the defect. The six affected members of generation IV are all sons of unaffected females of affected sibships and in each of these cases one member only of the sibship is affected; the individual cases are described as follows: IV. 97, aged 29 (1903), was a coal shoveller; a year ago he noticed that vision was dim in his left eye, objects in front of him could not be seen clearly with this eye though he could see objects at the sides; he had had toothache on the evening before he noticed the defect; the condition progressed and about six months later he noticed a similar defect in the vision of his right eye; a few weeks after this he was unable to read ordinary sized print; about this time he felt out of sorts and suffered from anorexia, feeling of weakness, frontal headache, occasional nausea but no vomiting; no nasal discharge; four months before he was examined he had been laid up for a week with "erysipelas" in the right foot. A year after the onset R. V. = fingers at four feet; large central scotoma for red with a large card the colour of which was only recognised at the lower and outer parts of the field; tension normal; pupils equal and contract to light; eye movements full; disc was too pale, a large circular cup with very pale floor, stippling well marked, edge of disc sharply cut, no white lines along retinal vessels which are not narrowed; yellow spot normal; L. V. = hand movements at one foot; eye movements full except on attempted convergence when this eye does not move inwards; fundus similar to that of the right eye except that the disc is much paler. This patient had always been strong and healthy, had no syphilitic history, no constipation, did not smoke and was temperate, had never been liable to headaches before the onset of the disease and had no history of giddiness or tinnitus; he was illegitimate and knew nothing of his father; his mother married and had at least two other children; an examination of the nervous system was almost negative though some rigidity in both legs and slight Rombergism are described. Subsequent examinations are described the latest of which in 1926 was twenty-four years after the onset; he was now aged 51, pupils were equal and contracted to light; eye movements were full except the left which did not move in much beyond the mid-line; there was no evidence of tower-skull or acromegaly; R. V. = fingers at one foot, L. V. = hand movements at six feet limited to lower-inner part of field; discs were very pale, greyish, edges sharply defined, retinal vessels not much narrowed; refraction was low hypermetropia in each; right field was much contracted peripherally and had an absolute central scotoma for white; the patient had never smoked and took no alcohol; general health was good; he had had three children of whom the youngest was a son aged 20 years; his daughter had had six children all of whom were young. Report of skiagram: "The sella is regular in outline, antero-posterior diameter = 13 mm., depth = 11 mm. The anterior clinoid processes are well formed, but the posterior ones are blurred and partly buried in what seems to be new bony growth. The sphenoidal sinus is well developed."

IV. 95, aged 22 years (1901), fireman on a locomotive, first cousin to IV. 97, had noticed his sight failing four months ago, his vision had gradually got worse for two months and then remained stationary; eight months ago he had passed the usual railway test for eyesight; some time before vision failed he had been troubled almost daily with headaches, mostly frontal, also with pain in stomach and dizziness; when smoking was discontinued two months ago the vision did not improve but it ceased to get worse and headaches also ceased; for the last five years the patient admitted having occasionally drunk too much but it never prevented him doing his work; he began to smoke at 16 years and smoked about three ounces of Irish twist weekly; no history of syphilis. Tongue and hands were tremulous but otherwise an examination of the nervous system revealed no defects; R. V. = L. V. = fingers at one foot; fields were full but absolute central scotomata for red were present; refraction was low hypermetropia; pupils were equal and contracted to light; eye movements were full; discs were normal or rather too red with deep physiological cupping; some of the smaller vessels were tortuous and possibly there were a few haemorrhages; the yellow spot and other parts of the fundi were normal. Six weeks later there was some indication of improvement and when seen in 1926 at the age of 49 vision had greatly improved and the improvement is said to have occurred during six months in 1902; now R. V. = $\frac{6}{60}$ or with + 1 D. = $\frac{6}{12}$; L. V. = $\frac{6}{60}$, with + 1·5 D. = $\frac{6}{9}$; he cannot recognise people in the street but can read very small print; fields of vision were full with large paracentral scotomata for red, green and blue above the fixation point; discs were pale with sharply defined edges, lamina cribrosa was much exposed; vessels were of good size with some narrowing of the inferior temporal artery on the right disc. This patient is not acromegalic and has no tower-skull; he has not again smoked a pipe but was smoking 70 cigarettes weekly; he takes no alcohol, was married at the age of 27 but has no children; general health was good; report of the skiagram states that "the sella is not quite regular in outline and its wall is thin; the clinoids are small and blurred; the sella measures 14 mm. antero-posteriorly and is 13 mm. deep; there is a blurred but quite distinct shadow lying free in the sella as if some mass, rather dense, was lying there." IV. 95 had one brother living, with good vision and normal fundi; one brother was dead but had apparently had no trouble with his eyes.

III. 10, Alexander Da., sixth born in a sibship of eight, aged 52 years (1909), was a pensioner; his vision had failed at the age of 25 years and had never improved; he smoked two ounces of tobacco weekly; vision was best in a dim light; R. V. = L. V. = hand movements at six feet; fields of vision were not contracted but an absolute central scotoma for white was present in each; colours were not recognised anywhere; pupils were equal and contracted to light; eye movements were full; media were clear, discs were pale, the retinal arteries were distinctly narrowed and the lamina cribrosa was exposed over most of the disc; there were no white lines along the retinal vessels, some vessels near the disc were more tortuous than usual. III. 10 was married to his first cousin, III. 26, who also had optic atrophy, but there was no issue; the patient died after operation for gastric ulcer in 1921. III. 7, William Da., aged 73 years (1926), was a retired coal miner; his vision became affected at the age of 20 years; he was now very deaf; R. V. = L. V. = hand movements at three feet; fields were not contracted but a central scotoma for white was present in each; no colours were recognised; the left disc was pale and retinal vessels of fair size; the right fundus could not be seen, pupils were small and examination difficult on account of the frailty and deafness of the patient; he smoked one ounce of bogie roll tobacco weekly; none of his ten children were affected. III. 9, John Da., became affected at the age of 18; he went abroad unmarried and had not been heard of since. III. 13, Robert Da., was a healthy coal miner when his vision failed at the age of 22 years, after which he became a pedlar; he had a twin son and daughter aged 21, his wife died at their birth; he died, aged 62, as a result of injury.

IV. 31, Hugh W., coal miner and son of the twin sister of III. 13, aged 42 (1926), became affected at the age of 21 years; he is strong, has had no illness, and formerly smoked heavily but has not now smoked for six years; he has had no alcohol for seven years but before this drank heavily once a week; he is liable to bilious attacks lasting for two or three days at intervals of from one to several months; he has four young daughters of whom the eldest is aged 6; R. V. = $\frac{3}{18}$ and 6 J.; L. V. = $\frac{3}{36}$ and 20 J.; fields of vision were full and no central scotoma for colour could be detected; right and left discs were pale, especially the left; lamina cribrosa was exposed; retinal vessels, of about normal size in the right, are rather diminished in the left eye; during fundus examination vertical nystagmus was observed in the left eye, not in the right; he said there was no miners' nystagmus amongst the men in his pit; he had one brother and seven sisters all unaffected. IV. 10, John P., coal miner, aged 40 (1926), does not admit that his vision is defective; R. V. = $\frac{4}{24}$, 16 J.; L. V. = $\frac{4}{12}$, 4 J.; refraction emmetropic or low hypermetropia; fields were full with no central colour scotoma in either field; pupils were equal and contracted to light; discs were pale with well defined edges, retinal vessels of good size, lamina cribrosa visible; a diagnosis of double optic atrophy with no evidence of previous neuritis was made. This patient gave the impression that he did not wish to acknowledge any defect of vision although it is well known to his relatives that his sight is very

Plate XLVIII.   DESCRIPTIONS OF PEDIGREE PLATES   359

bad;he wrote: "I really do not know when my right eye became defective; as far back as I remember there has been no difference; I am sure it has been the same all my life. I have smoked black tobacco, cigarettes, and also chewed tobacco since I was 14 years of age; I cannot remember it ever affecting my sight. I have also worked in the coal mines for 26 years using safety lamps and I think my sight is just as good to-day as ever it was." IV. 10 had one brother and two sisters who were unaffected, one sister died young; he was married and had three children.

IV. 87, William L., boxmaker, died unmarried, aged 33, after an operation for appendicitis; his vision failed in both eyes at the age of 25 so that he had to give up his work but he never became quite blind; optic atrophy had been diagnosed by an ophthalmic surgeon; he smoked in moderation; he had one brother and two sisters unaffected. III. 43, maternal uncle to IV. 87, a blacksmith, died aged 74 (1923), in a poorhouse, from "senility and cerebral haemorrhage of three days duration"; his sight failed at about the age of 35 but recovered sufficiently to enable him to get about and he gave up his work as blacksmith for that of night watchman; he was not a drinker; he had six unaffected sisters (three of whom had each an affected son) and eight unaffected children; an ophthalmic surgeon had noted the presence of double optic atrophy which did not clear up when smoking was discontinued. III. 60, aged 60 (1926), a street porter, became affected at the age of 20 years when his vision failed rapidly and worsened for about nine months; he thinks that during the last twenty years his vision has got very slowly worse; he smoked and still smokes one and a half to two ounces of bogie roll tobacco a week; always moderate with alcohol and was a total abstainer before the onset of the disease; he had good health but suffered from severe headaches in temples, forehead and occiput when vision failed; he had been twice married and had six unaffected children; he was intelligent and able to do his work which entails lifting heavy weights; R. V. = L. V. = finger counting at one foot; fields of vision were not contracted but large central scotomata for white were present in each field; red, green, blue and yellow were not recognised; pupils were equal and contracted to light, eye movements full, tension normal; discs showed marked pallor; lamina cribrosa exposed; edges of discs were well or sharply defined and retinal vessels somewhat narrowed; yellow spot was normal; refraction was low hypermetropia; III. 60 had one brother who died in infancy and two unaffected sisters.

III. 20, William Co., compositor, became affected at about the age of 25 years; his vision had formerly been good but it became very bad, though he was not blind, so that he was unable to work; his health was good; he smoked and was unmarried; he died, aged 65, in a poorhouse; Wassermann test was negative; there was no record of a thorough examination of his eyes; he was one of a sibship of nine of whom two died in infancy and four died young; two unaffected sisters had normal offspring. III. 39, William Re., coal carrier, aged 55 (1926), became affected at the age of 19; the right eye failed first, the left soon after; the defect became stationary in about six months and has remained unchanged since; neuralgia, attributed to teeth, accompanied the onset of the defect; he smoked three ounces of bogie roll tobacco weekly and still does so; he drinks beer and rum on Saturdays; he was married but had no children; R. V. = L. V. = fingers at one foot; fields of vision were not contracted but had absolute central scotomata for colours and white; discs were pale, edges well defined, lamina cribrosa exposed and retinal blood vessels showed some localised narrowings; in the left eye white lines were present along some of the vessels; refraction emmetropic. IV. 1, William Re., labourer, aged 52 (1926), became affected at the age of 38; the condition progressed for about twelve months and had since remained stationary; pain in his forehead accompanied the onset of visual defect; he was now able to see sufficiently to walk alone in quiet back streets; he had left off tobacco for a time without improvement of vision; smoked three and a half ounces of twist and drank one or two pints of beer weekly; R. V. = L. V. = finger counting at one foot; fields of vision were not contracted but central scotomata were present; large coloured objects were recognised nowhere; media were clear; refraction was low hypermetropia; discs were pale with well defined edges, lamina cribrosa exposed and retinal arteries slightly narrowed; yellow spot was normal.

III. 30, Mary Fo., aged 63 (1926), noticed that her vision was failing at the age of 31 years; at the same time catamenia ceased and never reappeared; health had always been good; R. V. = L. V. = finger counting at one foot; fields of vision were not contracted but absolute central scotomata for a large red object were present; refraction was low hypermetropia; media were clear, discs were pale with well defined edges, lamina cribrosa exposed and retinal arteries somewhat narrowed with no white lines along their edges; skiagram report reads: "Sella is too small and there is blurring of the posterior clinoid processes by bone, sphenoidal sinus is very large"; similar conditions were noted on another skiagram taken on a later day; III. 30 never smoked; she was married and had one daughter. III. 26, Aggie Da., aged 67 (1926), had been married to her affected first cousin for forty years but had no children, no still-births and no miscarriages; her vision failed at about the age of 33 years at which time she had much headache referred to the vertex; catamenia were regular until vision failed, they then ceased and never reappeared; always had good health and does not smoke; R. V. = little more than perception of light, L. V. = hand movements at one foot; fields of vision were peripherally contracted in all directions; a central scotoma was present in each field; media were clear, discs were pale with well defined edges, lamina cribrosa exposed and some narrowing of retinal arteries with no white lines along their edges; refraction was low hypermetropia. Skiagram report states that "the sella is rather irregular in outline, especially

towards the posterior part; it is 15 mm. in antero-posterior diameter, and 11 mm. deep; both clinoid processes are small and deformed and are partly obscured by new bony deposits."

For further information concerning unaffected members of the stock see the original history. No consanguinity. Bibl. No. 146.

Fig. 705. *Fleischer and Josenhans' Case.* Hereditary optic atrophy in seventeen males in a very extensive and fully worked-out pedigree. In the years 1917—18 four members of the pedigree, V. 36, V. 80, V. 87 and V. 104, consulted the recorders and were found to be suffering from hereditary optic atrophy; they believed themselves to be unrelated but since they came from the same district the recorders thought this fact should be investigated and with the help of the church registers succeeded in linking up all the members as shown in the chart; in the course of the investigation further cases of the defect were discovered and as many as seventy-five living members of the pedigree were examined. No female was found, or reported, to be affected.

IV. 42, aged 65, reported that he had seen badly since his 20th year; he could not read but was able to find his way in the streets; a central absolute scotoma was present in both eyes; in the left 5 cm. squares of colour were recognised in the periphery; in the right eye peripheral colour perception was not definite; both papillae were white, vessels were not changed; papillary margins were clearly defined. The patient's only brother, IV. 41, had become weak-sighted in the same way at an earlier age; his four sisters were free from the disease, but three of them who had sons transmitted the defect and one of them, IV. 36, had an early cataract.

IV. 76, an innkeeper, aged 62, stated that he had seen badly since his 23rd year; in other respects he had always been healthy; in both eyes central scotomata were present, vision was reduced to excentric finger counting at 1 m.; peripheral colour perception was intact; optic atrophy was noted; the papillary margins were clearly defined; vessels unchanged.

IV. 81, brother to IV. 76, went to the eye clinic at the age of 21 with the complaint that during the last six months his sight had diminished, first in the right eye and then in the left; in other respects he was healthy; he had no cerebral symptoms; vision in each was reduced to finger counting at $\frac{3}{4}$ m.; in each eye blue and yellow were recognised, red was uncertain and green was not perceived; both papillae were white and arteries narrowed; strychnine injections were given with no improvement of vision; pupillary reactions were normal. A third brother, IV. 80, was healthy; later he married abroad and was lost sight of. Two sisters were married and one of them, IV. 78, transmitted the disease to one of her five sons, V. 104.

V. 42, aged 53, nephew of IV. 42, reported that he had seen well up to the age of 50 when, following a cold, he noticed a rapid diminution of vision; he had had no other illness; vision was now reduced to finger counting with excentric fixation at 1 m.; the papillae were nearly white with clearly defined margins; arteries were narrowed; light reaction was prompt; no cerebral symptoms were present.

V. 47, aged 46, brother of V. 42, reported that his vision became markedly reduced at the age of 22; he had never had very good sight but had been able to read and in other respects had always been healthy; his vision now was reduced to finger counting at $\frac{1}{2}$ m.; refraction was hypermetropia, 3—4 D.; he had bilateral central scotomata so that only excentric fixation was possible; right papilla was yellowish white with blurred margin; vessels were tortuous; left papilla was a little pale with blurred margin; two months later some improvement was noted and the case was diagnosed as post-neuritic atrophy. Of the other males in this sibship V. 43 died aged 16; V. 50 died aged 36, he had good vision; V. 58, with good vision, died aged 25; their six sisters were healthy with the exception of one, V. 54, who was feeble-minded. The children of the next generation were mostly too young to have developed the disease; seven had died young and one girl had muscular atrophy of spinal origin.

V. 80, a gardener, aged 41, went to the eye clinic at the age of 39 with the statement that he had always seen very well with the left eye but less well with the right; with the right eye he could now only read large print; since eight weeks his left vision had also diminished so that he could no longer recognise people in the streets; vision was reduced to finger counting in the left at 1·5 m., in the right at ·5 m.; both papillae were rather cloudy with blurred margins; in the right the veins were dilated, in the left they were normal; there was some peripheral contraction of the visual fields for white and central scotomata were present; Wassermann test negative; no neurological defects; eight weeks later the papillae were pale and blurred and several small retinal haemorrhages were seen. Two years later vision was finger counting at 1 m. in each and the papillae were white. This patient had four siblings who had died young and three living brothers of whom two saw well and one, V. 82, was reported to have had weak sight since his 14th year. V. 80 had three children of whom one died young and two boys living were aged 11 and 13 years respectively.

V. 104 had always been healthy and had good vision until the age of 19 when he entered the Lancers; eight days later, following a cold, he noticed a diminution in his vision; nine months later he was discharged from the army. A year after the onset of the disease R. V. $=\frac{5}{60}$, L. V. $=\frac{5}{60}$; pupils reacted to light; bilateral central scotomata were present; colours were recognised at the periphery; papillae were very pale with slightly blurred margins; vessels were narrowed; patient showed slight infantilism; two years later his vision was reduced to finger counting at 2 m. in the left and at 3 m. in the right eye. One of the

Plate XLVIII.   DESCRIPTIONS OF PEDIGREE PLATES   361

patient's brothers was examined and had normal eyes; three other brothers, the youngest of whom was aged 21 years, also two sisters aged 31 and 17 years respectively, were reported to see well. V. 104 had two affected maternal uncles, IV. 76 and 81.

V. 87, a war pensioner, first noticed his eye disease whilst on active service in 1917 at the age of 28, earlier than this he had seen well; one month from the onset of the eye disease L. V. $= \frac{1}{60}$, R. V. $= \frac{6}{60}$; both papillae were pale; bilateral central scotomata were present; colours were not recognised. Six months later vision was reduced to hand movements and total bilateral atrophy of the papillae was present; no improvement was found after a further interval of fifteen months. The patient had two living children, a boy aged 6 who was normal and a girl aged 4 years also reported to see well. A third child had died in infancy.

V. 35 had good vision up to the age of 35 when he was in the army; he caught cold, following which his eye disease began; eight weeks from the onset the condition had progressed so that he could no longer recognise people in the streets. R. V. = finger counting at $\frac{1}{2}$ m.; L. V. = finger counting at $\frac{3}{4}$ m.; both papillae were pale and bilateral central scotomata were present.

V. 36, brother to V. 35, had good vision up to the age of 26 when he first noticed that he saw less well; a year from this time his vision was so much worse that he was unable to work; L. V. = fingers at 1 m. with excentric fixation, R. V. = fingers at 30—40 cm. with excentric fixation; both papillae were markedly pale; ten years later vision was reduced to finger counting at $\frac{1}{2}$ m. in each and bilateral severe atrophy of the nerve was noted. Another brother, V. 37, aged 32, was in America and was reported to have the same disease; three brothers aged 30, 26 and 22 years respectively, also a sister aged 29, were reported to see well. These three affected brothers had two affected first cousins, V. 42 and 47, also a first cousin in another sibship, V. 61, who were reported to see badly and to be unaided by spectacles; they were all nephews to the affected uncles, IV. 41 and 42. Of earlier members of the pedigree it was known that II. 3 (1781—1849) had seen badly and been unable to read, but none of his descendants were known to have had any defect of vision; it was also known that III. 27 (1816—1885) was nearly blind at the age of 40 and that his brother, III. 34 (1831—1897), had eye disease which spectacles did not help; none of the descendants of III. 27 were known to be affected.

The stock appears to be a healthy one and shows no significantly associated defect. No female member is known to have been affected but it appears probable that in every case the disease has been transmitted to the affected male by his mother. For further information see the original account. No consanguinity recorded. Bibl. No. 116.

Fig. 706. *Gould's Case.* Fifteen cases of hereditary optic atrophy in six generations. I. 1 was a sea captain, he became blind and deaf somewhat late in life; no more details could be discovered concerning his affection; his two sons, II. 2 and 3, became blind "from the same type of disease as that which has since appeared in the later generations"; the onset in the case of II. 3 was at the age of 40.

II. 2 had two sons and three daughters of whom the two sons, III. 2 and 3, were affected; III. 2 died aged 86; he had fourteen children and twenty-seven grandchildren all free from the disease; III. 3 was affected at the age of 25. Of the daughters of II. 2, one, III. 4, had "weak eyes" and persistent "watering" of the eyes but was not blind; she died, aged 62, having had ten children of whom three daughters died in infancy, one son, IV. 10, died aged 3, and one of the remaining four sons, IV. 11, became affected with the disease at the age of 40, his four children being normal. Both the married daughters, IV. 4 and 13, transmitted the disease to all their sons who survived infancy; thus IV. 4 had four sons who died in infancy, three sons, V. 4, 5 and 6, who became affected at the ages of 23, 28 and 33 years respectively; one daughter, V. 8, transmitted the disease to her only son who at the date of the enquiry had reached the age at which the condition was liable to appear. IV. 13 had three sons who became affected at the ages of 34, 28 and 23 years respectively, and one son, V. 41, who died in infancy. IV. 6, the normal son of III. 4, had a son, V. 13, aged 52, of whom we are told that "while chipping something, a small piece flew into the eye; the injury was slight, but blindness resulted; the other eye is now partially blind and failing." V. 13 had six brothers who reached the ages of 28—48, none of whom developed the disease but all of whom died in early or late middle life.

V. 8, aged 56, had seven children of whom one daughter, VI. 2, aged 36, has a "weak mind," a son and a daughter, VI. 3 and 4, died in infancy, a daughter, VI. 5, died aged 11, a son, VI. 6, developed optic atrophy at the age of 27, and two younger sons, aged 18 and 14 years respectively, have "chronically abnormal eye-grounds and optic nerve heads."

III. 6 became blind before her death at the age of 40, but she was "horned in the temple by a cow and one eye thus destroyed," blindness following in the other eye a few months later. III. 7 became blind late in life, the cause is unknown but the recorder suggests that as none of her children were affected she is unlikely to have had hereditary optic atrophy; three of her sons, however, died in infancy, three died at the ages of 47, 33 and 33 respectively and her only daughter died aged 26.

The recorder considers the disease to be typical white atrophy of the optic nerve; in his patient VI. 6 the vision, nine months after the onset, was so reduced that he could barely count fingers. Of other cases in the pedigree reports were obtained from hospitals or from other oculists who had examined the affected members; in a number of the cases the blindness is not absolute but some slight vision is retained through life. The recorder suggests that the histories given in the cases of III. 4, 6, 7 and V. 13 "show that normal vision or ocular health in the family was always on a precarious equilibrium, and when optic atrophy did not arise idiopathically, only a slight accident or exciting circumstance was needed to bring on a train of evil results." Attention should also be drawn to the heavy infant mortality and the incidence of early deaths in many members of the stock. No consanguinity recorded. Bibl. No. 40.

Fig. 707. *Hirsch's Case.* Ten cases of hereditary optic atrophy affecting males only in four generations. I. 1 and 2 died in old age with no eye affection; they had two sons and two daughters of whom II. 2, Alois St., became amblyopic in middle age; he was never quite blind up to his death at the age of 72; he was a moderate drinker; his children and their descendants were free from disease. II. 3, Rudolf St., became amblyopic at the age of 19; later he was operated on for senile cataract but saw no better for the operation; he was an immoderate drinker and died, aged 80, without descendants. II. 5 and her husband were healthy; their one son, III. 9, became amblyopic at the age of 20, he was unmarried. II. 6 and II. 7 were healthy; they had five children of whom III. 11, Heinrich M., became blind when he was young; the condition remained stationary. III. 11 was a heavy drinker; he had six children of whom five died young but his married son, IV. 10, had six healthy children. III. 12, Franz M., became almost blind at the age of 20; he also was a heavy drinker and died aged 37 in delirium tremens; one of his children, IV. 16, died young. IV. 19, also a drinker, died from suicide, leaving no descendants. IV. 17 had numerous children and grandchildren free from disease, though six children and six grandchildren died young. III. 14, Josef M., went to Roumania as a child and later became a hairdresser; he carried on his work to a considerable age but there is no definite knowledge of his vision or of that of his children. III. 16 became affected at the age of 20 and was only able to do rough work; he had two healthy married daughters one of whom had a son who died young; his two healthy sons were childless. III. 18 was a drinker; she died aged 47 leaving two sons and three daughters of whom IV. 27, Theodore E., hair-dresser, became affected at the age of 42; he was a great smoker; R. V. = L. V. = $\frac{6}{60}$ with correction for myopic astigmatism; central scotomata were noted; two of his children were examined, they and his married son saw well. IV. 28, Amalie, was very nervous and inclined to take too much alcohol; her husband was healthy; of their three children, Willi, V. 34, now aged 21, became affected at the age of 19; about two months after the onset the lateral halves of his discs were pale and large central scotomata were present. The brother of Willi, aged 19, and sister, aged 23, were examined and found to be normal. IV. 30, Emma H., and her three sons aged 18, 14 and 11 respectively, were all examined and found to be normal. IV. 32, Anna H., died aged 33 of tubercular disease; of her three children, V. 39, Trude H., aged 21, had an atypical distribution of the retinal vessels, similar in each eye. V. 40, aged 19, had normal retinal vessels but the papillae were rather blurred with indistinct margins; with some correction for myopia R. V. = $\frac{6}{18}$, L. V. = $\frac{6}{9}$. V. 41, Franz H., aged 13, had been under observation since the age of 6; he readily overtired and had a marked diminution of vision when fatigued; he had myopic astigmatism; the outer halves of the discs were very pale; no scotomata were present; the distribution of his retinal vessels was normal; R. V. = $\frac{6}{18}$, L. V. = $\frac{6}{9}$. IV. 34, Oswald E., was a great smoker; he became affected with retro-bulbar neuritis at the age of 20 and had central scotomata; Fuchs diagnosed Leber's atrophy in 1921 when his discs were markedly pale, especially the outer halves; there was some anomaly in the distribution of his retinal vessels; his three daughters aged 18, 16 and 15 respectively, and his three sons aged 14, 13 and 9 respectively, all had very good vision but had not yet passed the critical age at which the onset of Leber's disease is liable to occur. No consanguinity. Bibl. No. 126.

PLATE XLIX. Fig. 708. *Waardenburg's Case.* Hereditary optic atrophy in eighteen cases of five generations. The special interest of this pedigree arises from the marriage of an affected male, V. 31, with his first cousin once removed, VI. 14, who was also affected.

I. 1 and 2 were born about 1770; nothing was known of their vision; they had three daughters, II. 1 who was known to have always seen well, II. 3 who could see well and was married but childless, and II. 4 who lived in Utrecht and who had one daughter who was blinded in early childhood from some inflammatory eye disease. All the affected members of the pedigree arose from the marriage of II. 1. III. 2, eldest daughter of II. 1, saw well and was married to a normal man of unaffected stock; she had six children of whom two sons, IV. 2 and 5, were affected and had excentric vision; we are told that IV. 5 suddenly became blind and that afterwards no spectacles could help him; IV. 1, 4, 6 and 8 saw well though IV. 6 had high myopia. There was no knowledge of the descendants of IV. 1; IV. 2 had two normal daughters and three young grandchildren; IV. 6 had two normal daughters and a son who saw well up to the time of his death at the age of 25.

III. 3 had seven children of whom IV. 10, a sempstress, aged 59, saw well herself but had an affected son, V. 9; IV. 11 at the age of 42 saw well but had an affected son, V. 14; IV. 13 at the age of 69 saw well but had an affected son, V. 17; IV. 16 was affected at about the age of 24—25 and no improvement followed his treatment; he had five normal daughters and one normal son, also a number of grandchildren who had not yet shown signs of the disease. IV. 18 also became affected at about the age of 24—25 and the condition remained stationary; he was unmarried. IV. 19 was seen at the age of 83; she had suddenly

Plate XLIX.   DESCRIPTIONS OF PEDIGREE PLATES   363

lost her distinct vision at the age of 24 and had never since been able to see to read; she fixed objects excentrically and had absolute central scotomata with normal outer boundaries to her fields; she was never quite blind and could find her way about without aid; she had two sons of whom V. 30 died aged 24, and had good vision up to this time, whilst V. 31 became affected at the age of 20. IV. 21 was normal and had five normal sons. The husband of III. 3 was normal up to the time of his death at the age of 86.

V. 8 was unmarried; she was nervous and had convergent strabismus but a normal fundus. V. 9 was almost blind and could scarcely cross the streets without help; he had pale discs with sharp outlines and no alteration in the vessels; the onset was sudden in his case between the ages of 20 and 30 and treatment was unavailing; he had strabismus. V. 10 and 11 died young. V. 13 was normal and had a healthy young child. V. 14 became almost blind whilst on military service at the age of 22, ophthalmoscopic appearances were the same as for V. 9; he had convergent strabismus. V. 15 represents four siblings of V. 14 who died young. V. 16 was normal; she was married but had no children. V. 17 became almost blind at the age of 24; he was examined in Utrecht at the age of 55 when his vision had much improved and he had been able to carry on his work as a waiter; both discs were white and sharply outlined; his three daughters aged 17, 15 and 12 years respectively were healthy, also he had a healthy half-brother, V. 19, aged 46. V. 31 became affected whilst serving in the army at the age of 20; for a short time he was almost completely blind but his vision improved markedly after treatment in hospital; when examined in 1924 he had bilateral relative central colour scotomata, R. V. with $-1\cdot25$ D. $=\frac{2}{24}$, L. V. with $+0\cdot5$ D. $=\frac{2}{24}$; the discs were pale especially on the temporal side, vessels were normal. V. 31 married his first cousin once removed, VI. 14, who also became affected in 1921 at the age of 37, after the birth of her youngest child; her vision had rapidly diminished until R. V. with $+3\cdot5=\frac{5}{12}$, L. V. with $+3\cdot5=\frac{5}{18}$; she was again examined in 1924 and the condition was found to have remained stationary; Wassermann test was negative. These two affected parents had six children and there was one miscarriage; of these children VII. 3 died at 6 months and VII. 7 died at 4 months; the other members were all examined by the recorder and at the date of publication one son and two daughters appeared to be normal but none of them were beyond the age at which the disease might show itself. The second son, VII. 2, was in 1924, at the age of 21, brought to the recorder with the history that at first his right eye and about six weeks later his left eye had become weak-sighted and that for about three weeks he had been unable to carry on his work; he was found to have bilateral absolute central scotomata, the outer margins of the fields of vision were normal; slight bilateral optic neuritis was noted, there was no paleness of the discs, the margins were blurred and slight dilatation of the vessels was present; the patient recognised large coloured surfaces.

III. 5 was normal, he was married but childless. III. 8 was known to have been affected, he was married but had no children. III. 6 had always seen well herself but transmitted the disease to a number of her descendants; her three daughters all had affected sons and two of her five sons were also affected. Thus IV. 23 married her normal first cousin once removed and had the affected daughter, VI. 14, described above; an affected son, VI. 15, became blind at the age of 29 so that for a time he was unable to carry on his work, but later his vision improved and he was working at the age of 44, with ophthalmoscopic appearances of optic atrophy without marked changes in the vessels; he had at this time ten children. VI. 17 died aged 36, unmarried. VI. 18 was affected and became almost blind for a time, some improvement occurred but recovery was less marked than in the case of his brother. VI. 20 had normal vision; VI. 23 died aged $3\frac{1}{2}$ years, VI. 24 was normal. The husband of IV. 23 became blind at the age of 60 after an operation on his eye, he had seen well up to this period of his life and was not thought to have had optic atrophy.

IV. 24 was normal; IV. 25 and 26 became affected, according to report, at about the age of 30 and remained weak-sighted up to the time of their death at about the age of 60; they had excentric fixation but were not wholly blind and could carry on suitably chosen work. IV. 27 and her husband were normal; they had two sons of whom V. 34 died aged 7 and V. 35 became blind at 22; he said that he had lost his vision in a few weeks and that the condition had since remained stationary; he had at 47 large central scotomata but the outer limits of his fields were normal and he could see to go about alone; he could see large coloured surfaces; his normal daughter was aged 24. IV. 29 was normal. V. 30, his wife and his four children all saw well. IV. 32 and 33 saw well and six of their children with their descendants were normal; one son, V. 42, became blind at the age of 23—24, improvement occurred and at the age of 50 R. V. $=\frac{6}{60}$ with sph. $+1$ D. $=\frac{6}{30}$, L. V. $=\frac{6}{20}$ with $+1$ D. $=\frac{6}{10}$; he had relative small central scotomata and discs were pale. Consanguinity. Bibl. No. 131.

Fig. 709. *Alajmo's Case.* Hereditary optic atrophy in two females and six males of two generations. I. 1 was addicted to drink; he and his wife and known antecedents saw well to the end of their lives. I. 1 and 2 had five children of whom the first was a two-headed monster, the remaining four all had optic atrophy which developed between the ages of 19 and 26 in the different individuals. II. 3, aged 62, had no serious illness in her youth except frequent giddiness at about the age of 15 before menstruation commenced; she had 16 pregnancies, the first child was born prematurely and died in convulsions after twenty days, this was followed by two miscarriages at the third month; she had only seven living children of whom III. 3 and 4 were well, III. 5, 6 and 7 had optic atrophy; III. 8 was epileptic and III. 9 was well but aged 19 and still not beyond the period at which optic atrophy is liable to develop; the onset of the disease in II. 3 was at the age of 22 following some great emotional disturbance; she noticed a cloud before her eyes and had supra-orbital pain; a few weeks later her vision was reduced to the condition of only distinguishing people with difficulty at 1 m.; the patient was apathetic and of slight intelligence; response of pupils to light was sluggish; the papillae were white, the right disc uniformly so, the left disc more markedly white on the temporal side; the central excavation was accentuated; arteries normal, veins tortuous in each eye; central scotomata were present, absolute for red and green, relative for white; the peripheral fields for white were contracted and in the right eye the whole nasal half of the field was without perception; she was treated with no success.

II. 4, aged 54, had no serious illness up to the age of 25; menstruation started at 14 and was always regular; she had eight children seven of whom died young from acute infections, the only survivor, a son, became affected with optic atrophy at the age of 24. The patient was apathetic and intellectually rather feeble; at the age of 25 she suddenly noticed a cloud before her eyes; the condition rapidly progressed and in a few weeks she was unable to see to carry on her domestic work; she complained of pains in her head at this time and was able to find her way about but could not recognise objects; treatment met with no success; the papillae were uniformly white, arteries narrowed, veins tortuous; the left field had a marked concentric contraction and absolute central scotoma, the right field had perception of white over a small area only.

II. 6, aged 52, was never seriously ill up to the age of 20 when he had measles; he had broncho-pneumonia at 23; he had seven healthy children who saw well, the eldest daughter was aged 26; at the age of 25 he noticed one day a clouding of his vision and giddiness when in the streets, so that he had to be helped home; after an initial improvement a gradual diminution of vision occurred so that he was unable to carry on his work; he had some paresis of the right arm affecting abduction, reflexes were exaggerated; he was timid and irritable, also of poor intelligence; he smoked considerably, but had no venereal disease; R. V. = finger counting at 60 cm., L. V. = finger counting at 40 cm.; fields showed concentric contraction for white and he had no perception for red and green, central scotomata were absolute for colours, relative for white. II. 8, aged 39, was married but had no children; at 15 he had a venereal ulcer with affection of the inguinal glands, he said that he had no cutaneous symptoms at this time; he was excused from military service on account of organic weakness and neurasthenia; intelligence was poor and he drank and smoked to excess; reflexes were exaggerated; Wassermann negative; his vision suddenly became dim whilst he was at work at the age of 24 and he had to be helped home; for a few days he could only distinguish light and darkness; some improvement followed treatment for about three months, after which the condition remained stationary; he was never able to return to work; he suffered at the time of onset from very acute pains in his head; the temporal sides of the papillae were white, arteries were narrowed and veins tortuous, the whole fundus was greyish coloured; there was no contraction of the peripheral fields for white; central scotomata were absolute for colours, relative for white; R. V. = finger counting at 1·25 m., L. V. = finger counting at 70 cm.

III. 5, aged 39, was unmarried, he had convulsions from infancy which ceased with the onset of the eye disease; at 20 he was excused from military service on account of "cerebro-spinal neurasthenia"; reflexes were exaggerated, dermographism was present; he was impulsive and excitable and smoked and drank a good deal; Wassermann was negative; his eyes became affected at 24 when vision was reduced to perception of light, some improvement occurred and then the condition remained stationary; discs were wholly white, arteries narrowed, veins tortuous; the retina was of a uniform greyish colour; there was marked concentric contraction of fields for white and a still more restricted field for blue with an entire loss of perception for red and green; large central scotomata were present, relative for white; R. V. = finger counting at 30 cm., L. V. = finger counting at 40 cm.

It was not possible to see III. 6; he is said to have become affected suddenly at 19 and to have been unable to work since. III. 7, aged 26, was apathetic and of poor intelligence, reflexes were exaggerated; Wassermann negative; the onset of eye trouble was at the age of 19 when he became aware of clouds before his eyes; after a few weeks he was unable to carry on his work; the onset was accompanied by headaches; the whole discs were white with an accentuated central excavation; retinal arteries were narrow, veins were dilated and tortuous; the fields for white were normal, they were contracted for colours; central scotomata were relative for white, absolute for colours; R. V. = finger counting at 1 m., L. V. = finger counting at 40 cm. III. 11, aged 26, had pneumonia as a child and was excused military service on account of some deformity of the thorax; Wassermann was negative; he smoked a good deal and drank in moderation; at the age of 24 the patient had a severe illness which was diagnosed as encephalitis lethargica and after this he noticed a diminution of vision and clouds before his eyes; vision is now reduced to finger counting in each at 40 cm.; fields show some concentric contraction for white; absolute central scotomata are present; the discs are white on the temporal sides, the veins are dilated and tortuous; the patient is apparently almost stuporous and of slight intelligence. No consanguinity recorded. Bibl. No. 121.

Fig. 710. *Bramwell's Case.* Hereditary optic atrophy in three males of two generations. The patient, III. 12, aged 24, was a farmer living in a healthy locality; he had chorea at the age of 10; there was no

Plate XLIX.   DESCRIPTIONS OF PEDIGREE PLATES   365

history of syphilis or gonorrhoea; he was a very steady man, a moderate smoker and indulged in no form of excess; he was intelligent and in perfect health except for his eye trouble which he first noticed seven months previously; the onset was gradual and preceded by no illness or accident, but he had headache and occasional diplopia for three or four weeks before he noticed a diminution of vision; he had no vomiting or fever; the headaches were not every day, they varied in position and ceased after the diminution of vision developed; before the onset of his eye trouble he had been liable to occasional severe headaches associated with vomiting. Three months from the time of onset III. 12 was unable to see to read; discs were markedly pale on temporal sides; there were no indications of old neuritis; pupils were equal and reacted normally; R. V. = finger counting at 6 ins., L. V. = finger counting at 3 ft.; central scotomata were present, also some concentric contraction of fields, both more marked in the right eye.

The family were unusually healthy; the father died, aged 68, from influenza and heart disease, he was not blind; the mother, aged 53, was living and well; six siblings were in perfect health. An uncle, II. 2, became blind at the age of 28 and has continued so ever since; he is healthy in other respects; his blindness came on one day whilst he was sitting reading, a mist came over the print and he was unable to see; he had never had a headache in his life; vision was best in a dim light; he was a greengrocer and was unable to see to read but could tell the time by his watch. III. 6, cousin to the patient, became blind at 24; he was otherwise in good health; he had a cold in his head when the disease overtook him; some improvement occurred and he was able to read large print. No benefit to the patient followed his treatment.

A number of the members of generation III were still below the age at which affection occurred in their relatives; thus the eldest of the children of II. 2 was aged 28, III. 4 died aged 7, III. 7 was aged 24, III. 8 aged 22, III. 9 died aged 19; III. 13—20 were all under 24 years of age. We have been unable to hear of the subsequent history of this family. No consanguinity recorded. Bibl. No. 72.

Fig. 711. *Kropp's Case.* Hereditary optic atrophy in three males and one female of two sibships, the offspring of sisters. III. 1, Hans M., aged 28 (1927), was well and saw well up to the age of 20 when he complained of a slight diminution in the vision of his right eye; now pupils react sluggishly to light and convergence and R. V. = hand movements, L. V. = finger counting close to the eye; there was a bilateral slight concentric narrowing of the fields of vision and absolute central scotomata; Wassermann test was negative; light sense was only one-eighth that of the normal control; sella turcica was not enlarged; blood specimen was normal. III. 2, aged 26, became affected at the age of 24 when bilateral diminution of vision was noticed; the present state of disability was reached in two months, since when there had been no change; R. V. $= \dfrac{1 \cdot 5}{50}$, L. V. $= \dfrac{3}{50}$; slight concentric contraction of visual fields and absolute central scotomata were noted; light sense was slightly lowered; Wassermann test was negative; sella turcica was not enlarged; blood specimen was normal. III. 4, Heinrich K., aged 50, became affected at the age of 40 when he noticed a diminution of his left vision; right eye now presents a paleness of the temporal side of the disc, the left shows total optic atrophy; R. V. $= \frac{3}{50}$, L. V. $= \frac{1}{50}$; slight concentric contraction of the fields and absolute central scotomata are noted; light sense was lowered; Wassermann reaction negative; sella turcica was not enlarged and blood was normal. III. 5, Willi K., aged 38, became affected at the age of 29 following gas poisoning in 1917; pupillary action very sluggish and total optic atrophy now present in both eyes; concentric contraction also an absolute central scotoma in each field; R. V. = L. V. = hand movements close to the eyes; Wassermann test negative; blood normal. The ages of the unaffected members of the two affected sibships are not given; the onset was late in the case of III. 4 and it is possible that III. 7 is not beyond an age at which the disease may show itself. No consanguinity recorded. Bibl. No. 141.

Fig. 712. *Van Heuven and Oltmans's Case.* Four cases of hereditary optic atrophy in males of two generations. III. 11, G., at the age of 24 (Nov. 1922) complained that he saw very badly with his left eye; it was found that L. V. $= \frac{1}{50}$ (excentric), R. V. = 1; the left field had a scotoma between the macula and the blind spot, the right field was normal; the left papilla was swollen and the right papilla was also swollen to a less degree; whilst the patient was under observation the left scotoma became larger and the temporal side of the papilla became pale. In April 1923 R. V. $= \frac{1}{2}$, L. V. $= \frac{2}{300}$, and in May of the same year the right vision was further reduced to $\frac{1}{10}$ and bilateral absolute central scotomata were noted. III. 11 had two normal sisters; his maternal uncle, II. 3, J. D., aged 68, became affected very suddenly at the age of 27, now R. V. $= \frac{2}{60}$, L. V. $= \frac{2}{50}$; bilateral central scotomata were present and the ophthalmoscope showed atrophy of the optic nerve; there were signs of arterio-sclerosis. G. D., II. 6, aged 57, became affected at the age of 25—26; the left eye first became affected suddenly and later the right eye; R. V. $=$ L. V. $= \frac{2}{10}$; bilateral absolute central scotomata were present and the ophthalmoscope showed atrophy of the optic nerves; he had slight divergent strabismus, also some kyphoscoliosis; his two sons and a daughter were normal. There were four living and married sisters in generation II of whom two had each an affected son; possibly the youngest sister, II. 10, had sons who were still of an age at which they might develop the disease; we are not told how many sons she had or what were their ages. The eldest sister had sons and daughters of whom one son, J. B., aged 42, became affected at the age of 23; the visual disturbance appeared suddenly when he noticed a cloud before his eyes; R. V. $=\frac{2}{60}$, L. V. $=\frac{1}{60}$; bilateral absolute central scotomata were present and atrophy of the optic nerves. No consanguinity recorded. Bibl. No. 130.

Fig. 713. *Van Lint and Kleefeld's Case.* Hereditary optic atrophy associated with hypothyroidism in three siblings. I. 1 and 2 were normal and saw well, they had seven children who were all extremely nervous and of whom II. 2 was short but had good sight; he had three children of whom two died young, one of these had been very fat; III. 2, aged 7, was very fat, thyroid was imperceptible and her hair was short and dry; II. 3 was short and fat; his refraction was hypermetropic; of his seven children three died young; III. 4, aged 21, noticed a diminution of visual acuity at the age of 14 years when optic atrophy was diagnosed; vision was reduced to finger counting at 5 m. in the right and at 4 m. in the left eye; colour vision very defective, visual fields were very contracted but no central scotomata were present; divergent strabismus and horizontal nystagmus are noted; ocular reflexes were a little slow; cornea, iris and lens were normal in each eye. This youth was short and gave the impression of a child of 14 years; he had projecting frontal and temporal regions; skin was coarse, hair dry and friable with scarcely a trace of hair on face and little hair in the pubic or axillary regions; nails were striated and friable, dentition good; muscular system was badly developed and extremities were always cold; an absence of secondary sexual characters is noted with infantilism of the genital organs complicated by a left inguinal cryptorchidism; he was very nervous and emotional but of normal intelligence. III. 5, aged 16, had had a slow progressive diminution of vision since the age of about 11 years; vision was now very limited, colour vision was defective, visual fields were contracted but had no central scotomata; this patient had divergent strabismus but no nystagmus; some hypermetropia is noted, and white atrophy of the papillae was observed; stature was short, frontal region prominent; skin was smooth, hair was scanty, teeth good and nails normal; she was very fat but secondary sexual characters appeared with the onset of menstruation at the age of 13 and there was down in the pubic regions; nervous system and intelligence appeared to be normal. III. 6, aged 15, was short and fat; he had had excellent sight up to a year ago but could now see little; he had divergent strabismus; he was colour-blind; visual fields were only slightly contracted and no central scotomata were present; he had prominent frontal region, normal teeth, nails were striated and brittle; no trace of hair on axillary and pubic regions; genital organs still infantile; all reflexes were exaggerated and intelligence was mediocre.

II. 5 was of average height and had good sight; he had two children born at six months and five children who saw well; one of these, a male, aged 3, was very fat and very small, III. 9, aged 4, was thin and small, one of the siblings had heterochromia iridis. II. 7 was of average height and saw well. II. 8 and 9 were corpulent and wore glasses, the latter was short and thick set. No consanguinity recorded. Bibl. No. 105.

Fig. 714. *Van Heuven and Oltmans's Case.* II. 1 and 2 became affected with hereditary optic atrophy at the age of 20 years; they had two normal brothers, also three normal sisters, two of whom were married and had affected sons. Thus II. 3 had two sons who each became affected at the age of 20; II. 7 had six sons and three daughters, of whom one son, III. 5, became affected at the age of 20; III. 10, aged 17, was seeing badly with his left eye for which V. $=\frac{1}{10}$; the right eye still had good vision but the fundus showed early signs of trouble. No consanguinity recorded. Bibl. No. 130.

Fig. 715. *Kropp's Case.* Hereditary optic atrophy in a father and in two of his daughters. II. 2, Max W., aged 46, became affected at the age of 21; he had e i y been healthy and seen well; now R. V. $=\frac{5}{36}$, L. V. $=\frac{5}{36}$, or with correction R. V. $=\frac{5}{36}$, L. V. $=\frac{5}{36}$; the peripheral fields of vision were normal, relative central colour scotomata for green, red and blue were present; light sense was slightly lowered; Wassermann test was negative; blood was normal; there was no history of excess in the use of tobacco or alcohol. III. 3, Edith W., aged 21, was seen in 1919 at the age of 14 with her younger sister, then aged 7, who was similarly affected; there was at this time a suspicion of chronic arsenic poisoning from the use of preserved foods; however, no signs of arsenic poisoning were found but retrobulbar neuritis of doubtful origin was diagnosed; now bilateral optic atrophy was present; for III. 3 R. V. $=\frac{5}{60}$, L. V. $=\frac{5}{60}$; slight concentric contraction of the peripheral fields was demonstrated, also relative central scotomata for green and red. III. 4 at the age of 14 had R. V. $=\frac{3}{60}$, L. V. $=\frac{2.5}{60}$; her visual fields were similar to those of her sister; Wassermann test was negative for both sisters, blood specimens were normal, sella turcica was not enlarged in either case. The ages of the unaffected members of the sibship are not given but presumably III. 5 is younger than the age at which his father became affected. No consanguinity recorded. Bibl. No. 141.

Plate L. Fig. 716. *Meyer-Riemsloh's Case.* Twenty-five or twenty-seven cases of optic atrophy in five generations. Generations I to III are included to show relationships but there was no definite knowledge concerning the incidence of the disease in these generations. Of IV. 7 it was known that he had seen badly since his youth and that the condition remained unchanged until his death; he was the only male of his sibship and his sister, IV. 4, was the probable source of all other cases of the disease in the pedigree.

IV. 4 had twelve children of whom two males and two females died young, six females were normal themselves but transmitted the defect to their descendants, one female, V. 10, was affected and the only

Plate L.   DESCRIPTIONS OF PEDIGREE PLATES   367

male who lived to adult life, V. 8, was affected; thus all the children of IV. 3 and 4 who lived to adult life were either affected or were carriers of the disease. V. 2 was a carrier; she had one son, VI. 1, who had seen badly since his school days, spectacles did not help him and no improvement occurred. V. 3 died aged 2; V. 4 died aged 1 year. V. 5 was a carrier; she had six children of whom three sons were affected and two of her three daughters were demonstrated to be carriers, she herself remained unaffected up to the time of her death at the age of 77. V. 7 died young. V. 8 had been affected since his school days and never improved; spectacles did not help him. V. 10 married her third cousin on her father's side which was not known to be an affected branch of the family; she became affected at the age of 43 and was examined six years later when R. V. = finger counting at 1 m., L. V. = finger counting at $\frac{2}{3}$ m.; she had very severe headaches; pupils were normal; the papillae were markedly pale, margins not wholly clear; arteries were narrowed, veins normal; the visual fields showed absolute central scotomata with some concentric contraction of the outer limits; she was treated with strychnine, potassium iodide, inhalations of amyl nitrite and galvanisation, but after six months appearances were almost unchanged and R. V. = finger counting at $\frac{2}{3}$ m., L. V. = finger counting at $1\frac{1}{4}$ m.; the patient died at the age of 75 and saw badly up to the time of her death; she had seven children of whom the only two sons who lived to adult life were affected; two daughters died young and two daughters were married but childless, one of these daughters, VI. 19, was possibly affected. V. 11 died young. V. 12 was normal and had two normal daughters but it appears that she and both her daughters were carriers. V. 14 was herself normal but her only daughter had three affected sons. V. 16 was normal up to the time of her death at the age of 49 but she was a carrier, and of her two children the son was normal but had an affected daughter, VII. 32, and the daughter, VI. 29, was probably herself affected and had two affected sons; it is possible that the affection of VII. 32 did not arise through her father for in no other case in the pedigree has a male been demonstrated to transmit the disease and we know nothing of her ancestry on the mother's side. V. 18 died aged 75, she was herself normal and had a normal son, VI. 32, but one of her two daughters transmitted the defect.

VI. 3 was alive and seeing well at the age of 54 but she had an affected son. VI. 4 noticed a diminution of vision in his right eye at the age of 32 and the left eye became affected in the following year; he was then aged 62 and no improvement had occurred; he has a right divergent strabismus; R. V. = finger counting at $\frac{1}{2}$ m., L. V. = finger counting at 2 m.; pupils normal; the papillae are a greyish white colour clearly outlined; he has a bilateral absolute central scotoma; Wassermann reaction negative; he was married and had a normal son. VI. 6 died aged 52; she did not herself show signs of the disease but had two affected sons and two daughters who transmitted the disease. VI. 8 became affected at the age of 20, he was almost blind and lived in an infirmary; he was now aged 64. VI. 9 became affected suddenly at the age of 19 and saw very badly; he was at the time of enquiry aged 66 and occupied with agriculture but only carried on his work with difficulty. VI. 10, aged 56, was unaffected; she had one living son, VII. 18, aged 30, who had not yet become affected; three of her children died young and two daughters were apparently normal.

VI. 12 died aged 3. VI. 13 died aged 1 year. VI. 14, aged 53, became affected at the age of 46; he saw well in both eyes in November 1917, in January 1918 R. V. = L. V. = finger counting at 1 m.; pupils normal; the nerve was slightly pale on the temporal side and its margins were a little blurred; absolute central scotomata were present reaching to $10°-15°$ from the fixation point; peripheral limits of the fields were normal at this time but later there was some concentric contraction of the fields and vision was further reduced to hand movements only over a very restricted area; the pupillary reflex to light and accommodation was still present. At the age of 53 both nerves were white and sharply outlined, the arteries being very narrow; the nervous system was examined and was in other respects found to be normal. The patient was married and had two daughters. VI. 16, aged 51, became affected at 18 when he complained of a diminution of vision during eight weeks; the nerves were reddened and the margins slightly blurred; the patient was a painter and decorator, but showed no signs of lead poisoning, his nervous system was normal except for a sluggish patellar reflex; after two months of treatment with baths, hot packs and electricity R. V. with $+1·5$ D. $= \frac{5}{30}$, L. V. with $-2·5$ D. $= \frac{5}{30}$; after further treatment the patient improved markedly until at the end of three years from the onset R. V. with $+2·25$ D. $= \frac{6}{12} - \frac{5}{10}$, L. V. with $-4·0$ D. $= \frac{6}{20}$, the nerves were white with clear margins, arteries were narrowed and fields for white were full excepting a few small islands in the region of the fixation point. VI. 18 died aged 46; she was normal and married but had no children. VI. 19, aged 48, complained in 1897, when she was aged 20, of a sudden lowering of vision in the right eye; it was found that R. V. = finger counting at 2 m., L. V. with $+1·5$ D. $= \frac{5}{6}$; the right eye showed blurring of the margins of the nerve and marked venous congestion; there was a small retinal haemorrhage, but the condition responded to treatment and she regained full visual acuity and normal ophthalmoscopic appearances. In the autumn of 1898 she again had a diminution of vision in both eyes and R. V. = L. V. = $\frac{5}{6}$, and there were signs of optic neuritis, but again the inflammatory appearances cleared up and vision improved though the nerves were now markedly pale and sharply outlined, also the arteries were narrowed. In 1901, with correction of $+1·5$ D. in each, R. V. = L. V. = $\frac{5}{6}$; the fields showed signs of paracentral scotomata. The recorder suggests that the recurrence of symptoms in this case is in favour of their hereditary origin; the patient was married but had no children. VI. 20 died aged 1 year.

VI. 28 was normal and aged 60; his sister, VI. 29, died at the age of 62 and according to the statement of her daughter she had a sudden onset of eye disease at the age of 27 and saw badly to the end of her life; she was certainly a carrier and was probably also herself affected. VI. 32, aged 46, VI. 33, aged 55, and VI. 35, aged 49, were normal though VI. 33 transmitted the disease to one of her four sons.

VII. 1 became affected at the age of 16, he noticed whilst writing that he could no longer see; the condition remained unchanged and he had to give up his work as a joiner; at the age of 20 R. V. = finger counting at 2 m., L. V. = finger counting at $\frac{1}{2}$ m.; pupils were normal; both discs were white and atrophic; retina and retinal vessels were normal; absolute central scotomata were demonstrated; Wassermann test negative. VII. 3, aged 34, was unaffected and had a young son, VIII. 1, aged 6. VII. 5 died aged 33, she had two sons and two daughters of whom one daughter, VIII. 5, was affected. VII. 6 noticed on his way to school one morning, at the age of 11 years, that his vision suddenly became dim and when he reached school he was unable to see to read; some slight improvement occurred during the next year; he was now, at the age of 43, a basket-maker and R. V. = $\frac{5}{60}$, L. V. = finger counting at $\frac{1}{2}$ m.; discs were atrophic vessels perhaps narrowed; central scotomata were present of small extent in the right and large in the left eye; Wassermann reaction was positive; no other neurological defects were found. VII. 7 was normal and aged 42. VII. 9, at the age of 7, suddenly found that he saw badly at school; he was now aged 45, no improvement had occurred and R. V. = L. V. = finger counting at 3 m.; pupils reacted normally; discs were greyish white and absolute central scotomata were present; Wassermann test was negative. VII. 11, aged 34, was normal and had four young children then alive. VII. 13, aged 47, was normal but had an affected son. VII. 15 and 16 died young. VII. 18 was aged 30 and still unaffected. VII. 20, 21, 22 and 23 were aged 20, 18, 22 and 16 years respectively. VII. 26 and 27 were both affected but exact age of onset is not given, in one case it is said to have occurred in his youth, in the other case to have been after the age of 20. VII. 28, 29 and 30 represent three affected brothers, the onset was sudden in each case and occurred at the age of 12 in VII. 28 and at the age of 19 in his two brothers; all are said to see very badly. VII. 31, two sisters, aged 30 and 27 respectively, saw well. VII. 32, now aged 24, had suffered during the last five years from epilepsy attacks which at one time occurred every 8 to 14 days; for two years she was treated with bromide and luminal after which the frequency of attacks gradually diminished and no attack had occurred during the last five months; she had noticed that her vision was diminishing about two years ago but had not asked advice about it because she had no other symptoms, now R. V. = finger counting at $1\frac{1}{2}$ m., L. V. = finger counting at $\frac{1}{2}$ m.; pupils had a sluggish reaction to light; discs were pale, especially on the temporal side; bilateral central scotomata were present. The source of the defect in VII. 32 is uncertain in the absence of a knowledge of the family history of her mother, VI. 27; her only brother, VII. 33, was apparently normal up to the time of his death at the age of 26.

VII. 34 died aged 2. VII. 35, aged 49, was normal but had an affected son. VII. 37 was normal, aged 39, and had three young children. VII. 39 died aged 18; his sister reports that he became affected at the age of 12 and was almost blind from a disease of unrecognised nature. VII. 40, aged 43, was normal; she was married but childless. VII. 41, aged 41, became affected at 13 but was not wholly blind; he was in an institution for the blind for five years. VII. 43 and 45 were aged 36 and 32 respectively and were not affected; they each had young daughters. VII. 47 was aged 15. Of the four brothers, VII. 48—50, three were normal and aged 30, 25 and 19 respectively, the fourth, VII. 49, aged 23, suddenly noticed a diminution of vision in both eyes when he was aged 21, the condition progressed for a few days since when it had remained stationary; six months after the onset R. V. = finger counting in front of the eyes, L. V. = finger counting at $\frac{1}{2}$ m.; the right pupil reacted only slightly, the left pupil was normal; both discs were white with slightly blurred margins, arteries were narrowed; central scotomata were present in the fields with slight contraction of the outer limits; Wassermann test negative; examination of blood and of cerebro-spinal fluid revealed nothing abnormal. VII. 51 and 52, aged 24 and 20 respectively, were normal.

VIII. 1 was aged 6. VIII. 2, 3 and 4, aged 24, 22 and 20 respectively, were normal. VIII. 5, now aged 18, noticed suddenly when she was aged 12 that she saw badly with both eyes; according to the statement of her mother her right vision had definitely improved since that date when R. V. = L. V. = $\frac{1}{25}$; examined at 18, R. V. = $\frac{5}{20}$, L. V. = finger counting at $\frac{1}{2}$ m.; pupils were normal; the discs showed a medium grade of atrophy; small absolute central scotomata were present in the fields with concentric contraction of the outer limits to 30°—40°; Wassermann test negative.

VIII. 6, aged 16, VIII. 7, 8, 9, aged 24, 21 and VIII. 10, 11, 12, 13, aged 14, 12, 10 and 6 respectively, were none of them yet affected. VIII. 14 died aged $1\frac{1}{2}$ years. VIII. 15, aged 9, became affected at the age of 8; a few months from the onset papillae were pale on the temporal side and V. = finger counting at $1\frac{1}{2}$ m.; some improvement occurred and a year after the onset R. V. = $\frac{5}{30}$—$\frac{5}{24}$, L. V. = $\frac{1}{18}$; pupils were normal; discs showed a medium grade of atrophy. VIII. 16, aged 26, and three of his siblings, aged 19, 17 and 16 respectively, were still unaffected but one brother, VIII. 17, aged 23, became suddenly affected at the age of 18 and there had been no recovery since that date. VIII. 22, aged 16, became almost completely blind in eight days at the age of 7, some improvement had occurred since that time and at the age of 14 R. V. = $\frac{5}{25}$, L. V. = $\frac{5}{13}$; pupils were normal; discs showed white atrophy; Wassermann test was negative. VIII. 21, aged 19, was unaffected. Other members of this generation were all

Plate L.　　DESCRIPTIONS OF PEDIGREE PLATES　　369

quite young: VIII. 23 and 24, aged 12, VIII. 25, aged 3, VIII. 26, died aged 2, VIII. 27, aged 2½, VIII. 28, aged 1, VIII. 29, aged 8, VIII. 30, aged 4, and VIII. 31, aged 1½.

X-ray examination of the skull was made in the case of VI. 4, VII. 1, VII. 6, VII. 9, VII. 49, and VIII. 22; in all cases nothing abnormal was found and the sella turcica was normal. Abderhalden's reactions were examined for seven individuals as a possible means of determining whether there is any underlying defect of the internal secretions in these cases. The results are collected in a table: it would be of interest to have comparative observations on normal members of the stock and on an adequate number of individuals of the general population; no significant conclusion can be drawn from the values given. Consanguinity. Bibl. No. 135.

Fig. 717. *Taylor and Holmes's Case.* "C." Family. Eight cases of hereditary optic atrophy in an extensive pedigree of four generations; the disease occurred in males only but was transmitted through unaffected females of the stock. I. 11 suffered from occasional severe attacks of what was believed to be migraine, she died aged 71; I. 13 died aged 68, she had one healthy son, II. 25, who was the father of four healthy children; I. 17 is reported to have had bad eyes and to have been nearly blind, he was somewhat crippled with rheumatism; I. 11 had ten children of whom II. 11, Charles C., aged 55 (1913), became suddenly blind in the right eye in 1907, some months later the left eye became affected; vision improved a little within the first year, since when the condition had remained stationary; both fields showed large central scotomata; for four years this patient had complained of a steady aching pain in his right leg, also during the last year of slight numbness in his hands and fingers but no tingling or pain; he further had some difficulty regarding micturition; there was no history of excess in the use of alcohol and the patient smoked about one ounce of Navy Cut in a week. II. 14, Thomas C., now aged 49 (1913), at the age of 20 had suddenly noticed one day that "the road looked as if I could not get any further, as if it ended in the sky"; within a week he had to give up his work and has been unable to work since; he said that his two cousins, II. 35 and 36 who died aged 31 and 27 respectively, were "just like me, they could not see what they looked at"; 29 years after the onset II. 14 was examined and it was noted that both optic discs were pale, the vessels were normal; there was probably no peripheral contraction of fields but central scotomata were present; this man had suffered from severe periodic headaches for the past 15 or 20 years which were frequently unilateral but which were becoming less frequent; visual phenomena sometimes accompanied these headaches.

II. 20, Henry C., aged 43, had an operation for cataract at the age of 13, no improvement of sight followed. II. 23, Francis C., aged 36 (1911), had a history of headaches and optic neuritis in 1902; he was now found to have large central scotomata; optic discs were pale; the fundus was otherwise normal. II. 33, aged 56 (1913), was not quite blind; his vision had suddenly become affected 26 years ago; he also suffered from severe migraine with visual spectra; vision had failed in his two brothers at about the age of 17 years. III. 24, aged 43 (1913), was the only case of the disease in his generation; he could see quite well until the age of 30 when he suddenly became blind; the left eye was now quite blind and the right nearly so; he had been a soldier and had smoked heavily but had given up the use of tobacco for a considerable while; there was no history of venereal disease or of alcoholic excess; his sight had been unchanged for 13 years. III. 24 had two children of whom IV. 1, aged 21, had a high degree of myopia and IV. 2 suffered from migraine. The eldest son of II. 31 had always had poor sight and did not attend school after the age of 7 on this account; he and his brother, aged 31, were myopic.

The three eldest children of II. 11 were aged 32, 30 and 29 respectively, two of his later born children died in infancy. II. 14 had two children aged 24 and 22 respectively; the children of II. 18, II. 21 and II. 23 were all under 16 years of age; III. 21 represents five children who died in infancy; III. 22 had an orbital tumour and died aged 18; III. 27 died, aged 16, from phthisis; III. 31 died aged 14. III. 36 died aged 3 years. No consanguinity. Bibl. No. 100.

Fig. 718. *Waardenburg's Case.* Eleven cases of optic atrophy in three generations. I. 1 was deaf but saw well; his wife died rather young from disease of the breast; they had three children of whom two, II. 3 and 5, were believed to have had normal vision and one daughter, II. 2, was affected according to the statement of her daughter, III. 2. II. 1 had normal vision; II. 1 and 2 had 5 children of whom III. 2 suddenly became affected at the age of 19; no improvement had occurred in her vision since that time; she is now aged 55, has bilateral absolute central scotomata with normal peripheral limits to her fields; both papillae are white with clearly defined margins; vessels are normal. III. 4, aged 53, married a normal woman at the age of 25; he was himself blind from the ages of 28 to 34 years, after this improvement occurred; now his papillae were pale especially on the temporal side, vessels were unchanged, small paracentral scotomata were present and colours were seen better with the left than with the right eye; he had three normal children. III. 5 saw well but was deaf; he married a member of an affected stock (V. 16 of Fig. 708) but they had no children. III. 7, aged 48, was blind for five years from the ages of 12 to 17 but after this great improvement occurred and he was able to carry on work as a tailor; ophthalmoscopical appearances were the same as for III. 4; he was night-blind. III. 8, aged 46, was affected at the age of 18 but improvement had occurred; ophthalmoscopical appearances were the same as for his affected brothers.

II. 3 married a normal man who was still living and aged 72; he said that his wife, who died aged 52, had always seen well with the help of spectacles; they had seven children of whom III. 9, aged 45, was unmarried, he had been blind from the ages of 23 to 26 years, he was under treatment in Germany and lived too far away to be examined by the recorder, but he is said to have always been able to go about alone and to have improved so much that he was now able to read again. III. 11 was normal and had a healthy daughter. III. 13, aged 43, became blind suddenly at the age of 18; at the age of 20 gradual improvement occurred; he had a son whose age is not given but who had apparently not yet shown signs of the disease. III. 14 saw well. III. 16, aged 35, became blind at the age of 20; she has improved a little but is unable to read or do needlework; she can recognise people at a distance of 1 m.; she is married and has a son who has not yet become affected. III. 17, aged 35, sees well but is deaf. III. 19, aged 32, lost his distinct vision at the age of 19, in three weeks; three years before he had, following a fall whilst skating, been unable to read for an hour; he now has large absolute central scotomata with normal peripheral limits to his fields of vision; a severe grade of atrophy of the discs is present; he has three healthy small children.

III. 2 married a man with normal vision and had four children of whom two were affected and two daughters, IV. 4, aged 22 and 20 years respectively, were still normal and unmarried. IV. 2, now aged 26, became affected at the age of 20; she was never wholly blind and some improvement occurred but she remained unable to see to read or sew; she has a daughter aged 2 years. IV. 3, aged 24, became affected at the age of 20 whilst on military service in Utrecht; he has central scotomata but was never totally blind and some improvement has occurred. No consanguinity recorded. Bibl. No. 131.

Fig. 719. *Klopfer and Barth's Case.* Hereditary optic atrophy in seven males of a very extensive pedigree. The history, originally published by Klopfer in 1898, was greatly extended and brought up-to-date by Barth in 1921, who discovered two further affected members of the stock, VIII. 40 and VII. 41, and shows in his paper that all the affected members are amongst the descendants of IV. 20 and 21. We cannot be sure that all the affected members of the stock have been discovered; the stock founded by IV. 20 and 21 appears to be the source of the defect and we think it unlikely that the number of consanguineous marriages amongst the descendants of I. 1 and 2 has influenced the occurrence of the defect. The present pedigree of ten generations has been formed by combining the pedigrees given by Klopfer with information from five pedigrees worked out by Barth.

IX. 15, a clerk, noticed at the age of 21 that there was a cloud gradually becoming thicker before both his eyes; about a month later he was unable to carry on his work; there was no history of trauma or of acute disease or of syphilis to account for the origin of the disease; the patient drank only with moderation and smoked seldom; he was well at the time with a good appetite and no liability to headaches or fainting; he was treated with mercury and strychnine. Five months after the onset Klopfer saw IX. 15 and found that R. V. = finger counting at $\frac{1}{2}$ m., L. V. = finger counting at $1\frac{1}{2}$ m.; of colours only blue was recognised; no contraction of the peripheral boundary of the visual fields was found but a thick grey shadow appeared to overlay the whole field and central scotomata were present; the nerve was a little paler than normal; retinal vessels were normal and no signs of neuritis were present. Five years later there was no change in the patient's vision but now there was a marked atrophic discoloration and excavation of the optic nerve.

IX. 13 at the age of 24 went to hospital with the statement that since about 8 weeks he had noticed a very marked diminution in his vision; up to this time he had good sight and, as a soldier, was a good shot; his vision was now reduced to finger counting at 5 m. for the left eye and at 4 m. for the right; he recognised all colours; there was no contraction of the visual fields and no demonstrable scotomata; nothing abnormal appeared on ophthalmoscopic examination. Three years later he was again seen; he had not been ill since his first examination and reported that he had never had venereal disease and was a very moderate smoker and drinker; vision was now reduced to finger counting at 1 m. for the right eye and at 2 m. for the left; bilateral central scotomata were present and blue was the only colour recognised; the nerves were now white and atrophic. A similar history is given in the case of IX. 16 who became affected at the age of 20. IX. 6, first cousin to the three affected brothers, became affected with the same disease at the age of 20. VII. 27 became affected at the age of 23 years.

The stock in other respects appears to have been particularly healthy and vigorous; no disease of the nervous system or tuberculosis or other hereditary defect was known to have occurred in it; none of the cases improved with treatment. Consanguinity. Bibl. Nos. 56, 118.

Fig. 720. *Reeder's Case.* Hereditary optic atrophy in a mother and two daughters, two sons had normal vision; the patients were above the average in intelligence, they were well nourished and had no history of other hereditary defect; X-rays showed no abnormality in the skull; Wassermann reactions were negative. I. 1, Mrs R. W., aged 28 (1915), was first seen in 1915 when R. V. = $\frac{15}{100}$, or with -1.5 cyl. axis 180° = $\frac{20}{100}$; L. V. = $\frac{6}{200}$, or with -1.5 cyl. axis 5° = $\frac{30}{100}$; vitreous was clear, discs very pale with well defined margins, lamina cribrosa slightly visible; arteries and veins were very small; no macular or peripheral lesions were seen; fields were full for form but showed marked contraction for all colours with central scotomata for blue. In 1926, R. V. = L. V. = $\frac{5}{200}$, with correction R. V. = L. V. = $\frac{20}{200}$; discs were

Plate L.   DESCRIPTIONS OF PEDIGREE PLATES   371

very pale and blood vessels were more atrophic; fields showed paracentral contraction with no central vision for blue or red. II. 1, L. W., aged 14 (1926), had had rapidly failing vision during the past four months; she had always been a very robust child, periods commenced at the age of 13; she had had frequent headaches during the past few months and could now only read for a few minutes at a time; R. V. = L. V. = $\frac{6}{100}$; with + 2·0 sph. 0·5 cyl. axis 90° R. V. = L. V. = $\frac{20}{100}$; media were clear; discs were pale with well defined margins and slight central cupping; fields were full for form but contracted for all colours to within 10°. II. 2, F. W., aged 9 (1926), had complained of seeing badly for the past year; R. V. = $\frac{10}{200}$, L. V. = $\frac{2}{200}$, or with + 4·0 sph. R. V. = $\frac{20}{30}$—1, L. V. = $\frac{20}{200}$; media were clear, discs pale; vessels normal; fields were normal for form; for colours the right field was contracted to within 20° and the left to within 10°. We are not told the age of onset of the disease for I. 1, nor the ages of the two at present unaffected brothers. No consanguinity recorded. Bibl. No. 144.

Fig. 721. *Leber's Case IV.* Hereditary optic atrophy in II. 1 and in his two maternal uncles. II. 1 became affected at the age of 16 or 17 years, the condition progressed rapidly for about a fortnight since when it had remained stationary; central scotomata were present; the peripheral fields of vision were not contracted; ophthalmoscopic examination was negative when first seen, later white coloration of the optic nerve was noted. I. 2 saw well; her two brothers became affected at about the same age as II. 1; both were still living and their vision was said to have remained unchanged for a long period of years. No consanguinity recorded. Bibl. No. 8.

Fig. 722. *Mügge's Case.* Hereditary optic atrophy in two brothers; the parents were living and saw well; one brother, aged 21, saw well; two brothers, aged 10 and 11 years respectively, had not yet shown signs of the disease; one sister saw well. II. 1, George K., aged 23, did not know at what age he became affected but he had been unable to read easily at school; now R. V. = $\frac{1}{16}$, L. V. = $\frac{1}{16}$; slight improvement followed injections of strychnine; the temporal side of both discs was white; vessels were normal. II. 3, Frederick K., aged 19, first noticed a diminution of vision at the age of 12½; about two years later R. V. = L. V. = $\frac{5}{38}$; the discs were pale particularly in the temporal halves. No consanguinity recorded. Bibl. No. 93.

Fig. 723. *Pines and Tron's Case.* Hereditary optic atrophy in five of the six brothers of a sibship of thirteen; all the seven sisters had died under the age of 3 years from scarlet fever, measles, or inflammation of the lungs; all the brothers were of nervous and irritable temperaments; a maternal uncle had hereditary optic atrophy. The father, I. 1, died, aged 60, from typhus but was otherwise healthy; the mother, I. 2, was nervous but saw well and had normal fundi. I. 3 died aged 36, at the age of 12, his vision became so dim that he could not see to read or write and atrophy of the optic nerve was diagnosed by an ophthalmologist; during the three years following the onset of the disease considerable improvement in vision occurred and the patient could again see to read and write.

II. 1, Nikola, aged 40, had measles and scarlet fever in childhood; at the age of 28 years his vision became dim and atrophy of the optic nerve was diagnosed; strychnine was given without any result; hypnosis was then tried and was followed by improvement and now R. V. = L. V. = 1; refraction was emmetropic; media normal; the discs were white with sharply cut margins and narrowed arteries; fields for white were normal at the peripheral boundaries but a relative central scotoma was present; fields for colour were much contracted, especially for red. II. 2, Basil, aged 38, had seen badly since the age of 20; the onset of the disease was sudden; he now had lung disease but carried on his work; the ophthalmoscope showed atrophy of the optic nerve; he had central scotomata for red and green. II. 3, Paul, died aged 26 years; he began to see badly at the age of 14 when optic atrophy was diagnosed; the condition improved and he could see to read and write. II. 5, Peter A., aged 32, was born at term and appeared to be normally developed; he had scarlet fever, measles and diphtheria as a child and went to school at the age of 9 years; at the age of 14 he had an operation for strabismus; from the age of 23 he had had frequent headaches; since 1917 he had worked very strenuously in political movements for the Russian revolution and had had little sleep owing to much night work; he was on one occasion drunk for a month; at 28 he married but his wife had left him; he was very querulous and irritable and was sent to a psychiatrical department on account of temperamental difficulties. At the age of 31 he had typhus, and in the same year he noticed a cloud before his eyes on getting up one morning and could only see dimly; there had been no change in his vision in the last six months; syphilis was denied; he drank and smoked occasionally; refraction was emmetropic; R. V. = fingers at 35 cm., L. V. = fingers at 20 cm.; media were clear; the papillae were pale and sharply outlined; arteries were narrowed; temporal boundaries of visual fields were contracted and large absolute central scotomata were present; yellow, red and green were mostly not recognised. II. 4, Georg, aged 33, became affected at the age of 31; he had measles and scarlet fever in childhood and following these had some lung and kidney trouble; at 28 he had typhus; he had epilepsy with attacks once a month; refraction was emmetropic; R. V. = L. V. = 0·05; media were normal; the visual fields were contracted in the temporal region and relative central scotomata were present; green, red and yellow were not recognised. III. 6, Konstantin, aged 24, had normal vision and fundi but he was still below the ages at which three of his brothers had manifested the disease.

Three of the brothers had asymmetry of the face, three brothers had horizontal nystagmus and syndactylous toes. No consanguinity recorded. Bibl. No. 136.

PLATE LI. Fig. 724. *Worton's Case.* Hereditary optic atrophy in eleven males in three generations. II. 7 died unmarried; it was not known at what age he became affected with optic atrophy but the onset was believed to have occurred rather late in life; at the age of 60 he was drowned through walking into a pond; he had one brother, II. 5, who was unaffected, and had nine normal children, also three sisters, all of whom married and transmitted the disease. Thus II. 2 had eight children of whom III. 1, aged 64, became affected at the age of 25, III. 2, herself normal, transmitted the defect to three of her sons, and III. 4, aged 62, became himself affected at the age of 23; two sons and three daughters of II. 2 appear to have been normal and to have remained unmarried. II. 3 had a normal son, III. 11, whose children and grandchildren were likewise normal; a normal daughter, III. 12, who did not transmit the disease to her son or daughter; a daughter, III. 14, whose only son, IV. 22, was affected; a son, III. 16, aged 50, who became affected at the age of 24 and still had such bad sight that he was unable to work; a normal unmarried daughter, III. 18. II. 8 had a son, III. 24, aged 56, who became affected at the early age of 15 but whose sight had much improved; of the other children of II. 8, one son, III. 28, was normal and of the six normal daughters two were unmarried and one, III. 33, transmitted the disease. Of the three affected sons of III. 2, IV. 2, aged 44, became affected at the age of 30 and was now blind; IV. 4, aged 40, became affected at 32, the left eye was first attacked and the right a fortnight later; a few days after the onset he was unable to read large type and his vision steadily deteriorated for two years; now he sees so little that he has to be led about. At the time of onset, IV. 4 was smoking about one ounce of shag weekly and was a moderate drinker, but he discontinued these habits; he had influenza a month before the onset; his pulse was slow and he suffered from cold extremities; he had fallen three times, without losing consciousness, at intervals of about three years; R. V. = L. V. = hand movements; pupils reacted well but the reaction to light was not well maintained; discs were markedly pale, physiological cups more or less filled in; vessels were rather small. IV. 5, aged 30, became affected at the age of 17; he cannot now see well enough to work but is able to read large type.

IV. 22, now aged 35, the only son of III. 14, became affected at the age of 14; the left eye was first attacked and the right eye a few days later; he had always been in good health and was a non-smoker; pupils reacted well but response to light was not well maintained; now R. V. = L. V. = $\frac{6}{9}$; discs somewhat pale, physiological cups partly filled in; vessels were a good size; visual fields were full and no scotomata were found; this case, with a history of early onset, had thus regained normal vision. IV. 51, aged 19, son of III. 33, complained that his sight had become so bad that he had had to give up his work; he had first noticed a mistiness in the vision of the left eye four months before, which in a few days had become bad enough to prevent his reading large type with that eye; a fortnight later the right eye became affected and his vision was so much reduced that he was unable to go out alone; he was well nourished and had smoked cigarettes occasionally before his eyes became affected; he was practically an abstainer and had always had good health but suffered from cold hands and feet and chilblains in the winter. The parents of IV. 51 were not consanguineous and no epilepsy had occurred in the family; his blood pressure was normal, urine normal, nervous system normal; R. V. = L. V. = $\frac{2}{36}$, eccentric fixation; pupils reacted briskly but reaction to light was not well maintained; an absolute central scotoma surrounded by a partially scotomatous area extending to about 15° from the centre was present in each field; peripheral limits for white were normal; the ophthalmoscopic appearances were those of a mild neuritis; fifteen months from the onset vision was the same but slight atrophy of the discs was now present. IV. 52, brother to IV. 51, aged 17, became affected at the age of 9, his sight was bad for a year and then rapidly improved; he was a stout, ruddy, well-nourished youth; this patient suffered from cold feet and chilblains nearly all the year but in other respects had always had good health; he was an abstainer and smoked only a few cigarettes a week; nervous system was normal and urine normal; R. V. = L. V. = $\frac{6}{9}$ nearly; discs were a little pale; vessels a good size and physiological cups slightly filled in; there were marked shimmery reflexes seen all over the fundi which were more marked along the course of the vessels; no definite scotomata were found and peripheral limits of the fields were normal. The recorder concludes that early onset would appear to suggest a favourable prognosis. No consanguinity recorded. Bibl. No. 102.

Fig. 725. *Batten's Case.* This family has been under observation at various hospitals by Nettleship, Lawford, Worth, Batten and Paton since 1896 and members of it are still seen at intervals and have recently been reported upon. Five brothers of a sibship of eleven are affected with hereditary optic atrophy. I. 1 is reported to have lost his sight after a slight accident and never recovered it; I. 2 had a daughter who was blind and idiotic; I. 4 and 5, parents of the affected sibships, were believed to see well; they were still living when the case was reported in 1909.

II. 2, aged 58 (1925), had a son aged 13. II. 4, aged 56 (1925), became affected at the age of 27, the left eye was first affected and the right eye 5 months later; he used to smoke 3 ounces of shag a week and drank in moderation; there was a history of venereal disease seven years previously. II. 5, aged 54 (1925), had undergone treatment at Moorfields; he is reported to have lost his sight at the age of 33 years; he was

PLATE LI.   DESCRIPTIONS OF PEDIGREE PLATES   373

married and had one son, aged 28 (1925), and a daughter; the son was believed to be normal at this date. II. 7, aged 52 (1925), was examined at the age of 24 when his sight was normal; he writes that he lost his sight a day before he was 27 years of age; he has two daughters and a son, aged 26 (1925), not yet affected. II. 9, aged 49 (1925), was a heavy smoker; his sight began to fail at the age of 22, the right eye one month before the left. II. 10 died aged 12 years. II. 11, aged 44 (1925), reported that his sight had failed in both eyes fairly suddenly ten months ago; he had been subject to "nervous breakdowns" with severe headaches since the war; now vision in both eyes was reduced to hand movements; fields showed concentric contraction and discs were of a dead white pallor. II. 12, aged 42, had four children of whom the only boy was aged 10 years. II. 14 and 15 were aged 41 and 38 years respectively. The only unaffected male of this sibship was aged 34 in 1925 and thus was still below the age at which II. 11 became affected. The question of lead poisoning was raised, as at least three of the affected brothers were plumbers, but there was no decided evidence of plumbism. There was no recovery in any of the cases. No consanguinity recorded. Bibl. No. 85, p. clxxxi, with additional notes.

Fig. 726. *Jameson Evans's Case.* (Taken from Nettleship.) Leber's disease in seven males of three generations. No information could be obtained concerning the parents or ancestry of generation I. I. 2, 7 and 12 represent three affected brothers in a sibship of seven; I. 4 and 8 were two unaffected brothers whose children saw well; I. 5 and 10 represent two sisters who saw well. I. 10 had two daughters who saw well. I. 5 transmitted the defect to three of her four sons who reached adult life; one of her daughters, II. 9, had an affected son, III. 6. III. 5 died in infancy, III. 7, 8 and 9 were young at the time of the investigation. No information is given of the severity of the disease or of its progress, or of the age of onset, but III. 6 was aged 14, so that the age of onset in his case must have been relatively early. No consanguinity recorded. Bibl. No. 85, p. clxxxvi.

Fig. 727. *de Keersmaecker's Case.* III. 4, aged 19, reported that three months previously he had noticed a sudden diminution of visual acuity which had progressed in spite of treatment until, after six weeks, he had had to give up his work; the condition had remained stationary since; he complained of a large black spot which covered the centre of his visual field; on ophthalmoscopic examination it was found that the media were transparent, the papillae pale, the arteries narrowed, the veins dilated and tortuous; vision was reduced to finger counting with difficulty. The patient had not done work which exposed him to any kind of intoxication and there was no history of specific disease or alcoholism; his father was epileptic but had normal vision; his mother had good health and vision, her sisters also had normal sight but all her four brothers were amblyopic. II. 6, aged 40, had amblyopia which came on at the age of 20 years and had remained stationary ever since. II. 5, aged 45, never complained of his sight until the age of 40 when he had severe headaches for several weeks followed by a rapid failure of vision on account of which he had to give up his work; the condition had remained stationary. II. 3, aged 49, had violent headaches at the age of 32 years followed by a diminution of vision; after about six weeks there was some improvement and since then the condition had remained unchanged; he had a son, aged 29, with excellent sight up to the time of examination. II. 2 became similarly affected at the age of 37 years. The father of these four affected uncles was alcoholic and had had delirium tremens, he died aged 69. The patient's two sisters, III. 2 and 3, who were older than he, had excellent sight. No consanguinity recorded. Bibl. No. 20.

Fig. 728. *Hancock's Case.* Hereditary optic atrophy affecting males only and transmitted by females only in an extensive pedigree. I. 1 died more than 100 years ago (1808); it is known that in the third decade of life his sight failed very rapidly, and that after a long period it greatly improved. III. 2, a heavy smoker and drinker, had a marked failure of vision in both eyes between the ages of 20 and 30 which never recovered. III. 9, a very abstemious man with regard to the use of tobacco and alcohol, was also affected; after twelve to eighteen months from the onset he recovered his sight sufficiently to resume his work. III. 14, "not a careful liver," became affected between .20 and 30 years of age; his sight failed suddenly whilst working in his office and never recovered. Thus, all the males of this sibship were affected; they all married and had normal offspring. III. 16 became affected at about the age of 30 and did not recover. In the next generation there were five affected members. IV. 23 had excellent general health and took alcohol and tobacco in moderation, but the vision of both his eyes failed rapidly on returning from a holiday in 1906; in 1907, R. V. = L. V. = $\frac{6}{60}$, not improved by glasses; pupils were normal; the temporal half of each disc was pale, otherwise the fundi were normal; central colour scotomata for red and green were noted, no scotomata for white; peripheral fields were not contracted; strychnine with prohibition of alcohol and tobacco was prescribed, also a prolonged holiday. Six months later vision was the same; there was now a large central scotoma for white, pallor of discs was more marked, veins were tortuous and arteries narrowed. At a later date it was heard that this patient's vision had distinctly improved; he had three unaffected brothers. IV. 31 developed the disease at the age of 25; he was a heavy smoker and drinker; no recovery occurred though the patient was never quite blind. IV. 32, a fine athlete, neither smoked nor drank; he was overtaken by the disease at the age of 20 whilst in training for a race; he made a complete recovery after about a year. IV. 33, the third and only other male of this sibship, had a rapid onset of the disease at the age of 26; he reached his maximum disability in a fortnight when R. V. = L. V. = finger counting only; he had no headaches or pain; the left pupil was slightly larger than the right, both reacted sluggishly to light but briskly to convergence; the discs showed marked pallor, especially on the temporal side; retinal vessels were normal; central scotomata for white were noted, peripheral fields were full; this man had always smoked in moderation and gave it up entirely for six months; there was no history of syphilis; the patient had had occasional epileptic attacks since the age of 16 and had taken 90 grains a day of bromide; the bromide was reduced, smoking prohibited and a voyage advised; great improvement was noted. IV. 48 had a rapid failure of vision in both eyes at the age of 26 when he was suffering from tertiary syphilis; he was a heavy smoker but drank in moderation; great improvement was noted after 18 months of treatment; he had no headaches or pain in his eyes. The only sibling of IV. 48 was also affected. The sight of IV. 49 failed rapidly at the age of 31; the defect reached a maximum in ten days; he was a heavy smoker and a moderate drinker; six months later some improvement was noted; a year later R. V. = L. V. = $\frac{6}{9}$. V. 13 became affected at the age of 17; he never recovered but was not quite blind. Many members of generation V were still below the age at which they were liable to develop the disease. No consanguinity. Bibl. No. 79.

PLATE LII. Fig. 729. *Nettleship and Thompson's Case.* Eleven cases of hereditary optic atrophy occurring in males and two or possibly five cases in females in three or four generations. I. 2, Elizabeth A. (Mrs S.), was known by several descendants to have been blind from about the age of 30 till her death at the age of 80 years; she had an operation on her eyes at the age of about 30 and after this lost what sight she had. I. 3, Mrs B., was said to have had bad sight, but this was not confirmed and no detailed information could be obtained about it. No information was available of I. 1. II. 2 and her two brothers, II. 3 and 4, became nearly blind between the ages of 25 and 30 years; from the description given by III. 7 it was evident that the symptoms in his mother and at least one of her brothers were similar to his own, that their central vision was bad but the periphery of the field relatively good; II. 3 and 4 died unmarried at the ages of 56 and 90 years respectively. II. 5, Mrs L., had good sight and lived to be over 60; she had three children, one of whom, III. 14, was believed by III. 10 to be affected, but he could not be traced and there was no conclusive evidence of his affection. II. 2 lived to the age of 67; she married II. 1, whose sight was excellent, and had seven children of whom III. 1 died in early infancy. III. 3, with good sight, died, aged 60, of a fit, having had two previous seizures; her husband, III. 2, aged 77 (1912), had good sight. Of III. 4 it was reported that her sight failed at the age of 14—15 years and was bad for about a year, after which she made a complete and permanent recovery; the testimony of III. 7 in 1896 and that of III. 10 in 1912 are suggestive of amblyopia and not of accommodative failure; III. 4 was married but had no children; she died aged 76 (1912). III. 5, James L., was seen, aged 75 (1912), when he was at work on the road; his sight failed rather gradually at the age of 17; for a time he could not tell gold from silver and was quite unable to read but some improvement occurred so that he could read big letters; his vision was not tested, but evidently his peripheral vision was good; no ophthalmoscopic examination was made; he had either four or five sons of whom the youngest died aged 10, the others saw well and one at least was married and had some healthy children who also saw well.

III. 7, George L., aged 56 (1896), was Nettleship's patient; his vision was less than $\frac{6}{60}$, not improved by glasses; he had well-marked absolute central scotomata, pupils and ocular tension were normal; discs were pale especially on the temporal side; arteries were rather small in the right; his sight failed at about the age of 25, he was very temperate and began to smoke at about this time; when seen again by Thompson in 1912 the condition was unchanged; he had a son and three daughters of whom IV. 13 had to wear glasses but with them saw quite well. IV. 15 had four children, aged 27, 21, 17 and 15 respectively, who saw well.

III. 10, Job L., aged 58 (1901), was under the care of Lang for six months at this time and was told to stop smoking; he had smoked $\frac{1}{2}$ oz. a day; his vision began to fail at about the age of 30 but he could see to sharpen his saw and even to read until November 1900, when he rapidly became worse and could then only see to count fingers; refraction was emmetropic; central absolute scotomata were present; discs were atrophic, the outer halves white; in 1912 Nettleship saw this patient, now aged 69, when he was a healthy old man with sight as above. III. 10 was twice married; by his first marriage he had ten children of whom only three reached adult life, the others died aged 7 years, 6 weeks, and 8 months respectively, four were stillborn or lived for one day only; by his second wife III. 10 had three children one of whom was stillborn and the others died aged 3 and 2 months respectively.

III. 12, Albert L., died suddenly from heart disease at the age of 30—35; between the ages of 13 and 19 his sight became bad for about a year and then quite recovered; this account was given independently by III. 7 and III. 10 who were living at home at the time; III. 12 had two children of whom the elder died in her first confinement; the younger, IV. 33, a bricklayer, was known to have good sight. IV. 1 died, aged 39, of "sugar diabetes"; her sight became bad a year or so before death and she was quite blind the last day or two of life. IV. 3, Percy S., died, aged 43 (1907), from cancer of the throat, he married and left six children, aged 21—11 (1912), all reported to have perfect sight at this date; the sight of IV. 3 failed at the age of 28 and did not improve; he was a heavy smoker and drank freely. IV. 4, aged 45, had three children of whom V. 4 died aged 5, V. 5 and 6 were aged 9 and 5 years respectively. IV. 6, aged 42 (1912),

PLATE LII.   DESCRIPTIONS OF PEDIGREE PLATES   375

had a failure of vision at the age of 28, the defect reached its maximum in 2 weeks; he was smoking $\frac{1}{2}$ oz. black shag daily and had been losing flesh owing he thought to the nature of his work—he was a baker; the moon was never quite blotted out to him but he was unable to tell whether she were full or not; improvement occurred so that in 1912 he could see the stars, could write fairly well and with a + 3 D. lens he could read words of about 6 J.; he had a marked central colour scotoma; temporal half of each disc was pale; his vision ultimately improved to $\frac{6}{18}$ in the right, $\frac{6}{12}$ in the left; there was a slight general contraction of each field for white. IV. 8 and IV. 10, aged 39 and 36 respectively, saw well.

Attempts were made, with the assistance of one of the recorders, to get in touch with the family in 1923 and hear whether any further cases had occurred in generations IV and V, but my letters were returned by the dead letter office and the efforts met with no success. No consanguinity recorded. Bibl. No. 97.

Fig. 730. *Morlet's Case.* Twelve cases of optic atrophy in four sibships of two generations, one woman affected; unfortunately only two cases were examined as the family was much scattered but the recorder was in correspondence with all the affected branches of the family and was satisfied that the diagnosis was correct in each case. I. 1, A. P., a Chinaman, was married to an Irish woman; they had eleven children of whom II. 5 became blind at the age of 49; II. 6 died young; II. 7 became blind at the age of 45; II. 10 lost his sight at 21; II. 11 became blind at 24 and II. 12 became blind at the age of 20; one son was normal. Of the daughters of I. 1 and 2, three transmitted the disease and one, II. 14, Mrs T., had nine young children who had not yet shown signs of the disease. II. 2, Mrs R., had six sons of whom two died young, III. 3 became affected at the age of 25, III. 10 and III. 15 both became affected at 19; III. 16 had not yet shown signs of the disease but he was still too young to be confident of normality; Mrs R. also had one daughter, III. 8, who became affected at 30, one daughter who died young and four daughters who had normal vision. II. 3, Mrs F., had two sons and four daughters of whom one son, III. 24, became blind at 33. II. 8, Mrs T., had six sons and one daughter of whom III. 26 became blind at the age of 13, III. 27 became blind at 18, four sons were still of an age at which they might develop the disease but had not yet done so; one daughter was normal and had a young daughter.

III. 8 and III. 15 were examined; of the former we are told that she had always had good sight until at the age of 30, two months after the birth of her first child, the sight of her right eye began to get dim; within a few weeks the sight of both eyes became very bad indeed; she was seen four months after the onset when R. V. = finger counting at 30 cm.; L. V. = shadows only; wide dense central scotomata were present in each, pupils were dilated and reacted sluggishly to light; discs were pale and atrophic, left disc showed undoubted signs of a subsiding optic neuritis, the margin was blurred and the whole disc swollen. At a later date both discs were definitely atrophic and showed no signs of active neuritis.

III. 15 up to the age of 19 had good sight and was normally healthy though backward at school; two weeks before he was examined he had found difficulty in distinguishing the colours worn by the jockeys, the left eye was at first more dim than the right but vision in each had become worse every day; R. V. = $\frac{6}{60}$, L. V. = shadows only; very dense and extensive central scotomata were present; fundi were normal at this date but a few weeks later the condition had progressed and optic atrophy had become evident from ophthalmoscopic examination; this man had a slightly enlarged heart and a blood pressure of 160 mm. Hg.; Wassermann test was negative. No consanguinity recorded. Bibl. No. 120.

Fig. 731. *Hawkes's Case I.* Hereditary optic atrophy in seven males and one female of three generations. I. 2 had, by his first wife, five children of whom two sons became affected at the age of 30; his daughter, II. 4, married a man who was healthy and saw well; they had nine children of whom three of the four sons became affected and one of the two married daughters transmitted the defect; nothing was known of the vision of II. 6 and 7; by his second wife I. 2 had normal children and grandchildren. II. 2 was married and had normal children. III. 3 became affected at 48; he had children who were unaffected but still young. III. 4 had three sons of whom none were yet affected, but the eldest was only aged 19. III. 7 had five children of whom IV. 5 became affected at the age of 19; IV. 6 became affected at 18; IV. 7, a daughter, became affected at 14 when her vision rapidly diminished to $\frac{1}{60}$ and no permanent improvement had yet occurred. IV. 8 and IV. 9 were not yet affected.

All the affected members of this family who were examined had well-marked optic atrophy, vision of large objects only remaining; in other cases the diagnosis was made by ophthalmic surgeons; in three cases the disease was known to have begun as a retrobulbar neuritis; all cases give a history of very rapid failure of vision with little subsequent improvement. No consanguinity recorded. Bibl. No. 63.

Fig. 732. *Hawkes's Case II.* Hereditary optic atrophy in eight males of three generations and possibly in a female of the generation preceding these. I. 2 was reported to have become blind but no information is given concerning the age at which this occurred or its mode of onset; she had three children of whom two sons were affected; one daughter, who saw well, had four affected sons. These four brothers had a sister who saw well but transmitted the defect to her two sons. All the affected members of this family showed well-marked optic atrophy; their vision varied from perception of large objects only up to $\frac{1}{60}$; the onset in all cases was at about the age of 30. No consanguinity recorded. Bibl. No. 63.

Fig. 733. *Van Heuven and Oltmans's Case.* Hereditary optic atrophy in six males of three generations. IV. 2, aged 11, was undergoing treatment for scarlet fever when it was noticed that he saw very badly; on enquiry it was found that one to three months before his sight had suddenly become bad so that he could no longer follow the instructions given at school; an oculist was then consulted but he could find nothing to account for the lowered visual acuity and suspected that the child was malingering; he was again examined and now atrophy of the optic nerve in the right eye and slight neuritis in the left eye were noted; R. V. = $\frac{1}{5}$, L. V. = $\frac{1}{10}$; large relative and small absolute central scotomata were present; Wassermann test negative. IV. 2 had two sisters who apparently were normal; his parents and two maternal uncles were normal but six members of his mother's sibship had died young. II. 3, maternal great-uncle to IV. 2, aged 64, reported that at the age of 30 he had suddenly lost his good vision and the condition of his sight had since remained unchanged; now R. V. = $\frac{1\cdot5}{60}$, L. V. = $\frac{1}{60}$; the pupils were dilated but reacted slowly to light; the optic nerves were greyish white with large atrophic excavations; large relative and small absolute central scotomata were present in the fields.

III. 1, aged 40, became affected fully ten years ago; in 1919 R. V. = $\frac{3}{60}$, L. V. = $\frac{1}{60}$; the optic nerves were pale on the temporal side; Wassermann test in the blood was negative, rhinological examination revealed no defect; in 1924 the vision in the left eye was raised to $\frac{3}{60}$, in other respects the condition remained unchanged. III. 2 was also affected; the age of onset in his case is not given but bilateral optic atrophy was noted and R. V. = $\frac{6}{60}$, L. V. = $\frac{3}{60}$. II. 9 was almost completely blind but it was not known that optic atrophy was the source of his defect; his sister had one daughter who died young and three sons of whom two became affected at the ages of 18 and 15 years respectively; both these cases improved markedly and ultimately had fairly good vision. No consanguinity recorded. Bibl. No. 130.

Fig. 734. *Coste's Case.* Four cases of hereditary optic atrophy in males. IV. 2, A. R., aged 21, reported that six months previously he had first noticed a diminution of vision, the left side was first affected and the condition had progressed up to the present time when R. V. = $\frac{1}{60}$, L. V. = $\frac{1}{60}$; the media were transparent; the pupils were slightly dilated but reacted well to light and to accommodation; ophthalmoscopic examination revealed white atrophy of the optic nerve especially marked on the temporal side in each eye, the limits of the papillae were clearly defined; central scotomata were present, also some contraction of the visual fields; the patient was healthy, he had had typhoid fever at the age of 3 years and had not been ill since; at the onset of his visual trouble he had no fever or general symptoms but suffered from bad headaches for about a month which came on in the afternoon and lasted for from three to six hours; they were neuralgic in character and the pain was in the temporal regions. The father and mother of IV. 2 were living and well; the father, III. 2, had three brothers and a sister who saw well, his parents, II. 3 and 4, were first cousins; there was no history of eye disease in the antecedents of III. 2. The mother, III. 7, had three brothers of whom two, III. 4 and 8, were affected, also her first cousin, III. 10, was affected; each of these cases was investigated.

III. 4, Guillaume V., aged 58, refused to attend at the clinic because the treatment there had been unsuccessful in the case of his nephew; he became affected at the age of 23 and could not recall having had headaches at this time; he only allowed a very brief examination which showed paleness of the temporal portion of both papillae; there was said to be no central scotoma and his visual acuity is not given.

III. 8, Charles V., aged 48, became affected at the age of 35 and could not remember having had headaches; he had typhoid fever at the age of 10; no history of syphilis; had been a soldier; his wife and two children were in good health and saw well, but the eldest of his children was only aged 16; he himself had very good health. Report of his examination gives R. V. = hand movements at 0·40 cm., L. V. = hand movements at 0·10 cm.; white atrophy of both nerves is noted; visual fields were contracted on the temporal side. III. 5, the normal brother of this sibship, had three sons who saw well but the eldest was only aged 17. The parents of this sibship were normal, but the maternal aunt, II. 12, had an affected son.

III. 10, L. C., aged 53, was living in Algeria and reports his own case—he says there was no alcoholism; he had slight arterio-sclerosis; he had had a nephritic calculus 15 to 16 years ago; four years ago he noticed a diminution of vision; the left eye had always been weak and the eyelid tended to fall; central vision was lost and he could now see so little as to be scarcely able to go about alone. III. 11, aged 42, had pigmentary choroiditis; R. V. = $\frac{1}{10}$, L. V. with − 2 D. = $\frac{1}{2}$; he had no central scotoma. IV. 2 was born ten years after the marriage of his parents; IV. 1, born five years earlier, had good vision. Consanguinity. Bibl. No. 75.

Fig. 735. *Mügge's Case.* Hereditary optic atrophy in two brothers and probably in the brother of their maternal grandmother. III. 1, Wilhelm K., aged 27, became affected about ten years ago and was for a time almost completely blind; his brother Carl, III. 2, aged 26, became affected a year ago. Vision of III. 2 was now hand movements only in the left eye, the right eye could count fingers at $\frac{1}{4}$ m. I. 3 was said to have become affected with some eye disease shortly after his marriage, through which he was almost completely blind for four years; later he improved so markedly as to be able to carry on his work as a teacher up to the age of 56. III. 3, aged 21, had not yet shown signs of the disease. II. 1 was the only child of her parents. No consanguinity recorded. Bibl. No. 93.

Fig. 736. *Nettleship's Case.* Hereditary optic atrophy in three females and two males of two generations; other members of the stock possibly also affected. No information was available concerning I. 1 and 2; they had five children of whom II. 2 had bad sight and married a first cousin with bad sight; nothing was known of the nature of their defects nor of the sight of their twelve children. II. 3 had ten children of whom a son and a daughter had some defect of sight of which no details could be obtained. II. 5 had also some defect of sight, the nature of which was unknown. II. 6 was treated at Moorfields at the age of 14, when she became affected with Leber's disease; at the age of 61 her sight was not improved; she had ten children of whom six died young. III. 5 married at 18 but had no children; her vision failed at the age of 36. III. 8 became affected at the age of 26; her two children were below the age at which it is usual to show the defect. III. 10 was seen about nine months after the onset of the disease at the age of 22. II. 8 saw well; she had nine children of whom one son developed the disease at the age of 22 after influenza; the fifth born, a daughter, had fits. Consanguinity. Bibl. No. 85, p. clxxiii.

Plate LIII. Fig. 737. *Usher's Case.* Hereditary optic atrophy in seven males and one female of three generations. III. 9 had good sight and died aged 59 years, he was not related to his wife, III. 14, who also saw well; of their ten children three of the four sons became affected with hereditary optic atrophy. IV. 10, the second born, was the first to become affected and was seen January 28, 1899, when at the age of 21 years he complained that the vision of his right eye had commenced to fail three months ago and that of his left eye one month ago; he had had no illness, no headache, and felt perfectly well; there was no history of syphilis and throughout the winter he had bathed in the sea in the early morning; his grasps were equal, knee-jerks present, breathing through each nostril was present and there was no nasal discharge; pupils were equal and contracted to light; eye movements were full, nothing abnormal was felt in orbits; R. V. = finger counting at one foot; L. V. = $\frac{6}{60}$ not improved by spherical lens, reads 10 J. at nine inches, field of vision full; right disc was too pale, there was white along the edges of the vessels, the cup was filled in and the edge of the disc was blurred; the left disc was too red and the edge was blurred, white lines were seen along the vessels; under homatropine a few small haemorrhages were seen in the region of the disc in each eye, there was a black pepper appearance at the yellow spot and two black square patches of pigmentation are noted in the left fundus, whether in the retina or choroid was uncertain. Subsequent examinations of this case are described, the most recent of which was on December 18, 1909, when subjective sensations, dark or red, were found in the centre of the field; at this date R. V. = finger counting at two feet, L. V. = $\frac{1}{60}$ and discs were pale; absolute central scotomata for 20 mm. white square were present in each field and the periphery of each field was not quite full. The son and daughter of IV. 10 were school children with good vision and normal eyes.

IV. 9 was the second member of his sibship to lose his sight; at the age of 28 (1904) he complained of difficulty in reading during two months and in seeing at a distance for three weeks; he saw best in a dim light and had a full feeling in his brow; he smoked $2\frac{1}{2}$ ounces of a mixture, half of which was twist, and frequently drank five or six glasses of whisky in an evening; pupils were equal and contracted to light, eye movements were full; R. V. = $\frac{6}{60}$, L. V. = $\frac{4}{60}$; absolute central scotoma for a 10 mm. red square was present in each field; periphery of fields was full; discs were too red all over but especially at the temporal part; above and below each disc in the nerve fibre layer there appeared to be much dilated small blood vessels or minute haemorrhages; edges of discs were blurred; yellow spots normal; grasp was good, knee-jerks present, tremor of tongue but not of fingers; smell was normal; there was no nasal discharge, no tender spots on head or pain on pressure; the patient was an exceptionally strong man. Subsequent examinations are described and vision became worse though tobacco was discontinued; five months later R. V. = L. V. = $\frac{6}{60}$; fields were full with central scotomata, the outer part of each disc was too pale and edges less well defined than is normal; four years later his sister reported that his vision was no worse. IV. 9 was married but had no children.

IV. 15, aged 40 years (1924), was the third member of this sibship to become affected; his vision had gradually failed in both eyes during six months, left eye was first affected and he saw worse on a bright day; he was in good health but had been subject to headaches all his life; he had no giddiness and no sickness; tobacco had been given up for five months on doctor's advice; the patient had been worried and was working hard when the defect was first noticed; he experienced colour sensations when his eyes were closed; pupils were equal and contracted to light; tension was normal; R. V. = $\frac{1}{60}$, L. V. = $\frac{1}{60}$; absolute central scotomata for a red 20 mm. square were present and both fields showed irregular peripheral contractions; the right disc was too pale at the outer part, the left disc had a much better colour though the temporal third was too pale; blood was normal and Wassermann test negative; the sella turcica was 12 mm. in its greatest antero-posterior measurement and 8 mm. deep, its outline was regular and clinoid processes normal; a month later R. V. = L. V. = $\frac{1}{60}$. IV. 15 had two sons.

IV. 12, aged 29 (1908), complained of a floating black spot; she had no pain in her eyes and no headache; her vision was good and eyes were normal except that the left fundus showed pigmentation at the upper-inner and inner parts, most marked near the periphery but extending nearly to the optic disc; the pigment was not very dark and some of it lay in front of the retinal vessels; the vessels were normal, fields of vision full, no scotoma was present and no night-blindness. V. 8, the son of IV. 12, had good vision. IV. 14 died of typhoid, aged 21 years. IV. 17, aged 24 (1908), had good vision and each of her three children saw $\frac{6}{6}$ with each eye and had normal fundi (1926). IV. 19 and her three living children were abroad; the twins, V. 16, 17, died in infancy. IV. 21 and her son, V. 19, had normal vision and fundi. IV. 23, aged 36, and her three children were examined by Dr Ballantyne and reported to have no defect in colour vision and to have normal fundi and vision; they were all said to be thoroughly healthy and to present no anatomical defects. The paternal grandparents to this affected sibship, II. 1 and 2, saw well; they were consanguineous, but in a degree more remote than that of first cousins; I. 1, who died aged 104, could read to the last; information is given of the siblings of III. 9 and of their children, none of whom were affected or showed any visual defect. Five maternal aunts, III. 10, 15, 16, 17 and 18, had good vision but the only one of them to have children had an affected son, and one of them, III. 17, had a defective eye, the left fundus showing choroidal atrophy adjoining the disc and a few circular white spots in the posterior region; she attributed the defect to a blow with a snowball in childhood. A sixth maternal aunt, III. 12, an unmarried intelligent woman, aged 82 years (1927), with retentive memory, lost her vision in the space of a few months at the age of 45 years; she suffered much from headaches at this time; catamenia continued to appear for some years after vision had failed; drooping of the right upper lid occurred at the time of visual failure; she was now a healthy active woman with some ptosis of right upper lid; pupils equal and contract to light; tension normal; R. V. = L. V. = hand movements at three feet; both fields had an absolute central scotoma for a large white object and there appeared to be some contraction of the right field; no colour was recognised in either field but she knew whether a colour was light or dark; colour vision formerly was very good; media were clear; discs were pale but not markedly so; some narrowing of retinal vessels was noted; the edges of the discs were not sharply defined; no lamina cribrosa seen. The only brother of III. 14 died aged 47, married but without issue; at the age of 30 years his sight failed rapidly in both eyes at the same time; he, III. 13, was a big, strong man, a sail-maker, and though he continued to attend to his business he was very helpless to the end of his days. II. 3 drank heavily but had good sight. I. 3 and I. 4 had good sight.

IV. 26, aged 44, married with no children, wrote that his vision began to fail at about the age of 7 years; a certificate given to him by an ophthalmic surgeon in 1918 stated that there was marked atrophy of both discs and slight persistent nystagmus seen only on ophthalmoscopic examination: refraction was hypermetropic, 2 D. in each eye; at the age of 34 peripheral fields, tested with fingers, appeared to be quite full all round; patellar reflexes were normal. The two siblings of IV. 26 and their children saw well; V. 23 was aged 14 years, V. 25 was aged about 12 years and wore glasses.

II. 6, a farmer, died aged 67 years; his vision failed in both eyes at the age of 30 years and he could never read again; his defective vision was attributed to lifting heavy stones; he did not smoke much according to his son's statement; his eyes "quivered"; the defect of vision was said to be similar but more severe than that of III. 24; no direct descendants of II. 6 were affected.

III. 24, aged 65 years (1926), a retired schoolmaster, said that his vision failed rapidly at the age of 30, the left eye was first affected and the right eye failed one or two months later; he had never smoked much but gave it up entirely for a year with no improvement in vision; he was a healthy, intelligent man and said he could see as well as anyone at dusk; he could shoot birds on the wing and moving animals but not stationary objects; R. V. = $\frac{2}{60}$, L. V. = $\frac{3}{60}$; refraction was low hypermetropia in each; fields of vision were not contracted but large absolute central scotomata for red and green and smaller ones for blue were present in each field; media were clear; discs were pale but not markedly so; lamina cribrosa was exposed; retinal vessels of full size; edge of disc was well defined and macula lutea normal; he carried on his work as schoolmaster until the age for retiring; his four children by two wives, also his young grand-children, had good vision. IV. 31 had hair which was formerly very fair, now less so, irides were grey, pupils sometimes red, fundi normal and pale; no nystagmus was present. For further information see the original account of the history. Consanguinity. Bibl. No. 146.

Fig. 738. *Vogt and Schönenberger's Case.* This history was first published by Vogt in 1922; information was brought up to date and many cases examined by Schonenberger at a later date; no further cases of the disease had occurred in the interval of four years. III. 2 and 3 became affected at the age of about 20 years; III. 5 became affected at 22 years and died aged 75. III. 14, aged 67 (1926), had a diminution of vision at the age of 20 and now vision was reduced to finger counting in the right at $\frac{1}{2}$ m., in the left at 2 m.; the three married sisters of III. 5 and 14 had each affected offspring. Thus III. 6 had a daughter, IV. 8, with good vision who was married and had four sons and three daughters all of whom saw well but the eldest of whom was only aged 26 (1926); III. 6 also had a son, IV. 9, aged 37 (1926), who became affected at the age of 22 years. III. 10 had three sons and seven daughters of whom the youngest living was aged 31; only one of this family was affected, he, IV. 33, saw well until the age of 21 and now (1926), aged 37, his vision was finger counting in the right at 2 m., in the left at 4—5 m. III. 13 had five sons, all affected, and one daughter who saw well. IV. 37 became affected at the age of 18 and died aged 41 years.

IV. 38 became affected at the age of 36 and was now (1926) aged 48 years. IV. 39, aged 46 (1926), became affected at the age of 31 years; the discs are now white and sharply outlined, the vessels narrowed; vision is reduced to finger counting in the right at $\frac{1}{2}$ m., in the left at 1 m. IV. 40, aged 45 (1926), became suddenly blinded at the age of 40 and vision was now reduced to finger counting at 2—3 m.; the discs were greenish white, the vessels slightly narrowed and the peripheral fields of vision were intact; IV. 40 was married and had had two young daughters of whom one was living. IV. 42, aged 43 (1926), became affected at the age of 37 years; he now had greenish white discs and narrowed vessels; R. V. = finger counting at $\frac{1}{2}$ m., L. V. = finger counting at 1 m.; his two young daughters saw well. No member of generations V and VI was yet of an age at which he can be said to be free from the defect, excepting V. 32 and 34 who do not belong to the affected stock. Consanguinity. Bibl. Nos. 123, 138.

Fig. 739. *Leitner's Case.* (Taken from Nettleship.) Five cases of hereditary optic atrophy in males. I. 1 and 2 were normal; they had twelve unaffected children of whom nine were females and all were married; three of the daughters had affected sons. III. 1 became affected at 18, III. 2 at the age of 24, III. 3 at the age of 20. III. 5, affected at 18, was aged 24 at the time of publication. III. 15 became affected after the age of 32. The eldest child of II. 20 was aged 21; the eldest child of II. 22 was aged 24. III. 28 was aged 9 years. Thus other members of this generation were still of an age at which they were liable to show the disease. No consanguinity recorded. Bibl. Nos. 57 and 85, p. clxxvii.

Fig. 740. *Leitner's Case.* (Taken from Nettleship.) Hereditary optic atrophy in one female and four males of two generations. I. 1 and 2 were normal; they had six children of whom II. 7, the only son, became affected at the age of 25; II. 2, a daughter, became affected at the age of 39; she was married and had five children of whom three sons and a daughter were not yet affected but we do not know whether they had yet reached the age at which liability to the disease most commonly occurs; one son, III. 5, became affected at the age of 13. Two normal daughters of I. 1 and 2 were married and each had an affected son; thus II. 3 had a son who became affected at the age of 22 and a not yet affected daughter; II. 5 had three sons and three daughters of whom one son, III. 13, became affected at the age of 20. No consanguinity recorded. Bibl. Nos. 53 and 85, p. clxxvi.

PLATE LIV. Fig. 741. *Mooren's Case.* Hereditary optic atrophy in six males and one female. IV. 3 and 4 became affected at about the same time, the elder brother in his 22nd, the younger in his 18th year; two years later a sister, aged 28, also became affected. The eldest sister and both parents had good vision, but the father's brother, seen at the age of 60, had suffered from the same disease as his nephews since his 17th year. The diminution of vision in all cases appeared to remain stationary after its onset but the eyes of the younger generation when seen showed only slight atrophy of the nerve whilst in the uncle the condition was more advanced. A year after seeing these cases the recorder saw three brothers all of whom had lost their central vision at the age of 20; one sister of this sibship was not affected; these brothers were found to have the same great-grandmother as the first described sibship. Consanguinity. Bibl. No. 17, pp. 249—50.

Fig. 742. *Leber's Case I.* Optic atrophy in three brothers, in their two step-brothers by a different father and in two of their maternal uncles; the mother, II. 2, and both her husbands had good eyes; the grandparents, I. 1 and 2, were not known to have suffered from any eye disease but the two brothers of the mother, II. 3 and 4, suffered from a severe diminution of vision. The disease in III. 1, 2, 4, 6 and 7 developed at the ages of 20, 13, 28, 13 and 21 years respectively; in each case the affection quickly reached a maximum at which it remained stationary; all the brothers were now (1871) able to go about in the streets alone but could not see to read.

Leber reports that III. 8, the only daughter of II. 2, saw well, but Schilling (Bibl. No. 13) writing four years later states that she also had become affected but had not yet any demonstrable ophthalmoscopic changes.

III. 2, aged 33, was of a robust build but was of an excitable and nervous temperament; he suffered at times from giddiness; at the age of 13 years he developed, in four weeks, so serious a degree of amblyopia that he had to leave school; twenty years later he was seen to have bilateral central scotomata, on the left side small and defined, on the right side reaching as far as the periphery on the nasal side of the field; pupils were dilated and scarcely reacted to light; both papillae were white, arteries narrow, veins slightly dilated; the patient had two children under four years of age who saw well. III. 4, aged 32, suffered at times from slight fainting attacks; at the age of 18 he had suffered from palpitations; at 28 years he had a rapid diminution of vision which increased for about two weeks and then became more stationary, three or four weeks from the onset R. V. = finger counting at 6', L. V. = finger counting at 16'. Three years later the vision of the left had further diminished and was now the same as the right; severe colour-blindness over the whole of the visual fields was noted; he had a little daughter who saw well. III. 7, aged 21 (1871), had in childhood had some inflammation of his eyes following measles; a year ago he had Egyptian inflammation of the eyes; earlier he had complained of palpitations and giddiness; his present eye trouble appeared first in his right eye and eight days later in his left; three weeks after the onset the condition was progressing less rapidly; R. V. = finger counting at 2', L. V. = finger counting at 14'; a small scotoma was present in the right only; a severe degree of colour-blindness was present in the right eye, colour vision in the left eye was normal; signs of atrophy were present in the right disc and of neuritis in the left. Four months later both papillae were white; arteries narrowed; small scotomata were present in both eyes with no peripheral contraction of fields. No consanguinity recorded. Bibl. No. 8.

Fig. 743. *Raymond and Koenig's Case.* Optic atrophy in four males of three generations. I. 1 and 2 were first cousins; they had two children; a son, II. 3, who became affected suddenly with partial blindness at the age of 20, and a daughter, II. 2, who saw well. II. 3 had two sons who saw well but one of them died of phthisis at the age of 30. II. 2 had five children of whom two sons saw well, one son, III. 5, became partially blind at the age of 20; two daughters had each a son who similarly became partially blind at the same period of life; one of the daughters, III. 2, had two hysterical daughters. Consanguinity. Bibl. No. 86.

Fig. 744. *Bach's Case.* Optic atrophy in a boy aged 15, in his three maternal uncles and in his maternal grandmother. IV. 1, aged 15, the only child of his parents, had been affected for three months; a few weeks after the onset his vision was reduced to finger counting at about 3 m.; central scotomata were present, the peripheral fields had normal boundaries. The mother of IV. 1 was unaffected but her three brothers had all been examined by the recorder and suffered from the same disease with advanced atrophy of the nerve. The grandmother, II. 4, was believed to have had the same disease; her husband, II. 5, her father, I. 1, her sister, II. 2, and the three children of II. 2 were all reported to have healthy eyes. No consanguinity recorded. Bibl. No. 81.

Fig. 745. *Nettleship's Case.* Leber's disease in four males and one female of two generations. I. 1 and 2 had good eyes; of their children, II. 2, Mr H. of Birmingham, had a son, III. 1, who became affected at about the age of 40; II. 6, Mrs J., had a son, III. 4, who became affected so early that he never learned to read; II. 8, Mrs D., had fourteen children of whom III. 6 became affected at the age of 30. III. 7 married at the age of 22 and became affected at 33; she was seen soon after the onset of the disease. III. 9 and 10 were normal daughters of II. 8; III. 11 represents ten of her children who died quite young. II. 4, sister to II. 8, had a normal daughter, III. 3, whose only son, IV. 1, became affected early in life. III. 6 had five children of whom two died young. III. 7 had four children of whom two died young. Thus four children of I. 1 and 2 transmitted the defect though they were themselves believed to be normal. Nettleship was unable to discover whether there were other members of this sibship. No consanguinity recorded. Bibl. No. 85, p. clxxiii.

Fig. 746. *Nettleship's Case.* (Habershon's Case III.) Four cases of Leber's disease in a sibship of eleven. I. 1 died of cancer; his wife, I. 2, was weakly. Little was known of II. 1 but no cases of the disease were known to have occurred in her family. II. 2 died aged 55; he was one of a very large sibship of whom three males lived to adult life. II. 1 and 2 had eleven children of whom the eldest, a son aged 44, reported that he had had good sight until the age of 16 when within six weeks it failed and reached the present state; he described the defect as a cloud at the centre of the field of vision and said that he could see well round this; his perception of colours was defective, especially for red; discs showed white atrophy; this patient was a smoker but discontinued the habit one year after the onset. III. 2 died, aged 22, of phthisis; she saw well. III. 3 died, aged 20, of lung trouble; he was a smoker and saw well up to the time of his death. III. 4, aged 39, a non-smoker, became affected at the age of 15. III. 6 died, aged 24, of spinal disease; he saw well and never smoked. III. 7, aged 34, saw well. III. 8, aged 32, became affected at the age of 17 when he was not a smoker; he now smoked a good deal. III. 10, aged 30, was not affected; he smoked in moderation. III. 11, an affected male, aged 27, was a non-smoker at the time of the onset of the disease when he was aged 12 but smoked later. III. 12 died, aged 17, of phthisis; he never smoked. III. 13, aged 24, saw well. No consanguinity. Bibl. Nos. 29 and 85, p. clxv.

Fig. 747. *Buisson's Case.* Optic atrophy in two brothers. II. 2, aged 60, saw well; he was twice married, by his first wife he had one normal daughter who had five children; by his second wife he had three daughters with good vision and two affected sons, III. 3 and 9. III. 3, aged 31, became affected one year ago, now his vision is reduced to $\frac{1}{30}$ in right, $\frac{1}{10}$ in left; he has no pain; he was married at 20 and had five children of whom two died at 3 and 4 months respectively, three others are in good health, aged 9 years, 3 years and 7 weeks. III. 5, aged 26, had two healthy children; III. 7, aged 24, had two healthy children and one, born at the seventh month, had paraplegia of the lower limbs. III. 9, aged 19, reported the onset of amblyopia in the right eye three months ago, the left becoming affected a fortnight later; he was in good health and neither he nor his affected brother had ever been seriously ill or had syphilis; on Sept. 30, 1898, R. V. = $\frac{1}{30}$, L. V. = $\frac{1}{20}$; on Nov. 20, R. V. = $\frac{1}{30}$, L. V. = $\frac{1}{30}$; the condition progressed until when seen in June, 1899, R. V. = L. V. = $\frac{1}{120}$; central scotomata were present, discs were pale on temporal side, arteries a little narrowed, veins normal; red and green not recognised. The mother, II. 3, saw well up to her death, at the age of 45, from an abdominal tumour; her father, aged 86, saw well. III. 10, aged 17, saw well. No consanguinity recorded. Bibl. No. 59.

Fig. 748. *Posey's Case.* Hereditary optic atrophy in a male, in one of his maternal uncles and in one of his maternal great-uncles. I. 1 and 2 died at the ages of 60 and 75 respectively, both had good sight; of their thirteen children three sons, II. 2, 4 and 6, were normal and had normal children; three sons died young; four normal daughters had no offspring; one daughter, II. 11, had glaucoma, she had no children;

Plate LIV.   DESCRIPTIONS OF PEDIGREE PLATES   381

one son, II. 12, had hereditary optic atrophy and one daughter, II. 8, was normal herself but had a son and a grandson with hereditary optic atrophy. II. 12, aged 61, reported that his sight began to fail at the age of 30; the progress of the disease was rapid and he was soon unable to read; he denied syphilis; he began to smoke at the age of 15, for ten years had two cigars daily and after that five pipes daily; at the time of investigation R. V. $= \frac{3}{30}$, L. V. $= \frac{2}{10}$; discs were atrophied; vessels reduced in size; absolute central scotomata were present; pupils reacted sluggishly. .

II. 8 had three normal daughters and two sons of whom one was normal, the other, III. 12, aged 41, reported that his vision began to fail at the age of 24; the right eye was first affected and the left eye six weeks later; no history of syphilis; he was dyspeptic but otherwise had good health; at the age of 16 this patient smoked three cigars daily and up to the present time chews about two 'plugs' of tobacco weekly; now R. V. $=$ L. V. $= \frac{3}{10}$; discs show a greyish white atrophy; retina is hazy; vessels reduced in size; pupils react to light and accommodation; absolute central scotomata are present; blue is the only colour recognised in a 20 mm. square object. IV. 2, son of the only married daughter of II. 8, aged 25, complained that his sight had been failing in the right eye for three weeks; he noticed a mist before the eye and had slight pain; he had always been of a nervous temperament and dyspeptic, also there was a history of gonorrhoea eight years ago; for five years the patient had smoked five to eight cigars daily and chewed tobacco occasionally, he also took an occasional glass of beer or whisky; R. V. $= \frac{6}{30}$, L. V. $= \frac{5}{5}$; the right disc was hyperaemic with blurred edge; retinal vessels tortuous and full; the left disc showed an earlier stage of the same condition; three months after the onset R. V. $= \frac{1}{60}$, L. V. $= \frac{5}{40}$; central scotomata were present. Members of this family were nervous, easily excited and depressed, and most of them were dyspeptic. No consanguinity recorded. Bibl. No. 58.

Fig. 749. *Taylor's Case.* Optic atrophy in four brothers and in their maternal grandmother. I. 1 became nearly blind at the age of 40, eyes looking natural; she had three daughters of whom II. 2 and 4 had ten and five normal children respectively, II. 5 had eleven children and one miscarriage. II. 6, husband of II. 5, was a shoemaker, he saw well at the age of 47 but his eyes were weak and inflamed at times; he was subject to asthma and at one time had fits (? epilepsy); he was a great smoker and was inclined to drink too much. Of the children of II. 5 and 6, III. 3, Edmund S., born before the marriage of his parents, was seen aged 27 when he complained of "pins and needles" and numbness in his feet and hands and of cramp; no history of syphilis; his right eye became affected about 9 months previously and later the left also; he had occasional pain in the right frontal and temporal regions; vision was limited to hand movements only in the right, the left was a little better; visual fields were contracted and central scotomata were present; pupils reacted to light but not to accommodation; he was colour-blind to red and green; the discs were pale with a clear defined outline; the patient smoked $\frac{1}{4}$ oz. of shag daily and drank stout but no spirits. III. 3 died of inflammation of the lungs at the age of 37; he left one son, a soldier with good sight (1909), and five daughters.· III. 5, William S., was discharged from the army at the age of about 21 on account of his vision, he was then said to have optic neuritis; he began to smoke at the age of 16, as a soldier he had smoked about $\frac{1}{2}$ oz. shag and drank about four glasses of beer daily; at the age of about 21 he had a sudden pain in his forehead which caused him to close his left eye, then he noticed that he could not see with his right eye, three weeks later the vision of the left eye began to fail also; at the age of 25 pupils reacted to light, discs were pale, especially the outer halves, with slightly blurred margins, he could not recognise red or green anywhere in the field; there was some contraction of the visual fields, also central colour scotomata; he was married in 1909 and had five normal children; at a later date he complained of frequent cramp, his pupils reacted only slightly to light, discs showed a whitish yellow pallor and retinal vessels were of slightly less than normal calibre. III. 7, 9 and 12, three sisters, aged 23, 22 and 18 respectively (1892), were married and had children who were normal in 1909. III. 11, John S., aged 19 (1892), had his left eye only affected at the age of 6; he began to smoke at 15 and in 1892 was smoking two ozs. of shag per week and drinking half a pint of beer daily; the right fields were quite normal and R. V. $= \frac{5}{6}$, L. V. $= \frac{5}{6}$; he had no difficulty in matching colours; slight but distinct neuritis was noted in the right eye at this date, the left disc was pale; the left field had normal boundaries with a small central scotoma; in 1909 the right vision was still good but at a later date his brothers reported that he had had to give up his work as a shoemaker and that he was certain his right eye was then affected; he died of some acute lung disease. III. 14 and 16, aged 15 and 11 respectively (1892), were normal, they had good sight when last heard of, possibly about 1915. III. 15, George S., aged 13 (1893), had both eyes affected at the age of 6 when he was almost blind for about a year but improved after an operation for mastoid disease following middle ear suppuration; R. V. $= \frac{5}{6}$, L. V. $= \frac{5}{6}$; no peripheral contraction of fields, central scotoma present in right only; the discs were pale particularly the right, edges were clearly defined and vessels normal; (?) partial obliteration of the choroid over the area surrounding each disc. At a later date (?1915) III. 15 complained of cramp on rising in the morning; R. V. $= \frac{5}{6}$, L. V. $= \frac{5}{36} - \frac{5}{24}$; right pupil slightly wider than the left. III. 17 and 18, aged 9 and 7 years respectively, saw well. No consanguinity. Bibl. Nos. 38 and 85, p. clxvii, with some additional information sent by the recorder.

Fig. 750. *Norris's Case.* Leber's disease affecting males and females in five generations. V. 2, aged 49, a vigorous man who had been in the habit of taking neither alcohol nor tobacco, complained that he had been losing his sight for about a year; he had become so blind that he had some difficulty in getting about and had had to give up his work; pupils were normal but central vision was almost completely absent in both eyes; the right optic disc was greenish grey in colour and a trifle prominent; the retinal vessels had about their normal calibre; the patient was given strychnine and about a month later his peripheral vision showed a marked improvement. One of the brothers of V. 2 became affected at the age of 43; five of his eight siblings died in infancy. V. 11, aged 50, first cousin to V. 2, complained of a central clouding of his vision; irregular central scotomata, varying from 15° to 20° round the point of fixation, were demonstrated; the discs showed a greenish atrophic discolouration; there was little change in the calibre of the central vessels; this patient also showed marked improvement in his peripheral vision under treatment with strychnine.

IV. 2 after a period of blindness improved so markedly as to be able to resume his work. No consanguinity. Bibl. No. 23.

Fig. 751. *Kuhk's Case.* Hereditary optic atrophy in three brothers and their only sister, also in the sister's only son. III. 2, H. H. A., had had no serious illness up to the age of 22; he had in his youth frequent attacks of inflammation in his eyes but his vision remained good in both eyes. At the age of 22 years, after he had been standing in water for a long time washing sheep, he reports the sudden onset and rapid advance of a diminution in his visual acuity so that within fourteen days from the onset he was unable to read. On examination some infection of the conjunctiva was found; in both eyes the pupils were dilated and reacted feebly; the papillae were slightly blurred and the margins were indistinct; the blurring extended into the surrounding retina; the arteries were narrowed, the veins dilated and tortuous; the patient was treated with strychnine injections and discharged a month later with no change in his vision or in the appearance of the fundus. Twenty-two years later (1908) III. 2 was again examined; R. V. = finger counting at ½ m., L. V. = finger counting at 1½ m.; colour perception for red and green was absent and it was reduced for other colours; in the right field there was complete deficiency of the nasal half; in the left field peripheral margins were normal; the right pupil was larger than the left and bilateral complete atrophy of the optic nerve was present. In 1913 with the left eye large blue and yellow objects were distinguished but red and green were not recognised; with the right eye no colours were known; bilateral large central absolute scotomata were demonstrated. III. 2 was mentally fresh and alert and carried on with his work on the land; he was married and had a healthy daughter aged 18 years. III. 3, brother of III. 2, was born in 1871; as a child he was always healthy and had good sight in both eyes, but he suffered repeatedly from severe headaches; at the age of 20 years he had a severe wound at the back of his head due to a fall from a ladder but there was no loss of consciousness or fracture; at the age of 21, suddenly and for no apparent reason his vision became weak, the condition rapidly progressed and eight days later he was unable to see to read; he was examined and it was found that R. V. = finger counting at 40 cm., L. V. = finger counting at 20 cm.; fixation was excentric; bilateral large absolute central scotomata were present; atrophy of the optic nerve was present showing the typical appearance of the fundus; he was treated with salt and mustard baths and strychnine injections, with slight temporary improvement. Fifteen years later his vision was reduced to hand movements at 1 m. in both eyes; he could recognise blue and yellow but not red or green. Five years later again he could perceive only large blue objects with the left eye and no colours with the right.

III. 4, a factory worker, was born 1876; he had stammered since his earliest youth and had repeated convulsions during his first years, later he was always healthy. At the age of seven years he noticed at school that his visual acuity was rapidly diminishing, without any apparent cause, so that after a short time he was unable to recognise a clothes brush at a distance of ½ m. When seen in 1884 his pupils reacted well to light and convergence; in the upper and outer quadrant of the pupil a posterior synechia was present, also traces of a persistent pupillary membrane were noticed; vision was reduced to finger counting at 2 m. for the R. eye and at 3 m. for the L.; fields of vision were free and colour sense normal; papillae were pale, vessels narrowed and the retina round the entrance of the nerve was blurred and of a grey colour; the veins were not tortuous. The patient's condition at subsequent examinations is described; he was treated with potassium iodide and with strychnine; when last examined in 1908, L. V. = $\frac{6}{8}$, R. V. = $\frac{6}{18}$–$\frac{6}{12}$; colour discrimination was lowered; no central scotomata were present but there was slight peripheral contraction of the fields; some greenish grey atrophy of the optic nerve was present and the retinal vessels were narrower than normal. At a later date it was reported that his visual acuity remained good and that he was able to carry on his work.

III. 5, Charlotte W., sister to III. 2—4, had always been healthy and saw well until the age of 36 years when she had trachoma and was for a long time under treatment by different surgeons; soon after this she noticed a rapid diminution in her vision which in a short time reached a grade at which it remained stationary; when she was examined pupils were round, of normal size and reacted promptly; the papillae were white with sharply defined margins; R. V. = finger counting at 3 m., L. V. = finger counting at 1 m.; peripheral fields of vision were normal; in the R. a relative and in the L. an absolute scotoma for white and colours were demonstrated; in R. over the whole field only blue and yellow 20 mm. objects were recognised, in the L. only blue was distinguished. III. 5 married a healthy man, III. 6, and had one child, a son, IV. 2, who at the age of 15 years became affected with the same eye disease as his mother and her brothers. IV. 2

was born in 1893, he was a healthy boy but had inflammation of the lungs when he was quite small. At the age of 15 it was noticed that he frequently passed over words when he was reading and that blanks appeared in the lines; he had no headaches but eight days before the onset of the disease he had a severe nasal catarrh. On examination it was found that the left pupil was larger than the right; the papillae were slightly red with blurred margins; the veins were slightly hyperaemic, the arteries narrowed; myopia of 1·5 D was noted; vision was reduced to finger counting at 3 m. for the R. and at 1 m. for the L.; there was some contraction of the peripheral fields; perception of colours central and peripheral was absent except for blue. An account is given of the examination of the central nervous system; also repeated examinations of the eyes are described; the patient was treated with salicylates and mercury ointment and also with strychnine and electricity; considerable improvement was noted in 1913 when R. V. = L . V. = $\frac{6}{8}$ and a good colour discrimination was demonstrated.

III. 6 by his first wife had four daughters and three grandchildren with normal vision. The paternal grandparents of the four affected siblings, I. 1 and 2, were healthy and came of healthy stocks free from eye disease; their three children were healthy and no eye disease occurred in the children and grandchildren of their married daughter II. 2. The mother of the affected siblings, II. 5, suffered from night-blindness which appears to have been of the congenital stationary type for in good daylight her eyesight was good up to old age and ophthalmoscopic examination could detect nothing abnormal; her parents, I. 3 and 4, also her three siblings and the children and grandchildren of her only married sister, were normal. No consanguinity recorded. Bibl. Nos. 49, 104.

PLATE LV. Fig. 752. *Snell's Case.* Optic atrophy in two brothers and in one of their first cousins; parents and grandparents, aunts and uncles saw well except II. 5, the mother's brother, who had some trouble with his eyes after smallpox. III. 1, aged 36, reported that his sight began to fail at about the age of 24; he was examined then; now the discs were white, vision was reduced to finger counting at one foot; fields of vision were very limited and colour vision was defective; the condition had been stationary for about ten years. III. 6, aged 31, had noticed his sight failing for two or three months, up to this time he had seen well; now his discs were white and arteries narrowed; R. V. = finger counting, L. V. = $\frac{2}{200}$; visual fields were contracted. The patient's two brothers, III. 8, died aged 2 and 3 years respectively of croup; their five sisters aged 34, 32, 29, 25 and 18 respectively had good sight. The mother's sister, II. 6, had three sons aged 27, 23 and 16 and a daughter aged 12 who all had good sight; she had also one son aged 25 whose sight had been failing for a few weeks and now R. V. = $\frac{6}{12}$, L. V. = finger counting at one foot; large bilateral central scotomata were present with some contraction of peripheral fields. No consanguinity recorded. Bibl. No. 55.

Fig. 753. *Zentmayer's Case.* Optic atrophy in two brothers; they had another brother who died of typhoid fever and an unaffected sister. II. 1, J. C., became affected at the age of 30, he smoked moderately and took little alcohol; in February 1912 he accidentally discovered that the vision of his left eye was very poor, in August of the same year he had to give up his work; five years later R. V. = $\frac{1}{180}$, L. V. = $\frac{1}{240}$; excentric vision; visual reflexes were sluggish; absolute central scotomata were present; discs were a greenish grey colour, vessels contracted; X-ray showed a pituitary fossa enlarged both by deepening and in the antero-posterior direction. II. 3, aged 29, reported that his vision was failing; by the following week he could not see to read ordinary print; he had had congestion of the lungs in the spring of this year; he had smoked about 1 oz. of tobacco daily for several years and took no alcohol; he had one child living and well; R. V. = $\frac{20}{100}$, L. V. = $\frac{15}{100}$; scotomata were present, also slight contraction of the fields; X-ray showed possibly a slight deepening of the pituitary fossa. No consanguinity recorded. Bibl. No. 114.

Fig. 754. *Zentmayer's Case.* Optic atrophy in two brothers, and a sister presents symptoms suggestive of incipient pituitary disease; both parents were aged 53 and normal. II. 6, F. S., aged 26, fifth born in a sibship of nine, reported that his sight began to fail at the age of 12 and that six months later he was unable to read; optic atrophy was diagnosed at this time and his vision has remained stationary since; vision is excentric and for R. and L. = $\frac{1}{120}$; pupils were normal; his face was asymmetrical, the right side receding; his skull was high and narrow; both fields were contracted to some extent and central absolute scotomata were present; the patient had no colour perception; both discs were atrophic; vessels were normal in the right, slightly narrowed in the left; X-ray showed a large pituitary fossa on the border line of normality. II. 8, E. S., aged 22, seventh born in the sibship, reported that he had noticed two years ago that colours did not appear normal to him, at this time inflammation of the optic nerve had been diagnosed; now R. V. = $\frac{1}{60}$, L. V. = $\frac{2·5}{60}$; the X-ray shows a large pituitary fossa.

X-ray plates were taken of one normal male of this family and of one female, II. 4; the normal male had a much smaller fossa than his affected brothers; the female, aged 30, had a pituitary fossa which was on the border line of the abnormally large; she complained of headaches and sweating of the left side of her head, her vision was normal and right disc normal, the left disc was blurred and slightly prominent; she had small scotomata in both fields which also showed a decided concentric contraction for form and colour; II. 4 had had four children, two daughters were aged 8 and 9 respectively, one son was stillborn and one son died aged 8 hours. No consanguinity. Bibl. No. 114.

Fig. 755. *Batten's Case.* Hereditary optic atrophy in a mother and her three children, also in her brother and sister. I. 1 and 2 had good sight. II. 1, aged 51, remembered a rapid onset of defective vision at the age of 11; now R. V. $=\frac{6}{60}$, L. V. $=\frac{6}{36}$; the discs were pale and slightly atrophic but no gross changes were present; visual fields were practically normal with no scotomata. II. 2 died aged 33, she had been similarly affected and the disease in her case developed in the same rapid way in late childhood II. 4, Mrs Sarah P., began to lose her sight at the age of 12, the defect rapidly increased and then remained stationary; at the age of 48, R. V. $=\frac{1}{60}$, L. V. $=\frac{2}{60}$; discs were pale and somewhat atrophic, margins hazy, some cupping; there was slight contraction of the visual fields, no scotomata were demonstrated. There is no information of other members of this sibship. II. 4 had four children of whom III. 1 died aged 3; III. 2, Arthur P., aged 11, had, under atropine with correction of + 4·5 D., R. V. = L. V. $=\frac{6}{12}$; there was a concentric contraction of the fields and a paracentral scotoma in the left only; margins of disc were blurred and vessels were tortuous; at a later date vision was greatly improved but the condition of the discs remained unchanged. III. 3, Sarah Annie P., aged 9, had R. V. = L. V. $=\frac{2}{60}$; her discs were pale and atrophic; she did not recognise blue, red or green, yellow she called red; she had small scotomata and some contraction of fields. III. 4, Emily P., aged 8, had discs congested but no marked change except extreme redness and some enlargement of veins; under atropine and with correction R. V. = L. V. $=\frac{6}{9}-\frac{6}{6}$; colour vision appeared to be normal; two years later vision was reduced to $\frac{6}{12}$. No defect of vision was known to have occurred in any collateral branches of the family. An attempt to get in touch with the family again in 1923 was unsuccessful. No consanguinity. Bibl. No. 47.

Fig. 756. *Bruner's Case.* Optic atrophy in five males and one female of three generations. I. 2, aged 81, and her husband, I. 1, had normal vision; I. 3, aged 76, had been blind for years; he was told that the trouble was with the optic nerves and that treatment would not help him; he drank considerably; I. 4 went blind one night and committed suicide. I. 2 had two sons and six daughters of whom II. 1, aged 36 (1911), reported that he had worn glasses for nine years but had no difficulty until about four months ago when he noticed that his vision was blurred and he could only see part of an object; he had at this time some frontal and occipital headache but no vomiting or giddiness; two weeks ago he had severe headache for three days and his vision had been worse since; his general health was excellent but he had a history of gonorrhoea as a young man, no syphilis; he smoked and drank with moderation; he had been married for nine years, his wife had had two miscarriages and no living children; pupils were equal and reacted normally, discs were slightly oedematous on nasal side with hazy margin, pale on temporal side; veins were rather full; the patient failed to recognise red and green; central absolute scotomata were present. Lumbar puncture was made but the fluid was normal; X-ray showed nothing abnormal antero-posteriorly, but the lateral view showed much enlargement of the sphenoidal cells; De Schweinitz reported that a stereoscopic X-ray plate showed marked thickening either in the sphenoid region or in the neighbourhood of the sella turcica and suggests a family abnormality of skull interfering with the functioning of the pituitary gland as a possible source of the visual trouble; Dr Spiller considered that the plate showed a projection upwards of the floor of the sella turcica. An X-ray plate taken two months later showed no change. The patient became much worse and when he was almost completely blind a decompression was performed by Harvey Cushing, who found that he had an exceedingly oedematous brain, with great excess in the amount of fluid in the sub-dural space, under considerable tension; four weeks after the operation vision was limited to hand movements on the temporal side only for the R. and finger counting for the L.

II. 3 wrote that his vision failed at the age of 29, that within a few days everything looked hazy but "he could see an object from the outer circle of the eye"; his trouble was diagnosed as optic neuritis; he was a drinker; some improvement followed treatment with mercury, potassium iodide and strychnine.

II. 4, Mrs T. of Toledo, aged 41, had good eyes until the age of 34 when her sight gradually failed; the condition appeared to be stationary for three or four years since when she had noticed some improvement; she had been addicted to morphine at one time and after this to alcohol; R. V. $=\frac{1}{60}$, L. V. $=\frac{2}{60}$; discs were pale, especially the temporal halves, and arteries narrow; small central absolute scotomata were noted in each field with practically normal peripheral limits; X-ray plate showed much enlarged sphenoidal cells; she had been married twenty years and had a son, aged 18, and a daughter, aged 15, who both saw well.

III. 4, son of a normal sister of the affected siblings, was a doctor in Chicago, his vision became dim shortly after his marriage at the age of 22 and a few months later he became "entirely blind"; there was no history of syphilis; central scotomata were present; he was treated with mercury, potassium iodide, thyroid extract, pituitrin, strychnine, etc.; after a year he tried homoeopathic treatment and began to improve, now he has had $\frac{1}{4}$ normal vision for some years; X-ray plate showed much enlarged sphenoidal cells.

X-ray plates were taken, for comparative purposes, of the mother, I. 2, and one of her five normal daughters; they showed much smaller sphenoidal cells than those of the affected members. No consanguinity. Bibl. No. 95.

Fig. 757. *Snell's Case.* Optic atrophy in three brothers and in their maternal uncle. II. 2, John B., aged 62, had found his sight failing about ten years ago; the onset of the disease was gradual, the left eye first becoming affected and the right eye failing 8 months later, he thinks he sees more now than then; both discs are now white and arteries narrow; V. $=\frac{5}{60}$ in each eye; he had three sons who were still normal at

Plate LV.　　DESCRIPTIONS OF PEDIGREE PLATES　　385

the time of investigation. II. 4, William B., aged 57, said that his sight became impaired about ten years ago; now both discs were white, arteries a little narrow, V. about $\frac{4}{200}$ in each eye; he had been subject to fits, which occurred every four or five weeks, between the ages of 24 and 40; his son and five daughters were believed to be normal. II. 6, James B., aged 44, reported that his sight in both eyes had been affected for about 8 years; now both discs were white, arteries diminished and V. $= \frac{4}{200}$ in each eye. All the affected brothers had central scotomata in each and also peripheral contraction of fields; all were moderate smokers. The mother, I. 3, died aged 85, and the father died aged 67, both had good sight; one son, aged 43, and a daughter, aged 53, were unaffected; two daughters died in infancy; the mother's brother, a railway guard, became blind in middle age and never recovered his sight; the father's father lived to old age with good sight. No consanguinity. Bibl. No. 55.

Fig. 758. *Somya's Case.* Optic atrophy in five males and one female in three sibships of two generations. II. 1 was reported to have been blind and his brother, II. 2, to have been severely amblyopic; their mother's sister had four children of whom II. 4 became blind at the age of 28; II. 5 saw well; II. 7 became blind at the age of 34. II. 6 became amblyopic rather suddenly at the age of 18; his vision was reduced to finger counting in the R. at 5′, in the L. at 10′; he had central absolute scotomata and slight concentric contraction of the visual fields; many years after the onset he appeared to have post-neuritic optic atrophy, the papillae were pale, the vessels normal. II. 7 had a son Rudolf R., III. 1, who at the age of 19 noticed a gradual diminution of vision; he had always been healthy and no nervous or mental affections were known to have occurred in the family; his father's parents and siblings saw well; six months after the onset of the disease his vision was reduced to finger counting in the R. at 1·5 m., in the L. at 14″*; he had slight myopia; the papillae were pale especially in the temporal half; the vessels were markedly narrowed; bilateral large central and paracentral absolute scotomata were present but there was no contraction of the peripheral limits of fields; no improvement followed treatment by inunction and potassium iodide. No consanguinity recorded. Bibl. No. 37.

Fig. 759. *Lucas's Case.* Probably hereditary optic atrophy in five females of three generations. I. 1 had good sight. I. 2 became amaurotic at the age of 35. II. 2 lost her sight at the age of 19 but had some perception of light; she had seven children of whom III. 1 became amaurotic at the age of 13 and died two years later completely blind. III. 2 became blind at the age of 11. III. 3 also became affected at the age of 11; she was at one time unable to see to go about alone but the condition improved under treatment. The onset of the disease in all cases was characterised by headache, some strabismus, and a gradual diminution of vision until blindness became complete. III. 4 died aged 2 years when her vision appeared to be normal. III. 5, aged 13, had not yet shown signs of the disease. III. 6 and 7, two boys aged 3 years and 1 year respectively, could still see well. No consanguinity recorded. Bibl. No. 2.

Fig. 760. *Daguenet, Galezowski and Prouff's Case.* Hereditary optic atrophy in six males and probably one female of two generations. I. 1 and 2 had always seen well; they had three daughters and one son of whom II. 2, a daughter, died aged 52 having had six children, III. 1—6. II. 2 always saw well; her brother II. 3, aged 47, noticed at the age of 21 that his visual acuity was lowered, six months later he was unable to see to read; the defect is said to have reached a maximum two months after the onset and had since remained stationary; he had no headaches or nervous symptoms; he saw better in a dim light; at the age of 47 the papillae were pale with clearly defined margins, vessels were narrowed; vision was reduced to finger counting; fields were contracted and severe defects in colour vision were demonstrated, red, orange and green all appeared grey. II. 3 had one child who died aged 10. II. 5 saw well, she died aged 40, leaving two children, III. 8 and 9. II. 7 died aged 45, having for the last five years been able to see enough to enable her to go about alone; no further details are given of her defect; she had three children, III. 10—12.

III. 1 noticed a rapid diminution of vision at the age of 26, the condition progressed for two months and then became stationary; atrophy of the optic nerve following neuritis was noted five months after the onset; the papillary margins were still blurred, vessels were normal; only blue and yellow colours were recognised. III. 2, brother to III. 1, was healthy and saw well up to the age of 24 when amblyopia developed and the history given was precisely similar to that of III. 1, except that his colour vision was less markedly affected and he was able to distinguish all colours except green. III. 3 was similarly affected; he had headaches at the time of onset; colour vision was very defective. Of the other members of this sibship III. 4 died young; III. 5 and 6 were aged 19 and 15 respectively at the time of observation; the sex of these siblings is not given.

III. 8 had always been healthy up to two or three years before the onset of his defect at the age of 21 during which time he suffered from frequent headaches; the onset was rapid, progressed for about $2\frac{1}{2}$ months and then became stationary; about 16 months after the onset he had small central scotomata, all colours were recognised except green, optic atrophy was noted; the temporal halves of the papillae were rather pale, outlines clear; arteries were narrowed, veins were normal; vision was better in a dim light. III. 8 had one sibling about whom no information is given. III. 10, cousin to III. 8, became affected at

---

* [Measurements given in this way, partly in metres, partly in local inches (?), seem lacking in all scientific value. Cf. even Leber in the account of Fig. 742. Ed.]

the age of 27; the onset was rapid and the condition progressed for 6—8 weeks and then became stationary; he had no history of headaches but had nervous attacks with convulsions and colic, without loss of consciousness; no excess in use of alcohol or tobacco; he had concentric contraction of fields and severe defects of colour vision, he could only recognise blue; vision was better in the evening; six months after the onset optic atrophy was noted, the papillae were white, the veins were dilated and the arteries narrowed. The two siblings of III. 20 saw well. No consanguinity recorded. Bibl. Nos. 9, 10.

Fig. 761. *Fuchs's Case.* Optic atrophy in five brothers and in their two maternal uncles. I. 1 became affected at the age of 21, thirty years later his vision was so defective that he was scarcely able to go about alone; he was unmarried. I. 2, aged 49, also became affected at the age of 21, and now (1879) sees so badly that he only goes about alone with difficulty; his children were healthy. These brothers had four sisters who all had good eyes; one of them married I. 8, who saw well, and had six children of whom II. 2, aged 40, was at one time a butcher, but he had to give up his work on account of amblyopia; the onset in his case was at the age of 21. II. 3, aged 38, had seen badly since the age of 21, his sight was better in the evenings; seventeen years after the onset R. V. = finger counting, at short distance, excentrically, L. V. = finger counting at 1 m.; the left showed slight concentric contraction of field; red and green were not recognised; both discs were a greenish white colour, and vessels were narrowed. The twelve-year-old daughter of II. 3 saw well. II. 5, aged 33, complained of a very rapid diminution of vision three months ago; the onset was so sudden that after only eight days he had to give up his work as a hairdresser; R. V. = finger counting at 2 m., L. V. = finger counting at 3 m.; concentric contraction of fields was present; red and green were not recognised; signs of neuritis and of atrophy were noted in the papillae, arteries were narrowed and very tortuous; the son of II. 5, aged 3 years, saw well. II. 7, aged 32, and her three children saw well. II. 9, aged 24, had been amblyopic since the age of 20 and was exempted from military service on that account. II. 10, aged 20, was amblyopic. No history of syphilis in the parents or patients. No consanguinity. Bibl. No. 15.

Fig. 762. *Wilbrand and Saenger's Case.* Hereditary optic atrophy in two first cousins and two of their maternal uncles. III. 2, aged 33, had never seen very well in his youth but his vision had become much worse the last four weeks; he was neurasthenic and had a history of sexual excess, also of smoking and drinking a good deal; syphilis was denied and no signs of this disease were discovered; he saw better in a dull light but his visual acuity was markedly lowered in both eyes; on the right side the temporal half of the papilla was markedly pale, on the left the whole disc was paler than normal; the margins were not clear, the vessels were narrower than normal; the patient appears to have had scotomata since the age of 25. After persistent enquiry concerning the family history, information was given to the effect that II. 1, his maternal uncle, became amblyopic at the age of 18, he died, aged 60, and never became quite blind; II. 2 had bilateral scotomata at the age of 28; III. 1, his first cousin, had bilateral amblyopia at the age of 18. On the basis of this history the case was diagnosed as one of hereditary neuritis. Two years later III. 2 became father to a child who had congenital syphilis and died soon after birth; he was then given energetic antisyphilitic treatment under which his vision and also his general condition improved markedly. No consanguinity recorded. Bibl. No. 101, pp. 168—9.

Fig. 763. *Wilbrand and Saenger's Case.* Hereditary optic atrophy in two brothers and a sister. III. 1, aged 29, had always been healthy up to the age of 17, when his sight failed first in the left eye and shortly after in the right; fifteen weeks after the onset vision was reduced to perception of light in both eyes; the sister and brother of III. 1 were also amblyopic; three siblings had died from cholera, chest disease and teething respectively; an uncle of the mother was blind. The patient had drunk and smoked freely and his vision improved when he ceased to do either; both discs were atrophic; colours were not recognised; central scotomata, also some peripheral contraction of fields, were present. No consanguinity recorded. Bibl. No. 101, pp. 161—2.

Fig. 764. *Griscom's Case.* Fourteen cases of hereditary optic atrophy in three generations. The recorder examined six of the seven affected members of generation II and three of the six affected children of generation III; the patients were well-nourished and intelligent with no defect except the amblyopia which dated from early childhood in each case; externally the eyes appeared to be normal in all respects and pupils reacted normally.

Of those examined Mrs L., aged 46, had R. V. = $\frac{10}{20}$, L. V. = $\frac{10}{200}$, or with −1·00 cyl. ax. 180° R. V. = $\frac{18}{200}$, with − 3·00 cyl. ax. 180° L. V. = $\frac{20}{200}$; she had a few floating vitreous opacities; discs were pale with well-defined margins; arteries and veins very small; central scotomata were present; no peripheral contraction of fields; no recognition of colours. C. M., aged 36, had R. V. = $\frac{20}{200}$, L. V. = $\frac{20}{70}$, not improved by glasses; media clear; discs pearly white with well-defined margins; vessels normal; no peripheral contraction of fields for form; did not recognise green. Mrs P., aged 34, had R. V. = L. V. = $\frac{18}{200}$, with − 1·00 sph. R. V. = $\frac{20}{200}$, with − 1·00 cyl. ax. 90° L. V. = $\frac{20}{100}$ partly; both eyes had fine vitreous opacities; discs pearly white, margins clear; a well-defined complete narrow ring of choroidal atrophy surrounded the disc; vessels were thread-like; there was some pigmentary disturbance in the macular region and a few deposits of pigment in the periphery; central scotomata were present, peripheral fields for form were full; no vision for blue,

Plate LV.   DESCRIPTIONS OF PEDIGREE PLATES   387

red or green. C. M., aged 32, had R. V. = $\frac{20}{100}$, L. V. = $\frac{5}{300}$, with correction R. V. = $\frac{20}{50}$, L. V. = $\frac{20}{100}$; media clear; disc well-defined and pearly white on temporal side, pale on nasal side; vessels narrowed; granular pigmentation over whole retina; visual fields were full for form; no recognition of green. R. M., aged 30, had R. V. = L. V. = $\frac{10}{200}$, not improved by glasses; media clear; discs white with defined margins; vessels thread-like; retina finely granular with fine pigment deposits in the macular region; he had annular relative scotomata, fields slightly contracted at periphery; no recognition of green. Mrs G., aged 27, had R. V. = $\frac{20}{100}$, not improved by glasses; media were clear, discs very pale; vessels slightly smaller than normal; fields full; no recognition of green.

Of the parents of this sibship I. 1, the father, had poor vision; he was not examined; the mother saw well; all their three daughters and four of their six sons were affected. One affected daughter was married and had three normal children; all the sons were married and all transmitted the defect except II. 2, himself normal, who had six normal children.

Of the affected children of generation III, I. M., aged 8, female, had R. V. = L. V. = $\frac{20}{50}$, not improved by glasses; media were clear, discs very pale, especially on the temporal side, vessels normal. A. M., male, aged 6, had R. V. = $\frac{20}{12}$ = L. V., with appearances as for I. M. R. M., male, aged 6, had R. V. = L. V. = $\frac{20}{50}$, with slight pallor of disc on temporal side, margins well defined, vessels normal.

Wassermann was negative in all cases, heart, lungs and urine were normal in all but there was some evidence of tabes in R. M. In each case X-ray examination showed an entirely normal sella turcica and sphenoid with the exception of R. M. whose pituitary fossa was slightly enlarged. No consanguinity. Bibl. No. 119.

Fig. 765. *Lagrange's Case.* Optic atrophy in a male and in two of his three maternal uncles. III. 1 was seen aged 18 when his vision had been gradually diminishing for 18 months, in other respects he was healthy; now R. V. = $\frac{1}{2}$, L. V. = $\frac{1}{15}$; the discs were atrophic and uniformly white with clearly defined contours; vessels very narrow; the patient did not recognise green, fields for red were contracted; a radiograph showed normal sella turcica and sphenoidal cells; retardation of coagulation of the blood was noted. The patient's mother, her four sisters and one of her brothers saw well; two of her brothers, II. 1 and 2, suffered in the same way as III. 1, the onset in their cases being at the ages of 20 and 25 years respectively. No consanguinity recorded. Bibl. No. 122.

Fig. 766. *Mügge's Case.* Hereditary optic atrophy in two brothers; the onset in each case was sudden, at the age of 18 and 26 years respectively; the disease ran an acute course, there were marked neuritic signs in the papillae and vision was reduced to perception of light or knowledge of hand movements; then a gradual improvement occurred; in both brothers there was a severe disturbance of colour perception; large central scotomata were noted. It is stated that probably the brother of one of the grandmothers was similarly affected. No consanguinity recorded. Bibl. No. 90.

Fig. 767. *Westhoff's Case.* Hereditary optic atrophy in nine males of three generations. I. 1 and 2 had three children, a daughter, II. 2, and two sons, Jacob D., II. 4, and Jan D., II. 6. The eldest son, born 1820, a smith, began to see badly at the age of 25 when it was noticed that instead of putting the red-hot horse shoe on the hoof he put it on his hand which held the hoof; he was not absolutely blind at his death at the age of 65, he could go about alone, but could not read; he had four sons and one daughter of whom one son died aged 20; three sons saw well; the daughter and her son saw well. II. 6, born 1823, was also a smith; at the age of 20 he was unable to see to read but could go about alone; he died, aged 63, leaving three daughters and a son; they, their children and grandchildren all saw well. II. 2 saw well at the age of 60; she married twice, by her first marriage she had a son, III. 1, and a daughter, III. 3, of whom III. 1, a waggon-maker, lost his sight at the age of 20; at the age of 60 he was able to go about alone but could not see to read. III. 3 saw well but transmitted the defect to her sons; she had six children of whom IV. 2, Josef F., became blind at the age of 21; he was a smith, but had to give up his work; he was scarcely able to go out alone; his two healthy children were aged 3 years and 6 months respectively. IV. 3 saw well and had a son aged 3. IV. 5 was seen by Faber at the age of 22, who reported that he had a moderate degree of optic neuritis; six months later he had bilateral atrophy of the optic nerve with very marked lowering of visual acuity. IV. 6 was a tailor; at the age of 17 he complained of his vision but he improved after treatment when R. V. = $\frac{4}{24}$, L. V. = $\frac{5}{12}$; the temporal side of the disc was atrophic in the right and less severely affected in the left; he could read with the left eye and carry on his work, but not with the right. IV. 7, aged 6, a smith, complained that he had seen badly for about a week and was now unable to read his own handwriting; a year before he had been wounded in his left eye by an iron splinter; he was healthy and had never been ill; no excess of tobacco or alcohol; no trace of syphilis; both eyes looked healthy but there was a coloboma iridis in the left eye following his accident of a year ago when the iris had prolapsed and had to be excised; R. V. = $\frac{1}{8}$, L. V. = $\frac{1}{30}$; central scotomata were present in both; fields were slightly contracted for red, green and blue; media were clear; temporal half of disc was bluish white in both with clear margins.

By her second marriage II. 2 had two sons, III. 4 and 5, of whom III. 4 had seen badly since the age of 19; he worked at the age of 53 at the spool in a carpet factory and was able to go about alone but could not see to read or write; he was married but had no children. III. 5, aged 48, was with the army when his sight failed at the age of 19; he is now a basket maker and sees very badly; he is only able to go about with difficulty; he has a healthy child aged 3 years. No consanguinity recorded. Bibl. No. 46.

Fig. 768. *Jameson Evans's Case.* Seven cases of optic atrophy in males of three generations. V. 3, A. T., aged 11, was a bright intelligent boy; his mother had noticed some failure of his sight for three or four weeks; he complained of some pain over the left temporal and occipital regions; pupils normal; upper margin of right disc a little hazy, peripheral fields full, left disc a little hazy with a few minute haemorrhages on upper margin; R. V. $= \frac{6}{18}$ with $+ 1 \cdot 5$, L. V. = fingers at 1 ft.; large central scotomata were present; he was given iodide and strychnine, smoked glasses to wear, drops of cocaine and dionine in his eyes and galvanism; ten days later R. V. $= \frac{6}{30}$, L. V. = hand movements at 6 inches; this was on June 22. On July 30 R. V. = fingers at 2 m., L. V. = fingers at 30 cm.; pupils were dilated and hardly reacted to light; shortly after this the state of vision became stationary and remained so until March 28 of the next year when R. V. = L. V. $= \frac{6}{60}$; from this time vision steadily improved until September when it was $\frac{6}{8}$ in each, the discs however were pale and porcelain-like and arteries a little narrower than normal; colour vision was good, fine nystagmus was present. V. 3 had four siblings who were at this time normal; his mother saw well, but her three brothers, IV. 2, 6 and 7, were all affected. IV. 6, G. E., aged 20, had pains in his head for nine months which were now better but his sight had failed and R. V. = fingers at 1 m., L. V. = fingers at 6 inches; both discs were very pale and atrophic, arteries small; nervous system normal; he was given the same treatment as his nephew but no improvement followed and seven years later R. V. = fingers at 1 m., L. V.:=hand movements; fields were slightly contracted and central scotomata were present. The other affected members of the family, IV. 2 and 7, also their maternal uncles, III. 1, 3 and 7, all gave a similar history with regard to mode of onset, course and termination of the trouble, as in the case of IV. 6; thus failure of vision in all cases occurred at about the age of 20 and became permanently reduced to hand movements; also extreme pallor and atrophy of the optic disc was noted; one of the brothers of generation IV was a dipsomaniac and had been in a lunatic asylum for a few weeks. I. 1 was said to have been blind. No consanguinity recorded. Bibl. No. 109.

Fig. 769. *Haushalter's Case.* Hereditary optic atrophy in a female and in her three sons; her first cousin and a great-uncle were also affected. III. 2, aged 43 years, was the only child of a father who died young from some unknown cause and of a mother who was still living and well; she was intelligent and very impressionable; towards the age of 20 she had a rather rapid diminution of visual acuity which was said to be due to optic neuritis, the disease progressed for a year and had since been stationary; now, 23 years after the onset, she had perception of light; her great-uncle, I. 3, and her first cousin, III. 3, were also similarly affected; it is not stated whether these relationships hold through her mother or her father. III. 2 married a healthy man and had five children of whom IV. 1, female, died aged 13; she had had nervous anorexia for some time. IV. 2, male, aged 14, had a sudden onset of optic neuritis eight months ago; he cannot now read or recognise people in front of him; he is obese and rather capricious and lazy though intelligent, and he is subject to obsessions and phobiae. IV. 3, female, aged 12, was lively and intelligent but a little eccentric; she was a little obese. IV. 4, aged 8, became affected at the age of 6; he was normally developed and intelligent but nervous; vision was almost totally lost. IV. 5, aged 6, suffered from an onset of optic neuritis three months ago and already could hardly distinguish the large characters of a book. All three brothers were seen and treated by ophthalmologists but without any appreciable results. No consanguinity recorded. Bibl. No. 89.

Plate LVI. Fig. 770. *Jameson Evans's Case.* Hereditary optic atrophy in four males and one female of two generations; one case only examined. III. 1, E. G., a bright boy, aged 11, had a history of otorrhoea; just before the onset of the disease he complained of pain on the top and right side of his head and was liable to frequent vomiting; nine months later he had little pain, occasional vomiting and R. V. = hand movements at 3 m., L. V. = hand movements at 2 m.; discs were pale with well-defined edges, vessels small; slight peripheral contraction of fields was noted, also central scotomata; he was uncertain of all colours except blue; there was some improvement in the right vision three months later and scotomata were diminishing. The boy's maternal uncle, II. 3, also his three second cousins, two brothers and one sister, all appear to have developed the same complaint at the age of about 20 years. No consanguinity recorded. Bibl. No. 109.

Fig. 771. *Jakobsohn's Case.* Optic atrophy in a brother and sister. I. 1 was normal and had a normal daughter, II. 2, who at the age of 26 married II. 1, aged 28; he also was healthy and had no history of syphilis or of any serious illness; they had seven children of whom III. 1 died of bronchitis, aged 2 years, III. 2 and 3 were normal; III. 4 was well nourished and healthy when seen in 1883 at the age of $1\frac{1}{2}$ years but his mother had noticed for six months that the child was blind; he had marked atrophy of the optic nerve; pupils of medium size reacted slowly to light; no nystagmus; there was bilateral greyish white discoloration of the optic disc which had slightly blurred margins but in other respects the fundi were normal; the child died, aged $2\frac{3}{4}$ years, from inflammation of the lungs, no post-mortem examination was made. III. 5 and 6 were healthy. III. 7 became affected in the same way as III. 4 at the age of 5 months; she had greyish white discoloration of both discs, vessels were dilated; pupils were of medium width but

Plate LVI.   DESCRIPTIONS OF PEDIGREE PLATES   389

did not react to light; she was well nourished with no signs of rickets but had had some intestinal trouble during the first month of life. No consanguinity. Bibl. No. 26.

Fig. 772. *Leber's Case II.* Hereditary optic atrophy in three siblings. The father, II. 2, was dead but had seen well, the mother, II. 3, aged 59, suffered from "Kopfcolik" associated with sickness and fainting; sometimes the attacks recurred many times in a week, at other periods they were rare; she never had convulsive attacks; since about two years she had suffered from senile cataract, early in the right eye, more advanced in the left; no eye disease was known in other branches of the family and the grandparents on both sides were unaffected. II. 2 and 3 had six children of whom III. 1, female, aged 31, saw well but was very excitable and suffered from headaches and giddiness. III. 2, Friedrich B., aged 30, became affected with a sudden diminution of vision at the age of 17 so that after a week he could no longer read but was still able to go about alone; three weeks after the onset von Graefe noted severe amblyopia without ophthalmological changes; the patient was subject to epileptic convulsive attacks; 13 years later improvement in vision had occurred and he could read 3 J. with difficulty with the right and 1 J. with great difficulty with the left eye; at this time colour vision was normal, fields were full, the discs were a bluish white colour with marked atrophic excavation, the arteries narrow. III. 3, Emma B., aged 28, had a rapid bilateral complete blinding from no demonstrable cause; she had suffered from repeated headaches and had fainting attacks but no convulsions; vision was reduced to finger counting at 2' in the left and to no perception of light in the right eye; there was a severe contraction of fields and a slight degree of neuro-retinitis was noted; the patient improved and a fortnight after the onset could read 16 J. with the right, 15 J. with the left eye; there was said to be no central scotomata; colour-blindness was noted; a year later the whole papillae were white but the patient could read 1 J. with difficulty. III. 4, male, aged 25, was normal; III. 5, female, saw well. III. 6, Hermann B., became affected at the age of 19; fourteen days after the onset vision was reduced to 6 J. in the right and 16 J. in the left eye; large central scotomata were noted. This patient had been subject to attacks of giddiness at the time of the onset; eight months later some improvement occurred and he was ultimately able to read 1 J. with the right eye. No consanguinity. Bibl. No. 8.

Fig. 773. *Wagenmann's Case.* Optic atrophy in five males of three generations. III. 3, aged 21, had been affected for two years; his vision was excentric and equal to finger counting at about 3 m.; large central scotomata were present; colour vision was defective; slight improvement followed treatment with strychnine; the patient was in other respects completely healthy. The maternal uncle of III. 3, two of his maternal grandmother's brothers, and his mother's sister's son were also affected. No consanguinity recorded. Bibl. No. 80.

Fig. 774. *Ogilvie's Case.* Hereditary optic atrophy in three brothers; these were the only cases of the disease in a large sibship which was, however, characterised by a very heavy infant mortality. The father, II. 14, was an orphan whose family history was unknown, he at the age of 57 had good vision but showed early lenticular changes. The mother, aged 53, was the youngest in a sibship of 10 all of whom appear to have been normal. I. 1 and 2 died aged 80 and 82 respectively and had normal eyes. The three affected brothers were attacked by the disease in early adult life, at the ages of 24, 22 and 27 respectively; the onset was gradual in two cases, in III. 5 the disease reached its maximum in a single night, the other cases progressing gradually for three and six months respectively. III. 5 improved slightly and then remained stationary; he is now aged 33½. III. 12, aged now 28, improved distinctly and III. 17, aged now 24, remained stationary or became rather worse. The affected brothers drank no spirits but took beer in moderation; all smoked shag from the age of 18 but not in large quantities and III. 12 alone improved on stopping tobacco; there was no evidence of syphilis and no history of sexual excess. Headaches were absent in III. 5; they had occurred occasionally since childhood in III. 12 and were in this case associated with and relieved by vomiting; in the case of III. 17 headaches were associated with visual failure, they were severe in character and ceased when the visual failure had reached its maximum. There had been no significant past illnesses but III. 17 was hysterical.

There is no mention of other disease in the family except in the case of III. 18, aged 21, who had fits and had twice been admitted to a hospital for nervous diseases, also the retinal vessels were said to be tortuous throughout the whole family with the exception of the father.

On ophthalmoscopic examination it was noted that the optic discs were in all cases a good colour when first seen although the visual acuity was already greatly diminished, but they gradually became pale starting in the temporal half and there was some atrophic excavation. The retinal vessels, tortuous in all, were remarkably so in III. 12 and 17. The fundus generally was normal except for patches of choroidal atrophy in III. 17. The visual fields were full in III. 5 and 12, concentrically contracted in III. 17. Central scotomata were present in all cases. Colour vision was defective in III. 5, very defective in III. 17, normal in III. 12. No consanguinity recorded. Bibl. No. 50.

Fig. 775. *Doyne's Case.* (Published by Nettleship.) This very interesting case is unusual in several respects. I. 3 had some defect of sight but had not seen so badly as her daughter, II. 2; she could do needlework and read and her defect may have been only myopia; she had fourteen siblings; her first child was an illegitimate daughter, II. 2, aged about 71 when seen, whose sight failed in childhood and has remained the same ever since; symptoms and appearances were characteristic in her and the other cases of the pedigree, all of which were seen; she had been very deaf for many years. I. 3 afterwards married I. 4 and had by him two sons and four daughters all of whom saw well.

II. 2 married, apparently after 30; her husband, II. 1, of about the same age, subsequently lost both his eyes from a boiler accident; they had four children of whom III. 2, a son, aged 30, is normal and has one living child IV. 2, aged 8, who is also normal; III. 3, a son, aged 32, had three normal children, IV. 3—5, aged 5 years to 10 months. III. 5, a daughter, was seen by Doyne at the age of 20 and by Nettleship ten years later, she was "born with the sight as it is now," was married to III. 7, who was examined and found to be normal, and had five children, IV. 6—10, of whom three are affected. III. 6, a son of II. 2, aged 29, was also affected.

Of the children of III. 5, a son, IV. 6, was believed to have seen well till about the age of 3 years when he began to have "to look about for things"; at about the age of 8 the recorder found myopia of 7—8 D. in each eye, with 3 D. of astigmatism in the right; discs were pale; examined by Nettleship ten years later the condition was unchanged and he could read 3 or 4 J. slowly held very close. IV. 7, daughter of III. 5, saw well till she was aged about 4, at the age of 5 Doyne found discs pale, fingers were seen at 3 feet and refraction was hypermetropic, 2 D.; condition was unchanged when examined by Nettleship later. IV. 8, a son, died aged 9 months with good sight. IV. 9 represents a miscarriage. IV. 10 was noticed by his mother to see badly at the age of 2 months or earlier; at 6 months Doyne found irregular nystagmic movements and noted that the child did not follow a light; at the age of $1\frac{1}{12}$ years Nettleship found the disc decidedly pale on the temporal side and the mother said that he saw so badly that he would run against the table or chair and "had to look under the light to see." IV. 6—10 were all suckled and showed no other degeneracies; circumstances prevented a proper examination of the fields in any of these subjects but it was quite evident from the manner in which they looked at objects that sight was best towards the periphery; central vision was very bad in all, and all had more or less nystagmus; the discs were much alike in all, pale all over in the adults, but especially so on the temporal side; in the children the nasal side was fairly coloured but the temporal side quite pale. None of those affected, from the grandmother, II. 2, to the youngest member, IV. 10, are getting either worse or better. No consanguinity. Bibl. No. 85, pp. cxv—cxvii.

Fig. 776. *Rampoldi's Case.* This history is unsatisfactory as so few details are given and only one member of the family appears to have been examined; the recorder describes the condition as one of amaurosis due to optic atrophy in four generations. I. 1 was said to have been completely blind at the age of 35; she had three children of whom II. 2 suffered from no eye defect; his daughter, III. 1, died young. II. 4 became blind at the age of 35 from the same disease as his mother; he had two sons of whom III. 3 had no defect of vision up to the time of his rather early death when he had had four children. IV. 1 had good sight at the age of 33, his three siblings died young. III. 4, the recorder's patient, had optic atrophy in the right eye first and shortly afterwards in the left; when seen at the age of 67 the right eye was almost completely blind; he had a history of gastro-enteritis with some haemorrhage two or three years before his vision failed. The third child of I. 1 became blind between the ages of 35 and 40; she had two sons and one daughter of whom III. 5, had good sight; III. 7 was blind probably from the same disease as his mother; III. 8 was quite blind at 73 and her sight was said to have failed at the age of 65. III. 7 had a son, IV. 3, aged 31, who was nearly blind. No consanguinity recorded. Bibl. No. 21.

Fig. 777. *Leber's Case* (from Hormuth). Optic atrophy in four males of three sibships in the same generation. III. 2 was seen at the age of 56; he had noticed a diminution of vision in his right eye six months previously; his left eye became affected three months after the onset in the right; before this he had smoked a good deal; he was found to have R. V. = finger counting at 1 m., in the left eye central vision was still normal; the right field showed a large central colour scotomata; paracentral colour scotomata were present in the left; peripheral fields were not contracted; bilaterally the papillary margins were blurred, especially the left; the retinal vessels were dilated. A variety of treatments were tried including bleeding, sweating, inunction, potassium iodide, sodium salicylate, etc.; nine months after the onset vision was finger counting at 2 m. with + 6 D. in the right and at 3 m. with + 6 D. in the left

I. 1 and 2 had good eyes; they had three daughters, II. 2, 4, 6, who also had good eyes but all had one or more sons with hereditary optic atrophy. II. 2 was the mother of III. 2; II. 4 had one son, III. 4, whose central vision was lost at the age of 22, and a son, III. 5, who had severe amblyopia. II. 6 had a son, III. 9, who at the age of 40 was almost completely blind; he was alcoholic. All the affected cousins had normal siblings as shown in the pedigree. III. 2 had two sons aged 27 and 19 years respectively who saw well. No consanguinity recorded. Bibl. No. 64, pp. 158—60.

Fig. 778. *De Graaf's Case.* Hereditary optic atrophy in five brothers of a sibship of ten and in their maternal uncle. One of the brothers went to a clinic at Groningen to seek help because he had noticed a diminution of vision in his right eye only for the last fourteen days; there was no history of excess in the use of alcohol or tobacco; it was found that R. V. = $\frac{6}{30}$, no improvement with glasses, L. V. = $\frac{6}{8}$; colour perception in the right was markedly diminished, fields of vision were not contracted, a central scotoma for colours was demonstrated; an ophthalmoscopic examination was made and hereditary optic neuritis was diagnosed;

the patient reported that four of his brothers had lost a great deal of their vision from a similar defect which had begun in one eye and slowly progressed; he also said that a brother of his mother was similarly affected and that only males suffered in their family from the defect though it was transmitted by females; the onset of the disease occurred between the ages of 17 and 20 years and none of the children of the next generation had yet reached this age. No consanguinity recorded. Bibl. No. 103.

Fig. 779. *Usher's Case.* This case has been published before as Fig. 130 in *Albinism in Man* (Bibl. No. 98) but a number of additions have been made since the earlier history was issued; thus eighteen individuals in generation V, five individuals in generation IV and four individuals in generation II have been added to the original pedigree and another member, IV. 13, has become affected by Leber's disease. The following particulars of the new members are given: V. 1—5 have good sight; V. 8, aged 15, had a normal fundus; V. 9 died aged 6 weeks; V. 10, aged 12, iris green, hair brown, had a "muslin patch" on right optic disc, left fundus normal; V. 11, aged 10, iris blue, hair light brown, internal concomitant strabismus of right eye, hypermetropia estimated at 5 or 6 dioptres in each eye; V. 12, aged 9, iris brown, hair fair, fundi normal; V. 13, aged 6, fundi normal; V. 14, aged 2, iris brown, hair fair, fundi normal; V. 15, aged 9 months, iris blue, hair light brown, right optic disc seen was normal, media clear. IV. 1, 4, 5 and 7 all have good vision; IV. 2 was dead. III. 2 and her father had good vision. IV. 13 married his second cousin, IV. 1, and had eight children; he noticed his vision failing in the right eye at the end of 1916, in the left eye at the beginning of 1917, when he was aged 36; in July 1917 he was seen at the Aberdeen Royal Infirmary when R. V. $=\frac{1}{60}$, L. V. $=\frac{6}{60}$; peripheral fields were full and an absolute central scotoma for a 10 mm. red square was present in each field; he had smoked weekly two ounces of tobacco—Tam-o'-Shanter—for 16 years until three months ago when he gave tobacco up altogether, but, notwithstanding, his vision continued to get worse; in April R. V. $=\frac{1}{36}$, L. V. $=\frac{6}{12}$; nothing else was found to be abnormal in his nervous system, and nothing of note was found in ears, nose, accessory sinuses or throat; the radiographer reported pronounced thickening and prominence of both anterior and posterior clinoid processes which approach each other apparently to within a distance of 2 mm.; the widest antero-posterior diameter of the sella turcica is 13 mm. The Wassermann reaction was negative. In September 1920 the following note was made: iris blue, some stroma pigment, hair brown; R. V. reads letters about the size of 20 J., L. V. = finger counting; absolute central scotoma for red in each, peripheral fields full; optic discs are pale yet there is a fair amount of red, edges not irregular or too sharply defined, lamina cribrosa not conspicuous, retinal arteries of normal size, except a lower branch of each which is narrowed. IV. 12, seen on Oct. 24, 1899, aged 19, had been a healthy man though subject to nose bleedings; ten months ago he lost a lot of blood from a cut on his hand; nine months earlier, January 1899, his sight became defective and in a month's time vision had become as bad as at present; he smoked weekly 4 ozs. of strong tobacco—bogie roll—and sometimes he took too much alcohol; R. V. = finger counting at 6", L. V. $<\frac{1}{60}$, spelled words of 20 J. at 5"; right optic disc was of papery whiteness, slight tinge of red at outer part only, lamina cribrosa much exposed, margin of optic disc abnormally well defined, retinal vessels slightly narrowed, rest of fundus normal; left optic disc less pale than the right and the edge less well defined but otherwise conditions were the same as in the right eye; no nystagmus, irides blue, fields of vision full with a very large circular absolute central scotoma in each, nothing else found amiss in nervous system. This man is alive to-day, Dec. 22, 1923, with no apparent further change in his vision.

IV. II, seen on June 13, 1902, aged 28, had been always healthy; in August 1901 a mist came over his left eye and within a few weeks his right eye became affected; the sight gradually got worse and he had to give up his work as a butcher at the end of January; he had attacks of pain in both eyes, especially the left one, smoked 1 oz. of twist weekly and took very little alcohol; nothing abnormal found on general examination besides the fundus changes; R. V. = finger counting at 1', L. V. = perception of light; fields of vision full, absolute central scotoma in each; ophthalmoscopic examination showed marked contrast between the white outer parts and the red inner parts of the optic discs, edges of discs blurred, especially at inner parts; retinal arteries distinctly narrowed, margin of discs irregular; refraction hypermetropic, estimated at 1 D. in right eye and 5 D. in left; although he gave up tobacco vision did not improve and optic discs became paler; he was alive in 1923. IV. 24, hair brown, iris blue. V. 18, hair brown, iris blue. V. 17, hair very fair, iris blue, good vision. V. 16, aged 21 (1923), has good vision, iris blue. For description of the albinos in this pedigree, see the original account. In the case of III. 16 and 18, Leber's disease set in at about the age of 30 years. Consanguinity. Bibl. No. 97 and additional notes,

Plate LVII. Fig. 780. *Batten's Case.* Leber's disease in three generations. III. 17, aged 10 (1904), complained of rapid failure of sight for about a month, the mother had only noticed it for two days. On ophthalmoscopic examination the right optic disc was rather pale at the outer margin, the retinal vessels were not diminished; the retina was finely dotted—"red pepper"—the macula was somewhat oedematous, showing fine light rings; the left fundus was similar except that the optic disc appeared here to be normal. R. V. $=\frac{6}{60}$; L. V. $<\frac{6}{60}$. Later, after the vision had begun to improve, the discs were noted to be rather pale and excavated, the maculae showed slight pigment changes, there was no evidence of oedema. The patient was treated with arsenic and potassium iodide and his vision improved as follows: R. V. = L. V. =

$\frac{6}{60}$ (March 1904), $\frac{6}{36}$ (June), $\frac{6}{24}$ (July), $\frac{6}{18}$ (Sept.), $\frac{6}{12}$ (Feb. 1905), $\frac{6}{9}$ (March), $\frac{4}{12}$ (Feb. 1909). III. 13, aged 22 (1907), reported that his sight began to fail when he was about 16 years of age, the failure was gradual and associated with no illness. The optic discs were pale and atrophic, the retinal vessels not much reduced in size; in 1909 R. V. = $\frac{6}{60}$, J. 14 at 5 inches, L. V. = $\frac{6}{60}$, J. 20 at 6 inches; there had been no marked alteration since 1907, but the fields were slightly more constricted. In Nov. 1923, III. 13 reports that he is no better but that his brother, III. 17, is "quite all right." III. 1 was seen three weeks after his sight began to fail; he was found to have symmetrical retinal haemorrhages at the margins of the discs and "water silk undulations" of the maculae; he showed no improvement under treatment; the haemorrhages were absorbed and the discs became very white; R. V. = L. V. < $\frac{6}{60}$; later he developed nervous symptoms, cramp in both feet, numbness of his fingers and tremors of his lips; knee-jerks were absent, the pupils reacted well. Of other members of the pedigree, a maternal uncle, II. 4, and the maternal grandfather, I. 1, are notified as being affected. No consanguinity recorded. Bibl. No. 82.

Fig. 781. *Nettleship's Case.* Optic atrophy in four males and one female of two generations. I. 2, said to be "nearly blind," had children of whom no information was obtained. I. 4 was similarly affected and had an affected son, II. 2. I. 5 and I. 7 saw well but the latter transmitted the defect to two of her four sons. II. 10 became affected at the age of 12; no recovery had taken place when Nettleship saw the patient at the age of 49. II. 11 was also affected; no details are given of his case. II. 12 was unmarried. No consanguinity. Bibl. No. 85, p. clxxv.

Fig. 782. *Hormuth's Case.* Hereditary optic atrophy in a female and her two brothers; the maternal grandmother and her brother probably also affected. III. 3, Frl. Sch., aged 23, noticed that she could no longer see to read with the right eye, the left eye was at this time normal; nine months later the left eye also became affected; at this time the patient was very well nourished and did not suffer from headaches; R. V. = finger counting at 10', L. V. = $\frac{20}{30}$ to $\frac{20}{20}$; a small central scotoma was present in the right field; R. papilla was pale, vessels normal, L. papilla was normal, vessels dilated. III. 1, Richard Sch., aged 27, reported that at the age of 21 there was a gradual diminution of vision in his left eye which was not treated for six months, at the end of this time the right eye also became affected; he was treated by inunction and electricity but the condition remained unchanged for about eighteen months; after this a gradual improvement of vision, in the right eye only, took place; the patient suffered from headaches which were very severe at times. Five years from the onset of the disease R. V. = $\frac{20}{20}$, small central scotoma was present, L. V. = finger counting at 3—4', small central scotoma present; peripheral fields were not contracted; colour discrimination was uncertain in the left eye; the papillae were white especially so on the temporal side; arteries narrowed.

A younger brother, III. 2, aged 25, had suffered from the same disease since the age of 17; his visual acuity had improved but he was not able to read. The maternal grandmother had at the age of 27 been blind for half a year but had recovered later; a brother of this grandmother had also suffered from his eyes. No consanguinity recorded. Bibl. No. 64.

Fig. 783. *Heinsberger's Case I.* Retrobulbar optic neuritis in three brothers; one brother was young and might still develop the disease; two sisters, the parents and grandparents had never suffered from any eye disease. III. 5, Adam G., a carter, aged 20, noticed that his vision had become worse during the last month; he was small, of a robust build and florid complexion; pupils were equal and reacted well; R. V. = finger counting at 2 m., L. V. = $\frac{6}{60}$; media were clear; right papilla was very hyperaemic and showed deep physiological excavation; fundus pigmented; the left papilla was also hyperaemic; fundus was normal; no scotomata were present; at this date all colours were recognised; the condition progressed in spite of active treatment and four months later vision was reduced to finger counting at 2 m. in the right and at 2·5 m. in the left; green was not recognised in either eye and the right eye was also red-blind; the outer margins of the fields of vision were now contracted. III. 1, Philip G., aged 29, became affected with the same disease at the age of 21, he was treated in Wurzburg and in Wiesbaden. III. 3, Jacob G., aged 24, became similarly affected at the age of 20 and was treated in Heidelberg The youngest sibling, III. 6, had not yet shown signs of the disease. No consanguinity recorded. Bibl. No. 67.

Fig. 784. *Nettleship's Case.* Leber's disease in four brothers; their nephew and a maternal uncle were also affected. III. 1 became affected at the age of 14; he recovered sufficiently to be able to read. II. 2, 3 and 4 became affected at the ages of 33, 25 and 23 years respectively. II. 5, 7, 8 and 9 saw well. II. 5 had three children of whom III. 1 was Nettleship's patient at the age of 22. No further information is given. No consanguinity recorded. Bibl. No. 85, p. clxxiv.

Fig. 785. *Nettleship's Case.* Optic atrophy in three generations. III. 1 became affected at the age of 22 and was seen again seven years later. III. 4 became affected at the age of 17. These brothers had two unmarried sisters, also twelve siblings who had died young. The mother, II. 4, had two brothers, II. 1 and 2, who were also affected. The maternal great-uncle, I. 3, is also reported to have suffered from "the family blindness." II. 4 had two married sisters who were said to have normal children. No consanguinity. Bibl. No. 85, p. clxxv.

Fig. 786. *Nettleship's Case.* Leber's disease in a brother and sister. II. 2, aged 41, had noticed an

Plate LVII.   DESCRIPTIONS OF PEDIGREE PLATES   393

increasing weakness of vision in both eyes for four or five weeks; she was still suckling her baby aged 11 months; her vision was better in a dim light; she had had eight children and one miscarriage. At the onset of the eye trouble the patient was frequently giddy and vomited once or twice but had only slight headaches; no history of syphilis or other illness, the patient was now in good health; she could read some letters of 20 J. with the right eye and 19 J. with the left; the right disc was hazy and paler than the left, which showed only slight change; two months later vision was a little worse and colour sense very defective. II. 1 had defective sight from the age of 23 to the time of his death, from some chest complaint, at 40; his eye trouble was described as "weakness of the nerves of sight"; he was a non-smoker; this man was a gardener but could not tell the colours of his flowers. All other members of the family had good sight and were free from nervous affections. No consanguinity recorded. Bibl. Nos. 29 and 85, p. clxvi.

Fig. 787. *Higier's Case.* Optic atrophy in two brothers and in their maternal uncle; one sister suffered from migraine and epilepsy; the parents were healthy. II. 3, aged 20, complained that his sight had been getting worse for six weeks so that he could not now see to read; he had had not very severe headaches and giddiness; pupils were normal; R. V. $= \frac{1}{24}$, L. V. $= \frac{1}{16}$; central scotomata were present but there was no peripheral contraction of the visual fields; the discs were a little swollen and blurred, the temporal halves were a bluish white colour; vessels were normal: no other defects were found; there was no history of excess in the use of alcohol or tobacco. II. 2, a musician, aged 27, had been hindered in his work for many weeks and could only read his notes with difficulty; he did not smoke and drank little, but admits occasional sexual excess; he had three healthy daughters under five years of age. The vision of II. 2 was reduced to finger counting at $1\frac{1}{2}$ m. in the R. and at 1 m. in the L.; large central scotomata were present with no peripheral contraction of fields; the discs had blurred margins and were pale on the temporal side; veins were slightly tortuous, arteries narrowed; the condition remained stationary in spite of energetic treatment. I. 2 became affected at the age of 20. No consanguinity. Bibl. No. 52.

Fig. 788. *Schlüter's Case.* Hereditary optic neuritis in seven males of two generations. I. 2 was very short-sighted but in other respects had healthy eyes; her husband, I. 1, saw well; they had three children, Elizabeth, Caroline and Christian, of whom the two daughters, II. 2 and 3, were healthy, but their brother, II. 4, at the age of 25 became "weak-sighted." III. 3, the son of II. 4, aged 20, still saw well. Elizabeth N. married W. with good eyes and had two children, III. 1, the recorder's patient, and a healthy daughter. I. 4, sister of I. 2, and I. 5 had good eyes; of their four children the three sons, II. 6—8, now aged 50, 48 and 45 years respectively, all became "weak-sighted" at the age of 30; one of them was under treatment at the clinic but showed no improvement; their sister, II. 9, and her husband saw well but the two sons of these parents, now aged 21 and 30 respectively, had become "weak-sighted," III. 6 at the age of 17, III. 5 at the age of 20 years. III. 4 saw well.

III. 1, Hermann W., aged 20, reported that he had never been ill and had seen well up to eight weeks ago when he noticed some discomfort in his head and slight giddiness, associated with a diminution of vision which had gradually increased; vision was now reduced to finger counting in the R. at 8', in the L. at 10'; red and green were not recognised; absolute central scotomata were present but the peripheral fields were full; signs of optic neuritis were noted; the patient was seen from time to time but no improvement followed his treatment. No consanguinity recorded. Bibl. No. 19, pp. 46—49.

Fig. 789. *Habershon's Case I.* Optic atrophy in two brothers. II. 3, James N., aged 26, had suffered from imperfect vision since the age of 17 when his eyes became inflamed and vision dim; the onset was sudden, he was admitted to St George's hospital, cupped on both temples and treated with pilocarpine; optic neuritis was diagnosed; nine weeks later he left hospital with no improvement of vision and the condition had remained stationary since that time; he cannot distinguish people across the street and only reads the largest letters of print; he used to smoke $\frac{1}{4}$ lb. of Cavendish weekly but gave up smoking when his sight failed; he had also at one period been a heavy drinker of spirits but had been a total abstainer for the last two years; no history of syphilis or of sexual excesses or any previous illness. The father died from cancer of the tongue, the mother from phthisis, both had good sight. II. 3 had several brothers who all had good health and, with one exception, saw well. The patient's general condition was good; his pupils were large but reacted to light and accommodation; R. V. $=$ L. V. $=$ finger counting at 6'; refraction myopic, about 8 D. in the right and 6 D. in the left eye; discs were pale all over, vessels tortuous; absolute central scotomata were noted with no contraction of the peripheral fields; perception of red and green was impaired; a little improvement occurred under treatment with amyl nitrite.

II. 1, Michael N., aged 31, had had no serious illness; at the age of 22 he "found his eyes dazzled" one day, on reading the paper, so that he could not see the print; he was up to this time a heavy drinker of spirits and beer and smoked $\frac{1}{2}$ oz. of Cavendish a day; he married at 19 and had two children who saw well; he was now able to read about 19 J. in R. and 20 J. in L.; discs were very pale with edges a little blurred, pupils normal; central scotomata were present but no contraction of the peripheral fields. No consanguinity recorded. Bibl. No. 29.

Fig. 790. *Nettleship's Case.* (Habershon's Case IV.) Five cases of optic atrophy in males of two generations, the descendants of two normal brothers, I. 2 and 4. III. 2 was seen at the age of 34 one year after the onset of the disease; the right eye was first affected, the left eye failed five months later; the patient had been accustomed to smoke 3 ozs. of Wills's tobacco weekly since the age of 21; he had a history of slight syphilitic infection nine years before; no sexual excess; R. V. = 20 J. close, L. V. = 16—18 J. close; pupils reacted normally; discs showed a brownish pallor in the right eye, very little pallor but a hazy border in the left; vessels were normal; bilateral scotomata were present with no contraction of the peripheral fields. III. 2 was seen at intervals and the condition slowly progressed but three years later he was still able to go about alone; there was some defect of his colour vision, green was not recognised anywhere; his father had normal sons by his second wife. III. 3, first cousin to III. 2, was affected; the age of onset in his case is not given.

II. 7 became amblyopic at the age of 21; he was a smoker but gave up the habit for two years after the onset of the disease. II. 8 became amblyopic at the age of 60 and later developed diabetes. These two brothers had three sisters of whom one was unmarried; II. 11 had two healthy sons under 25 years of age; II. 9 had a son, III. 4, who became amblyopic at the age of 16. II. 3 and 4 had other siblings who died of phthisis. No consanguinity recorded. Bibl. Nos. 29 and 85, p. clxv.

Fig. 791. *Raymond and Koenig's Case.* Hereditary optic atrophy in three males of three generations. III. 1 noticed quite suddenly that he could no longer see to carry on his work; the same evening he had headache in the left temporal and occipital regions; reduction of central vision increased during several months and then became stationary; pronounced excavation and white atrophy of the papillae, also narrowing of arteries, were noted; central absolute scotomata were present; green was not recognised; vision was reduced to finger counting at 50 cm., using excentric vision; there was some dilatation of pupils which reacted to light and accommodation. Grandparents had normal vision but a brother of the maternal grandmother had a rapidly progressive diminution of vision whilst on military service; this man, I. 2, had two sons who saw well. The parents of III. 1 saw well but a maternal uncle, II. 3, died from an accident caused by amblyopia of the same nature. No consanguinity recorded. Bibl. No. 86.

Fig. 792. *Raymond and Koenig's Case.* Optic atrophy in a male and in two of his maternal uncles. III. 1, aged 20, noticed suddenly that he could not see to carry on his work; the condition progressed for a time and then became stationary, he is now able to go about alone but at a distance of 3 m. distinguishes neither people nor objects; excavation of the disc was noted, also white atrophy more marked in the temporal segment; retinal vessels were normal; central vision was diminished and colour vision for green was defective. The patient's maternal grandparents saw well; they had four children, II. 1—4, of whom II. 1 died of phthisis; II. 2, aged 48, had optic atrophy; II. 3 had optic atrophy which developed at the age of 25, II. 4, mother of the patient, died of phthisis. The maternal grandmother had a sister, I. 3, whose three children were normal; the daughter, II. 8, had a son with myopia. No consanguinity recorded. Bibl No. 86.

Fig. 793. *Raymond and Koenig's Case.* Optic atrophy in three brothers and in two of their nephews. I. 1 suffered from gout; he had ten children of whom four died young; the only three living sons, II. 1, 3 and 5, had optic atrophy; the only two married daughters had each a son, III. 2 and 4, with optic atrophy; in all cases the onset was sudden and developed at the same period of life; the ophthalmoscopic appearances were alike and typical in all. No consanguinity recorded. Bibl. No. 86.

Fig. 794. *Bride's Case.* Hereditary optic atrophy in three members of a sibship of four. III. 1, aged 15, showed well-marked optic atrophy in both eyes; her sight failed at the age of 9 years; she had suffered from epilepsy since the age of 11½ years. III. 2, Bruce E., aged 12, showed well-marked optic atrophy in both eyes; his sight failed at the age of 9; Wassermann reaction was negative and the child showed no other abnormality. III. 3, Robert Henry E., aged 8, showed well-marked optic atrophy in both eyes; his sight failed when he was aged 7; he showed no other abnormality; Wassermann was negative. There was no history of bad vision in the parents or any of their relations so far as was known; one brother, III. 4, had no ocular defect. No consanguinity. Bibl. No. 149.

Fig. 795. *Haswell's Case.* Hereditary optic atrophy in ten males and two females of three generations. I. 1 and 2 had excellent sight until their death but there was some indefinite history of blindness in the family of the wife, I. 2. All their four children suffered from optic atrophy; thus II. 2, Mary R., became blind at 48; II. 3, Richard R., became blind at the age of 9; II. 5, Charles R., became blind at 21 years and II. 6, Hannah, became blind at 14.

II. 2 married and had seven sons, of whom six were affected with the disease, and two daughters who each transmitted the defect. Thus III. 1, George J., became blind at 27; he had six children who were normal and of whom two daughters were married and had young children. III. 3, Jemima, was normal; she had several daughters with good sight and one son, IV. 4, who became blind at 23; IV. 4 had some young children. III. 5, John J., was normal and had four children with good sight. III. 7, William, became blind at 33; he had five children with good sight. III. 9, Annie, was normal; she had seven normal daughters, two of whom had young children, and one son, IV. 10, who was blind at the age of 17; IV. 10 had two young children. III. 11, Charles, became blind at 20. III. 12, Joseph, became blind at the age of 29; he had four children with good sight. III. 14, Walter, became blind at 18; his wife was blind from leucoma; they had three children one of whom was myopic; III. 16, Frank, became blind at 20; he had five children with good sight.

II. 3 married and had seven children with normal vision.

Four of the affected males were examined and all gave practically the same history, namely that at some particular age the sight was noticed to be dim, it rapidly became worse without pain or other symptoms being present; in a year from the onset the present condition was reached and had since remained stationary. In one case the left eye had been affected three months before the right; all had perception of light and two of the four could count fingers; the discs were atrophied in all cases and the vessels were small; the pupils were equal and reacted slowly to light. III. 14 had nystagmus. All the males were smokers. The children of generation V were below the age at which liability to the disease becomes manifest. No consanguinity recorded. Bibl. No. 30.

Fig. 796. *Lutz's Case.* Hereditary optic atrophy in seven males of two generations. II. 2 had two children, a son, III. 1, who became affected at the age of 30 and a daughter, III. 2, who had three affected sons. II. 3, sister to II. 2, had two sons, III. 6 and 8, who became affected at the ages of 27 and 20 respectively, and two daughters one of whom had no sons and the other, III. 9, had an affected only living son. III. 1, 6 and 8 were not examined but according to the report of members of the family they all suffered from disease of the optic nerve, though none of them were completely blind and they differed in the extent to which their vision was reduced and in their ability to carry on their work. All cases in generation IV were examined and all were found to be characteristic of retrobulbar neuritis; their vision was reduced to finger counting at 1—2 m.; the periphery of their visual fields was intact and large absolute central scotomata were demonstrated; there was a neuritic atrophy of the disc with no alteration of vessels; media were clear. IV. 1 became affected at 20, IV. 3 at 33, IV. 4 at 26 and IV. 15 at 20 years; IV 1, 3 and 4 had two unaffected brothers, IV. 15 had one brother who died aged 4. In each case the onset of the disease was sudden and no other disease was present at the time; the disease in each case attacked both eyes together or the second eye became affected a few days after the first; no improvement appeared to follow a variety of therapeutic measures prescribed. The brothers P., IV. 1, 3, 4, were indolent and not particularly intelligent; they were basket makers. IV. 15 was very excitable, on the other hand, and much more intelligent. No consanguinity. Bibl. No. 92.

PLATE LVIII. Fig. 797. *Waardenburg's Case.* Optic atrophy in six members of three generations. II. 2, aged 85 (1913), became affected at the age of about 50; there was no history of syphilis and no addiction to alcohol, urine was normal and nervous system was normal; ophthalmoscopic examination was made and optic atrophy diagnosed. III. 8, daughter of II. 3, aged 51 (1913), became affected at about the age of 38; papillae were white and clearly outlined; vessels were unchanged or perhaps slightly dilated; central colour scotomata were present; the patient was unable to see to read or do needlework; her two brothers were apparently unaffected by the disease.

III. 8 had ten children of whom four were affected. IV. 2, aged 28, became affected at the age of 15 when R. V. = $\frac{2}{300}$, L. V. = perception of light; the patient had had a blow on his eye a few months before and there was some haemorrhage into the macula; atrophy of the optic nerve was diagnosed; the margins of the papillae were blurred and the patient suffered from acute headache. IV. 6, aged 22, became affected at the age of 12; discs were white, especially on the temporal sides, margins clear. IV. 8, aged 19, became affected at the age of 11; he had large central scotomata but was never wholly blind and could go about alone; he had divergent strabismus. IV. 9, aged 17, had just become affected and the disease was seen in its early stages; central scotomata were present and slight optic neuritis; later, optic atrophy was noted. No consanguinity recorded. Bibl. No. 131.

Fig. 798. *Van Heuven's Case.* Hereditary optic atrophy in four brothers of a sibship of six; two sisters were themselves free from the disease but one of them had an affected son; the parents and paternal grandparents had had good vision; no information could be obtained concerning the vision of the maternal grandfather. III. 2, aged 64 (1925), had noticed a marked diminution in his vision at the age of 21 years, both eyes were affected and the condition had remained stationary in spite of all treatment since that time; now R. V. = $\frac{1}{50}$, L. V. = $\frac{2}{50}$; he had a concentric contraction of his fields in addition to bilateral absolute central scotomata; the ophthalmoscope showed a post-neuritic atrophy of the discs. III. 2 had one daughter with normal eyes. III. 3, aged 62 (1925), became affected at the age of 23 years and had remained an invalid since that time; he had three sons and three daughters all with normal eyes; one of the sons had two small boys who showed no eye defect. III. 5, aged 60 years, became affected at the age of 17 years; the right eye was first affected and the left eye became affected a year later. III. 6, aged 59, lost the vision of both eyes at the age of 21 years; he and III. 5 were unmarried. The sisters III. 7 and 8, aged 57 and 55 years respectively, had normal eyes; III. 8 had eleven daughters with normal eyes and one son who was affected. IV. 9 was examined; the vision of his right eye was first diminished and two months later the left eye became similarly affected; R. V. = $\frac{1}{50}$, L. V. = $\frac{6}{50}$; relative central scotomata were present in both eyes but there was no contraction of the peripheral fields; the ophthalmoscope showed optic atrophy. No consanguinity recorded. Bibl. No. 132.

Fig. 799. *Mansilla's Case.* Hereditary optic neuritis in four brothers and in the son of one of them. III. 4 became affected at the age of 24 years and though he never was quite blind, he died aged 45 with very little vision; one of his sons became affected at the age of 6 years. III. 1, aged 45 years, became affected at about the age of 10 years and worked in the fields with great difficulty. III. 2 was seen aged 29 years; he was an ill-developed youth of slight intelligence who worked in the fields; he had measles at the age of 18 and shortly after this noticed a marked diminution in his vision; now R. V. = finger counting at 2 m.; L. V. = finger counting at 30 cm.; colour vision was much altered; the peripheral fields were contracted in the upper parts and central scotomata appear to have been present; ophthalmoscopic examination showed a slight pallor of the discs and diminution of the vessels; radiographic examination showed dilatation of the sella turcica. III. 3, aged 25 years, was better nourished and much more intelligent than III. 2; he had good vision up to the age of 17 when he had measles and the onset of the disease followed; his affection was less severe than that of III. 2; his colour sense was normal; the peripheral fields were contracted in the upper regions; there was some dilatation of the sella turcica. III. 6 died young; III. 7, aged 21 years, had not yet shown any sign of the disease; III. 8—11 all saw well and those who were married had sons who also saw well. The parents and grandparents of this sibship were free from any ocular disease; there was no history of syphilis and no consanguineous marriages. Bibl. No. 134.

Fig. 800. *Taylor and Holmes's Case.* (The D. Family.) Three cases of hereditary optic atrophy in a sibship of nine. I. 1, aged 70, had good sight; I. 2 died twenty years ago (1913) from influenza; she had no ocular defect. II. 1 died of smallpox. II. 2 and II. 7 died from phthisis. II. 3, aged 47 (1910), the eldest living member of the sibship, has slight lack of control of the bladder sphincter and slight weakness of his legs; at the age of 43 he first noticed a failing in the sight of his left eye which rapidly became worse; about three years later the right eye also became affected; the patient had occasional attacks of giddiness at this period and was accustomed to smoke $\frac{1}{2}$ oz. of shag daily; now V. = $\frac{6}{9}$ in both eyes; discs were pale, vessels and retinae healthy; there was a central scotoma for white in the left and for colours in both eyes; there was no history of specific disease, no albuminuria or glycosuria. II. 4, aged 38 (1910), had had failing vision for eight years, the condition had gradually become worse and was associated with occasional attacks of giddiness; there was a history of a specific infection ten years ago and tabetic symptoms— sluggish reaction of pupils, absent knee-jerks, slight anaesthesia of lower limbs, etc.—were now present; there was no unsteadiness in walking; V. = $\frac{6}{10}$ in each eye; visual fields had central scotomata; the patient smoked $\frac{1}{4}$ oz. of shag daily. The recorders were of the opinion that II. 4 represents a case of Leber's disease complicating a case of tabes and not a case of tabetic optic atrophy.

II. 5, aged 33 (1910), noticed at the age of 27 that people walking down the street seemed suddenly to disappear as if in a mist; for three years the vision slowly deteriorated, then some improvement in the right eye was noted; the patient smoked $\frac{1}{4}$ oz. of shag daily and took an occasional glass of beer; now R. V. = $\frac{6}{9}$, L. V. = less than $\frac{6}{60}$; optic discs were pale, vessels normal; central scotomata were demonstrated in the fields. No consanguinity recorded. Bibl. No. 100.

Fig. 801. *Vossius's Case.* Hereditary optic atrophy in three brothers of a sibship of seven; their four sisters were free from disease; the onset was sudden in each case and in a short time vision was almost completely lost; two of the brothers became affected shortly after joining up for military service. No consanguinity recorded. Bibl. No. 113.

Fig. 802. *Thomsen's Case.* Hereditary optic atrophy in six brothers and in two of their maternal uncles; no information is given of other members of the family. Only one case appears to have been examined, he was now aged 39 and the onset of the disease was at the age of 21; he had been examined repeatedly and the condition remained quite stationary; bluish white discoloration of the disc, central scotomata with fairly good peripheral vision and red-green blindness are noted. The patient now, 17 years after the onset of the disease, was showing signs of some affection of the central nervous system associated with psychical disorder. No consanguinity recorded. Bibl. No. 31.

Fig. 803. *Sym's Case.* Leber's disease in a mother and her three sons. II. 5, aged 36, had always had good health except for occasional severe headaches, usually occipital; he is now almost blind; his sight was excellent until 1879 when it degenerated within a week to what it is now and has never changed for better or worse since; he was in Australia at this time and was aged 25; his headaches were then more frequent than usual; pupils were equal and dilated; media clear; optic discs perfectly white; arteries much diminished in size, veins moderately so; fundi were normal except for some slight disturbance of pigment immediately surrounding the discs; nystagmus was noted. The patient smoked in moderation and was strictly temperate; he showed no signs of syphilis. II. 1, aged 45, had always been subject to severe headaches, she lost her sight at the age of 51. I. 1, aged 77, saw well. II. 3, aged 47, had good health with no history of headaches but became blind after a severe attack of yellow fever at the age of 20. II. 4, aged 39, was strong and healthy with no history of headaches; he became blind at the age of 35. II. 2, aged 51, had good sight; she had four children, aged 12—18 years, who saw well. II. 5 had two sons, aged 6 and 8 years; he knew little of his grandparents or uncles and aunts but believed there was no case of

Plate LVIII.   DESCRIPTIONS OF PEDIGREE PLATES   397

blindness amongst them; a son of his mother's sister became blind at the age of 26; it was said to be due to a fall on the back of his head. The vision of other cases was not quite so bad as that of II. 5 and the onset was less sudden; all complained of a greyish cloud in the centre of the field, they rapidly became nearly blind but retained some peripheral vision. No consanguinity recorded. Bibl. No. 35.

Fig. 804. *Lawford's Case*. Four and probably six cases of optic atrophy in two sibships. I. 1 and 2 had seven children of whom II. 1, female aged 39, II. 2, female aged 37, II. 3, female aged 35 and II. 7, female aged 22, saw well; II. 4, James H., a police constable, aged 32, complained of a failure of vision during the last seven weeks; now R. V. = L. V. = $\frac{5}{6\cdot0}$; pupils reacted well to light and accommodation, fields were slightly contracted and discs pale; he had always had good health and had no history of syphilis; six months later vision was barely perception of light in each; pupils reacted well to light; discs were very white and vessels normal; II. 4 had always been colour-blind, his wife said he would mistake red for green or green for red. II. 5, Harry H., aged 28, was nearly blind; he was examined at the age of 22 when it was noted that his vision had gradually failed five years before, now advanced atrophy of the discs was present. II. 6, George H., aged 25, was nearly blind; the onset in his case was at the age of 19; in Sept. 1882 R. V. = L. V. = $\frac{6}{6}$; in Nov. 1882 V. = $< \frac{6}{6\cdot0}$ in each; in 1888 the discs were greatly atrophied and very white, retinal arteries diminished.

Three first cousins to this sibship, on the mother's side, were said to be nearly blind; one of these, a male, lost his sight gradually when about the age of 19; the other two, a male and female, "were said to be different." No consanguinity recorded. Bibl. No. 32.

Fig. 805. *Müller's Case*. Optic atrophy in three brothers. II. 1, aged 25, first noticed a diminution of vision at the age of 21; the onset of the defect was gradual and since a year ago he had only recognised people and colours with difficulty; pupils reacted normally; the papillae were atrophic and sharply outlined; vessels not narrowed; R. V. = L. V. = finger counting at 30 cm.; visual fields showed a severe concentric contraction but no central scotomata; colour sense was defective and blue only was recognised. II. 2, C. R., aged 23, had noticed for six months that his vision was failing, he now recognised people with difficulty; ophthalmoscopic appearances were as for II. 1; R. V. = $\frac{1}{2\cdot4}$, L. V. = $\frac{1}{1\cdot8}$. II. 3 was under treatment elsewhere for the same condition. Three younger siblings, aged 9 to 13 years, still saw well. The parents and their siblings were healthy and knew of no other cases of eye disease in their families. No consanguinity recorded. Bibl. No. 41.

Fig. 806. *Lor's Case*. Hereditary optic atrophy in three siblings. II. 3, female aged 28, was seen about a month after the onset of the disease when R. V. = $\frac{1}{3\cdot3}$, L. V. = finger counting at 50 cm.; central scotomata were present, absolute in the left eye, for colours only in the right; the patient complained of frequent headaches not definitely localised. II. 2, male aged 32, had had similar symptoms for 12 years; for him R. V. = $\frac{1}{7\cdot0}$, L. V. = $\frac{1}{1\cdot5}$; the discs were atrophied. II. 4, female, became affected at the age of 8 years. One sister was normal. This sibship was from the second marriage of the father who had a normal daughter from his first marriage. No consanguinity recorded. Bibl. No. 54.

Fig. 807. *Mooren's Case*. Optic atrophy in two brothers and a sister. II. 1, aged 22 (1859), came up for treatment; he improved greatly so that he was ultimately able to read medium-sized print; he needed strong convex spectacles. II. 2 saw well. II. 3 became affected when she was away from home and was not seen by Mooren until the disease was fairly advanced and there was grey discoloration of both nerves; after two years' treatment her vision was reduced further than on the first examination, but she was very persevering with her treatment and three years later was able to read J. 2. II. 4 became affected at 16; he also, after a long treatment, improved and was able to read the finest print without difficulty. The parents were unrelated and saw well. No consanguinity. Bibl. No. 17.

Fig. 808. *Kowalewski's Case*. Optic atrophy in three siblings and in their maternal uncle. I. 1 and 2 saw well. I. 3, aged 55, became affected whilst in the army at the age of 20, vision had remained stationary with no recovery since that time. I. 1 and 2 had four children, II. 1—4, of whom II. 1 became affected at the age of 20 when onset was rapid; the condition then remained stationary up to the time of his death from dropsy, at the age of 32; he had absolute central scotomata with normal peripheral fields. II. 2, aged 35, became affected at the age of 25; she had central scotomata with normal peripheral fields; all colours were recognised outside the scotomatous areas; she had been married seven years but had no children. II. 3, aged 26, was healthy and saw well. II. 4 became affected at the age of 21 when he suddenly noticed a cloud before both eyes and a marked diminution of vision; he had central scotomata with normal peripheral fields; he had an asymmetrical skull, also slight proptosis from shallowness of orbits; no syphilis or excess in use of alcohol or tobacco. No consanguinity recorded. Bibl. No. 74.

Fig. 809. *Leber's Case III*. Hereditary optic atrophy in a brother and sister; two sisters and the parents saw well. Pauline P., II. 2, aged 27, complained that her right eye became blinded at Christmas and her left eye had been weaker since Whitsuntide; the patient had had no illness and had had a headache since the previous day only; she was rather anaemic; R. V. = hand movements, L. V. = 10 J., with + 10 D., with difficulty; the right papilla was pale over the temporal half, the left papilla was normal when first seen but a few days later showed signs of neuritis; the condition progressed and four months later R. V. = hand movements with hesitancy, L. V. = finger counting at $\frac{1}{2}$ foot. II. 3, Alexander K., aged 23, had suffered for two years from amblyopia and the condition had slowly progressed; now R. V. with + 6 D. = 16 J., L. V. = 17 J.; he had bilateral large central scotomata; over a zone surrounding the scotoma vision was relatively normal but towards the periphery there was further defect in the fields. No consanguinity recorded. Bibl. No. 8.

Fig. 810. *Gunn's Case.* Optic atrophy in a mother and two of her three children. I. 1, Mrs C., aged 39 (1907), said that her sight had been bad ever since she could remember but that it was now better than it used to be; R. V. = $\frac{6}{36}$; central scotoma was noted for red and green; L. V. = $\frac{6}{9}$ with no central scotoma; fields showed marked peripheral limitations; the discs were greyish white, vessels normal. I. 1 married her first cousin and had three children. II. 1, Doris C., aged 8, had R. V. = $\frac{6}{12}$ partly, L. V. = $\frac{6}{18}$, her vision had been known to be defective since she was aged 5; no scotomata were present but fields showed great peripheral contraction; discs were very pale, the margin of the left being somewhat blurred. II. 2, Leo C., was aged 4; his mother considered that his vision had been defective for at least a year, probably longer; the discs were very pale, vessels normal. II. 3, aged 2$\frac{1}{2}$ years, had excellent sight and was always asked by the brother and sister to look for things for them. There was no history of defective sight in the family of either parent. Nettleship was unable in 1909 to obtain any further information of this family. Consanguinity. Bibl. No. 76.

Fig. 811. *Fuchs's Case.* (M Family.) Optic atrophy in three brothers; one brother, aged 49, and four sisters, aged 44, 37, 28 and 27 respectively, saw well; the parents were healthy and had no history of syphilis. II. 3, aged 43, became affected at the age of 32; he is now (1879) able to read very large print. II. 5 became affected at the age of 25; at 33 he was able to see to read very large print. II. 8, aged 26, became affected at the age of 22; two years later both discs were pale, especially in the temporal halves. In each case neuritis was noted at the time of onset. No consanguinity. Bibl. No. 15.

Fig. 812. *Fortunati and Mingazzini's Case.* Hereditary optic atrophy in a brother and sister; five sisters and one brother were unaffected; the parents saw well, they were consanguineous; the father died from cerebral haemorrhage, the mother from cardiac disease. II. 2, aged 22, became affected at 20; he had no syphilis and took alcohol in moderation. II. 8, aged 19, became affected at 16. Consanguinity. Bibl. No. 78.

Fig. 813. *Hutchinson's Case.* I. 1 and 2 were first cousins; there was no history of blindness or insanity in their families; they had three children, a boy, who died aged 4 months, and whose sight was believed to be good up to this time, and two girls, aged 4 and 1$\frac{1}{2}$ years respectively. II. 1 and 2 were both quite healthy, the eldest did not walk until the age of 2 years, the younger could now just stand, they were quite intelligent, clever children; II. 1 only saw enough to avoid large objects and would run against a chair; II. 2 could see the clock, but her mother believed her vision to be getting worse and was of the opinion that she could see well until six months ago; neither child was yet absolutely blind; in II. 1 both discs were perfectly white, the vessels shrunk to an extreme degree; in II. 2 the discs were white and the vessels very small but less so than in her sister. Consanguinity. Bibl. No. 6.

Fig. 814. *Wilbrand and Saenger's Case.* Hereditary optic atrophy in two brothers. The father, I. 1, had died 5 years ago from an undiagnosed disease; the mother, I. 2, had never had trouble with her eyes; two sisters, II. 1 and 2, had passed the age of 20 years and saw well. II. 3, J. Sch., aged 17, gave a history to the effect that two years ago his vision had suddenly diminished in both eyes, and the defect progressed for some time; he had, during this time, headaches and giddiness; the papillae now were white with blurred margins; vessels markedly narrowed; bilateral central scotomata were present, the left peripheral boundaries and colour fields were normal but in the right eye there was peripheral contraction of fields and colour-blindness over the whole field. II. 4, S. Sch., aged 12, said that the vision of both eyes had been diminishing for a year and a half and that during this time he had suffered from frequent headaches; both papillae were white; bilateral central absolute scotomata were present, peripheral fields were normal. No consanguinity recorded. Bibl. No. 101, p. 148.

Fig. 815. *Sedgwick's Case.* A man, whose brother became blind in both eyes between the ages of 55 and 60, had ten children, seven sons and three daughters. The eldest son, II. 1, became amaurotic in both eyes at the age of about 56. II. 2, aged 63, was normal. II. 3 died from paralysis at the age of 56. II. 4, aged 60, was partly paralysed. II. 5, aged 56, was normal. II. 6 died from paralysis; he became amaurotic in both eyes at the age of 48. II. 7 became amaurotic in the left eye at the age of 46. II. 8 became amaurotic in both eyes at the age of 42. II. 9, and II. 10 aged 38, were free from disease. We include this history with our cases of hereditary optic atrophy, following Nettleship and others, though there is uncertainty about the nature of the condition in the absence of clinical details and ophthalmoscopic examination. No consanguinity recorded. Bibl. No. 4.

Fig. 816. *Behr's Case.* Hereditary optic atrophy in two brothers; two maternal uncles had seen badly since the age of 21 years, otherwise there had been no eye or nerve disease in the family; three brothers, aged 30, 28 and 19 years respectively, saw well. II. 3, aged 26 (1909), became affected at the age of 24; II. 4, aged 23, became affected a few months ago (1909): in both cases vision was reduced to hand move-

Plate LVIII.   DESCRIPTIONS OF PEDIGREE PLATES   399

ments at 1—2 m.; large absolute central scotomata and slight peripheral contraction of the visual fields are noted in each brother; the discs showed atrophy of the temporal halves with slight neuritic signs and narrowing of vessels; in each case both eyes were affected at the same time; no nervous symptoms were present; there were no signs of syphilis; treatment led to no improvement in vision. No consanguinity. Bibl. No. 83.

Fig. 817. *Alexander's Case.* Optic neuritis in three b he   and in their maternal uncle. II. 3, Ludwig E., aged 20, had seen badly for four weeks; $V. = \frac{14}{200}$ with $+$ 10 D.; fields of vision were full and no scotomata were demonstrated; the papillae were blurred and margins indistinct, veins were dilated and tortuous, arteries normal; the patient had never been ill or had trouble with his eyes before, he was a non-smoker and drank little. II. 1, aged 29, had noticed diminution in his vision for four weeks, he was neither a drinker nor a smoker and had up to this time always seen well. $V. = \frac{14}{70}$ with $+$ 10 D.; no scotomata were present and the peripheral fields were full; ophthalmoscopic appearances were those of retrobulbar neuritis; three months later $V. = \frac{14}{200}$. II. 2, Hubert E., aged 23, came the same year complaining of the same difficulty as his brothers; ophthalmoscopic appearances and visual fields were found to be similar to those observed in their cases; $V. = \frac{10}{200}$.

A brother of the mother, I. 4, had been myopic and weak-sighted for a number of years and several different surgeons had treated him without improvement showing; he had been acutely ill three years ago and after this his sight became much worse. No other cases of similar eye disease had been known to occur in the family. No consanguinity. Bibl. No. 11.

Fig. 818. *Nettleship's Case.* Optic atrophy in four males, the sons of two sisters. II. 1, Mr F., a tutor, aged 28, had perfect sight until six months ago when his sight failed rapidly; the defect reached a maximum in 4 or 5 weeks and had since remained stationary; $V. = \frac{6}{70}$ in each eye and 16 J.; discs were sharply defined and rather pale on temporal side; retinal arteries were rather small. The patient reported that two sons of his mother's sister were similarly affected, both were heavy smokers and had drunk too much; the onset in one, a shopman, was at the age of 25—30, in the other, a small farmer, at the age of 35; the former had to give up business and never recovered, the farmer had bad vision for two years and was then said to have recovered his sight completely.

In 1902 Doyne wrote to Nettleship to enquire about II. 1, whose brother was under him and had reported that II. 1 had recovered; his vision had begun to improve nine months after the onset, in a few months he could see to read and now was headmaster of a large school and saw as well as ever he had seen; he resumed smoking within two years of his failure; his brother, II. 2, was a non-smoker.

II. 2, aged 25, noticed a defect in his right vision one month ago; now R. V. = finger counting at 3 feet. L. V. = $\frac{6}{9}$; pupils react readily, fundus normal or perhaps some lack of definition in the right disc. No consanguinity recorded. Bibl. No. 70.

Fig. 819. *Wilbrand and Saenger's Case.* Optic atrophy in two brothers. II. 1, J. H., aged 16, complained of a diminution of vision in both eyes which had been progressing for three months; he had been quite healthy during the last few years but had suffered from headaches during the time that his eyes had troubled him; there was no suspicion of infection or intoxication; general nervous system was normal; the temporal areas of the papillae were pale, peripheral fields were normal; no change was found after six months. II. 2, T. H., aged 13, had a similar defect of vision four years ago; he complained of headaches and giddiness; the whole papillae were pale and especially so on the temporal side. Two other siblings had healthy eyes. No consanguinity recorded. Bibl. No. 101, p. 147.

Fig. 820. *Behr and Takashima's Case.* Hereditary optic atrophy with associated defects of the central nervous system in three siblings of a sibship of six. This case was first described by Behr in 1909 when II. 3 and II. 5 were examined. II. 4 became affected at a later date and her condition is described by Takashima in 1913. II. 3 had learned to walk and to speak at the usual age and had never been seriously ill; he was now (1909) aged 13, and was said to have been weak-sighted for some considerable time and to have always had an unsteady gait; he attended a school for defective or backward children; at the age of 5 years he had suffered from night-screaming and was wet day and night; he was quarrelsome and subject to fits of temper; there was no history of fainting or of headaches; horizontal nystagmus was now present; the papillae were bluish white on the temporal side; vessels and periphery of fundus were normal; it was not possible to test the boundaries of the fields but bilateral central scotomata for colours were noted; R. V. = L. V. = $\frac{6}{10}$—$\frac{6}{35}$; refraction was emmetropic; he had now nocturnal enuresis and slight incontinence during the day; gait was stiff. II. 5, aged 11 (1909), walked and talked at the age of 2 years and had never been seriously ill; R. V. = L. V. = $\frac{6}{35}$; bilateral atrophy of temporal halves of discs is noted; he had slight horizontal nystagmus; relative central scotomata were noted in the fields, with no peripheral contraction; there was a definite hypertonus in all his extremities; reflexes were irritable and gait was unsteady. II. 4, aged 17 (1913), had no history of convulsions, she had occasional headaches and was backward at school; there was no incontinence of urine; she had always had weak sight and had not noticed it get worse at any time; R. V. = L. V. = $\frac{6}{15}$; some horizontal nystagmus was present on looking towards the right; atrophy of the temporal side of the disc is noted, vessels were normal, margin of disc was slightly blurred; gait was normal when her eyes were open but there was definite uncertainty and slight swaying when her eyes were closed; there was no definite hypertonus and no ataxy of the lower extremities. I. 1 was a drinker; I. 2 died from phthisis; II. 1, 2 and 6 were normal; there was no knowledge of nerve or eye trouble in the ancestry of this affected sibship. No consanguinity. Bibl. Nos. 83, 99.

Fig. 821. *Velhagen's Case.* Optic atrophy in three brothers, the only living children of parents who saw well and had never been seriously ill; there had been many other children who died young. II. 1 became affected at the age of 19; three weeks from the onset his vision was so diminished that he was unable to carry on his work; he was under treatment for three months but showed no improvement and from this time the condition remained stationary for $1\frac{1}{2}$ years; after this there was some improvement; no history of syphilis; the patient was not a drinker and smoked little; he complained of frequent headaches and loss of appetite; at the age of 27, R. V. with $-2 \cdot 0$ D. $= \frac{2}{20}$, L. V. with $-1 \cdot 0$ D. $= \frac{2}{20}$; discs were pale on the temporal side, retinal arteries very much narrowed; vision of red and green was defective; central scotomata were present but peripheral limits of fields were normal for white and blue. II. 2 became affected at the age of 25 when he noticed a rapid diminution of vision; seven months from the onset R. V. = finger counting at $2\frac{1}{2}$ m., L. V. = finger counting at 4 m.; central absolute scotomata were present and the patient was red-green blind; peripheral limits of fields were normal; atrophy of the optic nerve was noted, especially on the temporal side; the arteries were narrowed; the disease progressed for about three months and then became stationary; the patient was a moderate drinker; the condition did not respond to treatment. II. 3 was not examined but his brother reported that he had to give up his work as a seaman at the age of 20 on account of a sudden diminution of vision. No consanguinity recorded. Bibl. No. 51.

Fig. 822. *Lawford's Case.* A single case of optic atrophy in a sibship of seven of whom five died in infancy; the father was healthy; the mother had a history of three epileptic fits at long intervals but was healthy in other respects. II. 1, Walter H., aged 20, saw well until two years ago; now his vision was reduced to hand movements only; reaction of pupils to light was scarcely noticeable and advanced atrophy of the discs was noted. II. 2 died, aged 2, of "consumptive bowels"; II. 3 was healthy and intelligent; II. 4 was still-born; II. 5 died, aged one year; II. 6 and 7 died, aged one year, from diarrhoea. No consanguinity recorded. Bibl. No. 32.

Fig. 823. *Dodd's Case.* Hereditary optic atrophy in two sisters. I. 1 never had eye trouble, he was addicted to excessive alcoholism, as his father had been before him; I. 2 died, aged 54, from pneumonia; she was myopic but had otherwise no eye trouble. These parents had six daughters of whom three died in infancy, one was living and healthy and had never suffered from eye trouble; II. 3 became affected at the age of 12; the onset was associated with severe headaches and a progressive diminution of vision, which improved to some extent at a later date and then remained stationary until her death from accident at the age of 34. II. 4, aged 14, reported that about two months ago she began to have severe frontal headaches, two or three times a week; about one month later she noticed the sight of her right eye was failing and a few days later the left eye began to grow dim; R. V. $= \frac{12}{200}$, L. V. = finger counting at one foot; visual fields showed some contraction, perception of colours was poor; slight congestion was noted in the right eye, faint pallor of the temporal part of the disc in the left; large deep physiological cupping of the discs was present; eight months later R. V. = L. V. = finger counting at 3 feet; the discs were paler and the whole nerve was now atrophic though the condition was more marked on the temporal side.

No other member of the family was known to be affected. No consanguinity recorded. Bibl. No. 44.

Fig. 824. *Behr's Case.* Hereditary optic atrophy in two step-brothers who had the same mother; two sisters and a younger brother (aged 20) saw well; it is not clear to which sibship the two sisters belong. II. 1, aged 33 (1909), became affected at the age of 18; II. 4, aged 28 (1909), was affected at 24; vision in each case was reduced to finger counting at 1—3 m. No consanguinity recorded. Bibl. No. 83.

Fig. 825. *Fuchs's Case.* (W. Family.) Optic atrophy in three brothers. II. 3, Michael W., aged 49, complained that he had seen badly for about six months, he saw better in the evening; R. V. $= \frac{6}{9}$, L. V. $= \frac{6}{8}$; some concentric contraction of fields was noted, also central scotomata for red; outer halves of both discs were a little paler than normal. A few days later his brother Heinrich, aged 53, came for advice; the conditions found were identical in the two cases. Both brothers said that in America they had a brother, aged 59, who ten years ago had written that his eyesight was gradually diminishing and that he was afraid he would become blind; he had not been heard of since. No information is given of parents or other siblings. No consanguinity recorded. Bibl. No. 15.

PLATE LIX. Fig. 826. *Snell's Case.* Optic atrophy in three males and two females of a sibship of eight. The parents and grandparents of the affected siblings were known to have good sight. III. 1, male aged 33, was unaffected. III. 2, female aged 32, had R. V. $= \frac{3}{20}$, L. V. $= \frac{3}{20}$; discs were pale; colour sense feeble. III. 3, male aged 31, had good vision and normal fundi but he was colour-blind; he confused dark greens with reds and pale blue with pink. III. 4, aged 29, had R. V. = L. V. $= \frac{8}{200}$; he said that so far as he could tell his sight had always been the same; both discs were white, vessels were normal; he smoked one ounce of honeydew a week; his three young children saw well, and one of them, IV. 2, aged 3 years, was examined by the recorder. III. 6, aged 27, had R. V. = L. V. $= \frac{6}{9}$ with -1 D.; discs were pale, especially on the temporal side; colour vision weak. III. 7, female aged 25, was unaffected. III. 8, male aged 24, had R. V. = L. V.

Plate LIX.   DESCRIPTIONS OF PEDIGREE PLATES   401

$= \frac{6}{60}$; discs were pale and colour sense defective. III. 9, female aged 21, had R. V. = L. V. = $\frac{6}{24}$ with $- 6$ D.; discs were pale; crescents were noted; colour sense appeared to be normal.

All the affected members of this pedigree had had amblyopia from their earliest recollections; no scotomata were demonstrated and no contraction of the visual fields. No consanguinity recorded. Bibl. No. 55.

Fig. 827. *Knapp's Case.* Hereditary optic atrophy in three generations. II. 2, J. D. S., a German, aged 67, had emigrated to America at the age of 12; at the age of 24 he noticed, whilst driving a truck, that he could no longer see the street signs; from this time his sight gradually diminished until he was unable to see to read; during the last ten years it had again improved so that he can now see to read with the aid of glasses; R. V. = L. V. = $\frac{10}{200}$; he has central scotomata for white and colours, peripheral limits of fields normal; the temporal half of both discs was atrophic, nasal halves were discoloured and ill-defined; he smokes, but rarely takes alcohol. The parents, two brothers and three sisters of J. D. S. had normal vision; one of his siblings died aged 17, one at 30, one at 67; two were still living (1904). II. 2 had eight children of whom three sons died young, one daughter, III. 6, saw well; two sons, III. 2 and 3, and two daughters, III. 4 and 5, all became affected with optic atrophy during their early school years. III. 2 had two sons with normal vision; III. 5 was married but had no children; III. 4 married the son of her father's brother and had six children of whom three became affected. III. 4 was examined at the age of 33 when V. = $\frac{20}{200}$ in each; she had concentric contraction of fields but no central scotomata; no colour perception; discs were atrophic, especially in the temporal half. IV. 2, Henry S., aged 12, IV. 4, John S., aged 10, and IV. 5, Willie S., aged 8, all became affected at an early school age; in 1904 all had V. = $\frac{20}{200}$ in each; pupils normal; concentric contraction of fields; no colour perception; discs showed pronounced atrophy in the temporal areas, the nasal half in each was pale and ill-defined; the children were in other respects perfectly healthy, they had no central scotomata and retinal vessels were normal; they were of normal intellect and had no history of convulsions; they had all started to attend school at about the age of 6 when the defect was discovered. IV. 7 died aged 4, he had good vision up to this time. IV. 3 and 6 had good vision in 1909 when they were aged 15 and 9 respectively. Consanguinity. Bibl. Nos. 73 and 85, p. cxviii.

Fig. 828. *Du Seutre's Case.* Ten cases of hereditary optic atrophy in three generations. I. 1 became affected at the age of 40, she was in good health at the time; the disease made rapid progress; she died aged 70; both her sons and three of her five daughters became affected. Thus Paul, II. 2, became completely blind following a sudden onset at 46; he died from an aneurism at 75, leaving three daughters who saw well. Emma, II. 3, was less severely affected, the onset in her case was at the age of 30 but the progress of the disease was arrested after a few weeks, leaving her with enough vision to go about alone and look after her house; she died at 70 from tumour of the stomach. II. 4, Berthe, died at 70; she and her two sons saw well. II. 6, Alcide, became affected at about 16, the condition was very severe in his case and vision was reduced to perception of light; he had good health and died at 60. II. 7, Zilda, became affected at 35, she was able to see to go about alone and look after her house; she died at 60, was married, but had no children. II. 8, Alice S., had a progressive diminution of vision which set in at about the age of 28, six months later the condition became stationary; she could not see to read but could go about alone; she died, aged 63, from pleurisy; of her five children four became affected. II. 10, Celine, aged 68, saw well.

Of the children of II. 8, the eldest, III. 8, Gustave, aged 39, saw well up to the age of 33 when his vision diminished without apparent cause; the defect progressed for two months and then became stationary; he had to give up his work but could read large characters and tell the time by his watch. III. 9, Marcel M., aged 37, was always healthy and saw well up to the age of 21 when he became affected, he saw better in a dim light but three months after the onset had to give up his work as a tailor; vision was now reduced to perception of light in both eyes; he could not go about alone unless the road was familiar; pupils reacted normally; discs were white, edges not very well defined; veins were dilated, arteries a little narrowed; radiograph showed a normal sella turcica. III. 10, Hélène, aged 33, had good health and normal vision; her three children were healthy, but still young. III. 12, Alice, aged 30, had influenza, and a month later noticed a diminution of vision; the condition progressed for four months and then became stationary; she now, aged 31, can tell the time by her watch but cannot read and can only go about with difficulty; she has four children; one little girl complains of headache. III. 14, Albert, aged 24, had always been healthy but became affected with the family disease at the age of 17 and could now read and write with difficulty; he had severe headaches in childhood and these became worse at the time of the onset of the disease; the condition progressed for two months and had since been stationary; he had to give up his work but could see to go about alone; he was totally colour-blind, pupillary reflexes normal; fields showed no peripheral contraction; relative central scotomata in right, absolute in left; the discs were of a uniform greyish white colour with well-defined edges; veins normal, arteries narrowed; Wassermann test negative. III. 8 married his first cousin III. 5, daughter of the affected II. 2; his only child, a son, was still young. Consanguinity. Bibl. No. 117.

Fig. 829. *Snell's Case.* Optic atrophy in two males and one female of a sibship consisting of four males and two females; the parents and grandparents had good sight; there were other children of the affected sibship who died in infancy. III. 1 and III. 3 were seen in 1883 and in 1896, at the latter date they were aged 40 and 32 respectively. III. 1 had V. $= \frac{7}{300}$ in each eye; his sight began to fail at the age of 13 or 14 but the condition had now been stationary for some years; discs were white; vessels slightly narrowed; fields showed concentric contraction as well as central scotomata; he was colour-blind and matched greens with greys, pinks with light blues, reds with browns and purples; he was married but had no children. III. 3 also had V. $= \frac{7}{300}$ in each eye and pale discs, but colour vision was normal; she was married but had no children; her sight had been good up to the age of about 13 and the condition had now been stationary for some years. III. 5 was said to be similarly affected, the onset in his case also being at about the age of 13; he was married and had three children who saw well. The unaffected siblings, III. 2, 4 and 7, had children whose eyes were normal so far as the recorder was able to discover. No consanguinity. Bibl. No. 55.

Fig. 830. *Hensen's Case.* Hereditary optic atrophy in six males. II. 1, aged 70 (1916), had seen well up to 1870 when, at the age of 24 after a fatiguing march with the army, he suddenly became affected with severe bilateral amblyopia; he was under treatment for a long time but there was no improvement; now he had large bilateral central scotomata; papillae were absolutely white; R. V. = L. V. = finger counting at 1 m.; the patient had no headaches but complained of bright spots and lights before his eyes. One brother and three sisters of II. 1 apparently saw well or were not known to have been affected. The three sisters were married, none of them had sons and none of their daughters appear to have been themselves affected, though four of them had affected sons. Thus IV. 1, Franz K., aged 27, had always had healthy eyes and had been on active service from 1909—11; he had served again in the army from Aug. 1, 1914, and kept well until Oct. 1916, when he caught cold and then noticed that his vision had become so bad that he could not see to read; he was treated in several hospitals and for some time malingering was suspected; there was no history of excess in the use of alcohol or tobacco; no syphilis; the patient had suffered from headaches since the onset and complained of bright spots and lights before his eyes; vision was reduced to finger counting in the right eye at $\frac{5}{4}$ m., in the left at $\frac{1}{2}$ m.; the temporal halves of papillae were pale and atrophic, margins slightly blurred; veins were dilated and tortuous; slight peripheral contraction of fields and large central scotomata were demonstrated; after four months' treatment and seven months from the onset the defect had increased. IV. 2, the only brother of IV. 1, Wilhelm K., aged 24 (1916), had seen well up to about 1903 when he became affected; he was almost completely blind for some time but after a year a progressive improvement set in, especially in the left eye; the condition had now been stationary for some time, R. V. $= \frac{4}{60}$, L. V. $= \frac{6}{12}$; papillae were markedly pale; vessels normal; a ring scotoma and peripheral contraction were noted in each field.

IV. 3, Leopold B., aged 27 (1916), saw well up to Aug. 1912, when after a fatiguing march he became suddenly affected with a severe amblyopia, and was almost blind for a time; the condition progressed for eight months, then became stationary and later showed some improvement; R. V. = L. V. $= \frac{6}{24}$; slight peripheral contraction of fields was noted; papillae were pale, temporal halves white; vessels normal. IV. 3 had two brothers, one of whom died young, the other was not yet affected.

IV. 11, Robert M., aged 14, was affected; R. V. = L. V. $= \frac{1}{24}$, he had not improved under treatment and nerves were almost white; he had three sisters and one brother who had not yet become affected. IV. 16, Bernhard R., aged 16, was affected; he had a sudden onset and showed an improvement after five months' treatment; he had never been ill and had seen well up to this time; vision was reduced to finger counting in the left at $\frac{1}{2}$ m., in the right V. $= \frac{6}{60}$; bilateral central scotomata were noted. The parents and siblings of IV. 16 were healthy. No consanguinity recorded. Bibl. No. 111.

Fig. 831. *Wagenmann's Case.* Optic atrophy in twin brothers and in their maternal uncle. II. 1, aged 16, complained of diminution of vision; it was found that R. V. $= \frac{6}{24}$, L. V. $= \frac{6}{12}$; fields were full, colours were recognised, retinal veins were tortuous; in other respects the ophthalmoscopical appearances were normal. A month later R. V. = finger counting at 6 m., L. V. $= \frac{6}{12}$; no scotomata were present. Nine months later the patient's twin brother came, complaining also of amblyopia; his colour vision was normal and fields were full; the papillae were reddened. At this date the first brother had V. = finger counting at 5 m.; his colour vision for red and green was now defective; papillae were whitish on the temporal side. In other respects both brothers were healthy; they had ten healthy living siblings; their parents were dead. An uncle, whilst serving in the army, had developed amblyopia and had to leave the service. No consanguinity recorded. Bibl. No. 80.

Fig. 832. *Strzeminski's Case.* Hereditary optic atrophy in two females and five males of three generations. II. 2, aged 58, looked healthy; her pupils were dilated and reacted fully to light, normally to accommodation; she had central scotomata in each field, also some peripheral contraction; no perception of colour; L. V. = R. V. $= \frac{1}{30}$; both papillae were bluish white with blurred contours; considerable narrowing of vessels; atrophy of the optic nerve following neuritis with an onset at the age of 25 was noted. The mother of II. 2 died twelve years ago; she was reported to have had a sudden diminution of vision at about the age of 25 years and to have been unable to read though she could go about alone without difficulty. II. 2 had two daughters who were perfectly healthy and saw well, and five sons who were all amblyopic and of whom one was epileptic, another was mentally defective. III. 2, a Russian priest, aged 36, complained

PLATE LIX.   DESCRIPTIONS OF PEDIGREE PLATES   403

of amblyopia which had come on twelve years ago; pupils were equal and dilated, reactions were feeble to light, normal to accommodation; the fields had normal boundaries with central scotomata; L. V. = $\frac{1}{15}$, R. V. = $\frac{1}{15}$; within the scotomata no colours were recognised, outside green and violet were not recognised; temporal half of disc was completely white in both eyes, contours were blurred; vessels were narrowed; the patient suffered from migraine but had no other pains in eyes or head; he could not see to read or write but later some improvement allowed him to do so with difficulty; he was not a smoker and took a very moderate amount of alcohol; no history of syphilis or of any serious illness except pneumonia at the age of 16; he was married and had healthy children under the age of 15. III. 4, aged 35, also a Russian priest, was very similar to his brother with regard to general health and the state of his eyes though he did not suffer from migraine; pupillary reactions, visual fields and ophthalmoscopic appearances were all as described for III. 2; R. V. = L. V. = $\frac{1}{15}$; no history of syphilis or excessive use of alcohol or tobacco; the onset in his case was at the age of 25; he also was married and had healthy children under the age of 15. No consanguinity recorded. Bibl. No. 61.

Fig. 833. *Buisson's Case.* Optic atrophy in a mother and in all her three living children. I. 3 died, aged 35, of phthisis; her sister, I. 2, died blind and paralysed at 50; II. 4, daughter of I. 3, aged 58, had a progressive failure of vision which commenced at the age of 48; at 50 she had an attack of hemiplegia; she was found to have double optic atrophy, pupillary reactions normal; II. 3, sister of II. 4, died blind at 58, she had some cardiac affection; either she or another sibling had a son who was blind at 30. III. 3, daughter of II. 4, became amblyopic at 33; several months after the onset R. V. = $\frac{1}{15}$, L. V. = finger counting at 1 m.; two years later R. V. = finger counting at 2 m., L. V. = finger counting at 1 m.; discs were white, pupils reacted normally; she had central scotomata with normal peripheral fields; red-green blindness was noted; this patient had two children, aged 8 and 7 years respectively. III. 5 became affected during military service and recovered. III. 6 became affected at 27; two months after the onset R. V. = $\frac{1}{3}$, L. V. = $\frac{1}{15}$; discs were a little blurred and oedematous; veins tortuous, arteries rather narrow; he did not recognise blue or yellow; slight deafness was noted in left ear; the one daughter of III. 6 died young. Five further members of this sibship died young, two were still-born. No consanguinity recorded. Bibl. No. 59.

Fig. 834. *Ginzburg's Case.* Hereditary optic atrophy in five males and four females of three generations. I. 2 lived to old age and was twice married; by his first wife he had one son and five daughters of whom the son, II. 2, and one daughter, II. 4, were amblyopic; by his second wife he had many children of whom one daughter, II. 9, was amblyopic; there was no knowledge of her siblings. II. 2 had a granddaughter, IV. 1, who was night-blind. II. 4 married II. 5 who died aged 76; II. 5, his brother, II. 6, and his five sisters always saw well. II. 4 and 5 had four children, of whom III. 5, Samuel S., aged 60, had been amblyopic since his youth, and vision was now reduced to finger counting at 1·5 m., not improved by glasses; paleness in the temporal half of the right disc was noted and a bluish white atrophy of the whole of the left disc, margins of discs were clearly defined; vessels were narrowed; there was some contraction of the peripheral fields but no central scotomata for white or colours. III. 7, Rosa, died aged 50, she was married but had no children; she had been amblyopic since her youth and had been treated with injections of strychnine for atrophy of the optic nerve. III. 8, Raisa, had been amblyopic since her youth but during the climacteric her vision had certainly become worse; now R. V. = 0·1, L. V. = fingers at 2 m., not improved by glasses; discs were greyish white with clear margins; vessels narrowed; peripheral fields contracted, central colour scotomata in left only; III. 8 was married to III. 9, who died, aged 43, from typhus, he had always seen well; their only child, IV. 6, was still-born. III. 10 died at the age of 6 years.

III. 5 was twice married, by his first wife he had two sons and by his second wife one son, he was not related to his first wife, his second wife was a daughter of his cousin; his three sons, Boris, aged 26, Leo, aged 22, and Israel, aged 15, all suffered from partial atrophy of the optic nerve with marked lowering of vision.

IV. 3, aged 26, noticed a diminution of his vision at the age of 20, now temporal halves of papillae were conspicuously pale with clear outlines; vessels and peripheral fields were normal; no central scotomata were found. IV. 4, aged 22, noticed a diminution of vision at the age of 8, a further rapid degeneration occurred between the ages of 13 and 16; he was examined at the age of 12 when he suffered from headaches; now V. = fingers at 2 m., not improved by glasses; discs were pale and clearly outlined, vessels narrowed; fields for white were normal, fields for red were diminished and green was not recognised by central vision. IV. 5, aged 15, noticed his vision failing at the age of 7 to 8 years, now R. V. = fingers at 1·5 m., L. V. = fingers at 2 m., not improved by glasses; discs were pale, especially their temporal halves, margins were clear; fields for white and red were contracted; small relative central scotomata for red.

X-ray photographs were taken of the three brothers; in IV. 3 the base of the skull appeared to be normal; in IV. 4 the fundus of the sella turcica was wider than normal, in IV. 5 the sella was very small and its entrance narrow. III. 6 was examined and found to be normal. All the patients examined were quite healthy. Consanguinity. Bibl. No. 125.

Fig. 835. *Lauber and Guzmann's Case.* Optic atrophy in four brothers and two sisters of a large sibship. I. 1 was known to have been blind from his youth; the four grandparents of the affected sibship

saw well. III. 2, the father, aged 73, saw well. III. 3, the mother, died at 53, from a disease of the liver·
Three brothers, IV. 10, died at the age of a few months; IV. 11 died aged 11, IV. 12 died aged 15 months
and IV. 13 died aged 13 years. IV. 1, female, aged 53, saw well. IV. 2, J. B., born 1860, became affected
1882, when on military service; the condition progressed for five months and then became stationary; in
1911 both discs were white; arteries very narrow, veins tortuous, peripheral limits of fields normal; R. V.
= L. V. = hand movements. IV. 3, A. B., born 1862, became affected 1883; in 1911, R. V. = finger counting
at 50 cm., L. V. = finger counting at 1 m.; pupillary reactions sluggish; discs were white with blurred
margins, arteries narrow, veins normal; peripheral limits of fields normal. IV. 4, female, aged 47, saw well.
IV. 5, K. B., born 1868, became affected 1895; after four months, during which time he was treated with
mercury and potassium iodide, vision was reduced to hand movements at $\frac{1}{2}$ m.; in 1911 V. = perception of
light; neuritic atrophy was noted. IV. 6, aged 44, had always seen well until five months ago when she
had a sudden diminution of vision; she had rachitis as a child and rheumatism since but was otherwise
healthy; her five children were healthy and saw well; R. V. = finger counting at 30 cm., L. V. = finger
counting at 20 cm.; temporal halves of discs were white, margins blurred, arteries narrowed; central
scotomata were demonstrated for all colours with normal outer limits of fields. IV. 8, female, born 1872,
became affected in 1902 in the left eye only, on Oct. 2, R. V. = $\frac{6}{5}$, L. V. = $\frac{6}{9}$, on Oct. 18, L. V. = $\frac{6}{12}$, Oct. 29,
L. V. = $\frac{6}{24}$, Oct. 30, L. V. = $\frac{6}{36}$, five weeks later, L. V. = $\frac{6}{60}$, the lateral half of the disc was pale and there
was marked concentric contraction of the field; right eye was normal; two years later the vision in the left
eye was as good as in the right; a year later again IV. 8 had a still more marked lowering of vision in the
left eye which improved as before and she was now able to see to read with her left eye. IV. 9, born 1876,
became affected in 1898; in 1896 he was examined and his vision was normal, in 1899, R. V. = $\frac{1}{3}$, L.V. =
finger counting at 2 m.; the discs were a whitish green colour, the arteries narrower than normal; large
central scotomata were present; peripheral limits of fields normal. No consanguinity recorded. Bibl.
Nos. 68, 96.

Fig. 836. *Mathieu's Case.* Hereditary optic atrophy in five males and five females of three generations.
II. 3 had excellent vision up to the age of 50 when she became amblyopic in both eyes and was unable to
see to sew, but could go about alone; the condition remained stationary until her death at the age of 69;
her parents saw well, but a brother of her father had bad eyes; she had five brothers and two sisters who
all saw well, but one of her sisters, II. 7, had affected sons. II. 3 had six children of whom III. 2 was
born several years before her mother's marriage and nothing was known of her father; she saw well up to
the age of 40 when she suddenly became amblyopic in the left eye only, the right eye became affected eight
years later; she had good general health but when seen at the age of 58 it was impossible for her to sew
and she could scarcely see well enough to go about alone; her pupils were dilated and neither reacted to
light nor to accommodation; atrophy of the optic nerve was noted, discs uniformly discoloured, arteries
narrowed; R. V. = finger counting at 50 cm., L. V. can scarcely see fingers; right eye recognised blue, red and
yellow, left eye recognised no colour. III. 3 died aged 2 days; III. 4 died aged 34 when her vision was just
beginning to fail. III. 5, now aged 51, reported that he had a sudden onset at 22, both eyes became affected
at the same time, he saw better in a dull light; pupils, now slightly dilated, reacted very sluggishly to
light, more definitely to accommodation; there was bluish grey discoloration of the discs, especially in the
temporal sections; arteries were narrowed; R. V. = finger counting at 20 cm., L. V. = finger counting at 30 cm.;
right eye recognised blue, left eye recognised yellow and blue. III. 6, female, aged 45, began to lose her
vision six years ago, the defect progressed for six months during which time she had very severe temporal
headaches, later she complained of giddiness; she saw better in a dim light; pupils were normal and showed
normal reactions; discs were bluish grey, especially in the temporal section; arteries were narrowed, veins
normal; vision reduced to finger counting in the right at 30 cm., in the left at 20 cm.; blue was the only
colour recognised. III. 9 had normal vision but one of her sons was affected.

II. 7, sister to II. 3, had two illegitimate sons, III. 12 and 14, by different fathers, who were affected;
she also had two normal sons, III. 11 and 13, who were soldiers, and a daughter, aged 27, who was still
normal; the exact parentage of these siblings or half siblings is obscure. The mother, II. 7, had good eyes
at the time of her death at the age of 64. III. 12, aged 47, became affected at the age of 32, the condition
progressed for a year and had since been stationary, he now saw better in a dim light; pupils were dilated
and reacted feebly to light and accommodation; atrophy of the disc was present; vessels normal; R. V. = $\frac{1}{10}$,
L. V. = $\frac{1}{9}$; both eyes became affected simultaneously. III. 14, aged 43, became affected in the right eye
only at the age of 28, the left eye became affected two or three years later; pupils slightly dilated, reaction
to light scarcely perceptible, no reaction to accommodation; discs were white, especially so in the temporal
section, very marked narrowing of arteries is noted; absolute colour-blindness; vision in both eyes was
reduced to hand movements. All the affected members of this generation had pterygium.

III. 2 had fourteen children of whom three boys died young, four girls were dead at the time of the
record, three sons and two daughters saw well, and one son, IV. 2, and one daughter, IV. 8, were affected.
IV. 2, aged 32, had a sudden onset in both eyes at the age of 18; no history of headaches; pupils dilated,
reacting feebly to light, not at all to accommodation; discs were pale, arteries slightly narrowed; R. V. =
finger counting at 15 cm., L. V. = finger counting at 10 cm.; right eye recognised blue and red, left eye

perceived blue only; the patient was married and had three healthy children. IV. 8, aged 23, had a sudden onset in both eyes at the age of 19, with no associated pain in head or eyes; she had suffered from arthritis of the knee at the age of 18 for three months but had no history of other illness; pupils dilated; vision became very bad and remained so for about five months after which the left eye improved, now R. V. = finger counting at 20 cm., L. V. = 1 m. ; right eye recognises blue and red, left eye perceives all colours except green; edges of both discs were blurred and surrounded by exudate. III. 6 had six young children, the eldest boy, aged 15, suffered from epilepsy. III. 9 was married twice and had seven children of whom one son and two daughters died young, two daughters, aged 25 and 20 respectively, had good sight, one son, IV. 16, was affected, and a son, aged 10, was not examined but was reported to have defective vision. IV. 16, aged 23, had excellent sight as a child but he had a sudden onset of amblyopia at the age of 15 associated with severe headaches, and movement of head or eyes made the pain worse; vision diminished for one year and then some improvement occurred during the next two years, especially in the left eye; pupils were normal with a normal reaction; discs pale especially in the temporal section; arteries very narrow; R. V. = finger counting at 25 cm., L. V. = finger counting at 1 m.; defective perception of all colours in each eye. The father of IV. 16 had good eyes. No consanguinity recorded. Bibl. No. 66.

Plate LX. Fig. 837. *Hogg's Case.* Hereditary optic atrophy in twenty-five males and two females of five generations. The recorder describes the cases as "retrobulbar neuritis followed by atrophy of the papillo-macular fibres"; there is no definite tendency to nervous disease in the stock but some of the patients have suffered periodically from frontal headaches. This pedigree has not been used in any statistical analysis of cases for there was difficulty in obtaining information of some of the families and we are told that there may be more persons affected than are here given; moreover, the ages of individuals are not given, so that there is no means of determining which members may still develop the disease as they reach the critical age; the age of onset is given in no case. All the males of generations II and III are affected and all the females of these generations transmit the defect; every case in the pedigree has arisen through an unaffected mother. The points specially requiring verification are the unaffectedness of all the children of III. 5 and of IV. 11 and the number of unaffected sons of III. 15 and III. 17; we need further to know the ages of unaffected members of generations V and VI. No details of any individual cases are given. No consanguinity recorded. Bibl. No. 151.

Fig. 838. *Schönenberger's Case.* Hereditary optic atrophy in nine males and one female of three generations. I. 1 died aged 58, at which time he had good vision; he and I. 2 had four sons and four daughters of whom II. 2, born 1828, lived in America, but was said to have had good vision; II. 3 was affected and lived to the age of 81; II. 4 died aged 76, having had good vision, her three children were unaffected but her only daughter had affected sons. II. 6 was affected; he died aged 81. II. 7 died, aged 70, with good vision. II. 8 died aged 28; she saw well but both her sons were affected. II. 10 died aged 74; he is entered on the chart as an affected member but is also said to have seen well. II. 11 died aged 67 and saw well herself but had four affected children. In generation III there were four affected members of whom III. 10 died in 1912; he had seven children of whom IV. 9 died aged 14, IV. 11 was examined and had good vision, IV. 12 died aged 2 years and IV. 13 died aged 1½ years; IV. 8, 10 and 14 were said to see well. III. 11 became affected at the age of 28 years; he had always been delicate; his optic discs were greyish white and atrophic, the vessels were narrowed and he had a bilateral scotoma for green; R. V. = L. V. = $\frac{1}{24}$; he is by an error entered in the original chart as unaffected. III. 11 had three adult children who were examined and who saw well. II. 11 had four children of whom IV. 15 and 17 were examined and saw well. III. 16, Sophie Hi., became affected at the age of 24; her discs were greenish white; arteries and veins markedly narrowed; R. V. = L. V. = hand movements at 4 m.; this patient had nystagmus and a divergent concomitant strabismus. III. 18 was affected but no information is given of his case. Other affected members of the family are IV. 2, Adolf E., who became affected at the age of 20; his pupillary reactions were normal; R. V. = L. V. = $\frac{3}{60}$—$\frac{3}{60}$; the discs were markedly pale, especially in the temporal quadrants. IV. 4, Julius E., was affected; he died, aged 51, leaving four children, who saw well at ages varying from 27 to 8 years; one of his children had died aged 9 years. IV. 6, Karl E., became affected at the age of 12 years; his discs were pale, greenish white, and clearly outlined; the vessels were much narrowed; R. V. = L. V. = $\frac{4}{60}$, not improved by glasses; he had two children, aged 17 and 18 years respectively. No consanguinity recorded. Bibl. No. 138.

Fig. 839. *Schilling's Case.* (Taken from Nettleship.) I. 2 was twice married; by her first husband she had three sons who became affected with hereditary optic atrophy at the ages of 14, 10 and 29 years respectively; by her second husband she had two sons who became similarly affected at the ages of 11 and 20 years respectively, and a daughter, II. 6, who at the age of 20 became extremely amblyopic in both eyes; her vision was reduced to finger counting at 12 inches, visual fields were contracted, no ophthalmoscopic changes had occurred; she recovered perfectly and Nettleship suggests that the condition was probably a hysterical amblyopia. No information was given concerning the vision of the parents. No consanguinity recorded. Bibl. No. 13.

Fig. 840. *Favier's Case.* Hereditary optic atrophy in three or probably four males and in two females

of three generations. III. 1, Lucien T., aged 19 complained that his vision had diminished during the past month; examination revealed a severe grade of amblyopia; the right eye could detect hand movements only, the left eye had a fiftieth of the normal vision; pupils reacted normally, the periphery of the visual fields was normal; the fundus presented discs which were a little pale with slightly blurred margins and narrowed vessels; a number of tests were made, the results of which were all negative and retrobulbar neuritis of unknown cause was diagnosed; treatment was carried on for a year with no improvement and at the end of this time R. V. = L. V. = $\frac{2}{100}$; the peripheral fields of vision were unchanged, but large central scotomata were present. Shortly after this the man died from encephalitis lethargica; the recorder was away on holiday at the time and no post-mortem examination was obtained. Three years later III. 3, Gaëtan T., aged 20, complained of a diminution of vision during the last month; vision was found to be $\frac{1}{100}$, peripheral visual fields were unaffected and the appearances of retrobulbar neuritis were present.

The parents of III. 1 and 3 had thirteen children of whom III. 2, III. 4 and III. 7 died young; III. 5 and 6 were two living females, aged 18 and 16 years respectively, other living members of the sibship were aged 14, 12, 11, 8, 6 and 5 years respectively; thus no other member of the family had yet reached the age at which the disease most commonly manifests itself. The father, II. 4, was an inveterate drinker; he had three brothers and one sister living and normal, and one sister had died of whom no information was available. The mother, II. 5, appeared to be quite normal; she had two sisters who were dead, but she could not say from what cause. The mother's maternal aunt, I. 4, married to a drinker, had three children of whom a son, II. 8, now aged 50, had at the age of 20 years become affected in the same way as III. 1 and 3; his vision had always remained very weak with scarcely appreciable variations. II. 9, aged 49, became affected at 47 years and II. 10, aged 43, became similarly affected at the age of 42 years. The mother's maternal uncle, I. 3, now dead, was reported to have been similarly affected but the recorder had been unable to verify this report sufficiently to be quite sure of the nature of the defect in this case. The patient, III. 3, received rather drastic treatment but no improvement of his visual troubles followed. No consanguinity recorded. Bibl. No. 140.

Fig. 841. *Schönenberger's Case.* Hereditary optic atrophy in a brother and sister; no other members of the family were known to have suffered from eye disease. The two affected siblings were examined by Vogt, but the condition found is not described and the age of the patients is not given, nor the age at which they became affected. The brother, IV. 2, was married and had three unaffected children, but we have no means of judging whether they had reached the age at which liability to the disease becomes manifest. The sister, IV. 3, married her third cousin and had two children, a son who died aged 21 years and a daughter who died aged 12. Consanguinity. Bibl. No. 138.

Fig. 842. *Leitner's Case 1.* (Taken from Nettleship.) Hereditary optic atrophy in six males of two generations. I. 1 and 2 were normal; they had three sons who became affected at the ages of 23, 24 and 25 respectively, also one normal daughter, II. 2, who married and had three affected sons and one normal son. III. 2, 3 and 4 became affected at the ages of 23, 24 and 25 respectively. No consanguinity recorded. Bibl. Nos. 53 and 85, p. clxxvi.

Fig. 843. *Baudot's Case.* Hereditary optic atrophy in five males and one female of three generations. I. 2 had a son, II. 3, who became affected at the age of 33, and a normal daughter who had however an affected son. I. 3 was affected but we are not told the age of onset of the disease in his case. I. 4 had a son, II. 6, who became affected at the age of 25 and a daughter, II. 5, who became affected at 24. Thus all members of generations I and II were either themselves affected or they transmitted the defect. II. 5 had a son, III. 4, who became affected at the age of 13. II. 2 had three children of whom only one was at present affected; the age of the two unaffected siblings is not given, but they are probably still of an age at which the disease might become manifest and cannot be regarded as definitely normal. III. 2, aged 23, was the only case examined; he complained that his vision had progressively diminished during the last two years and that now he had to be led about; vision was reduced to perception of light; the papillae were greyish white; arteries were diminished in size; X-ray of sella turcica and sphenoidal cells revealed no abnormality; the patient was normal in other respects and there was no history of sexual excess or abuse in the use of nicotine or alcohol; he improved with treatment and after six months R. V. = $\frac{1}{25}$, L. V. = $\frac{1}{30}$. No consanguinity. Bibl. No. 127.

Plate LXI. Fig. 844. *Fisher's Case.* Five cases of hereditary optic atrophy in two generations. The recorder suggests that the disease may be due to an inherited tendency to disorder of the hypophysis. A. G., II. 1, aged 14, was quite well up to his 12th year, when his sight rapidly failed so that he had after this to be taught in schools for the blind. V. = $\frac{6}{18}$ for right eye, $\frac{6}{60}$ for left; peripheral fields full but central scotoma in each; optic discs very pale; X-ray of sella turcica normal; Wassermann test negative. R. G. II. 2, aged $11\frac{1}{2}$, had rapid onset of failure of sight in 1915. V. = $\frac{6}{60}$ for each eye; R. optic disc a little hyperaemic, L. disc a trifle pale; no peripheral limitation of fields but central scotoma in each. In 1916 all hyperaemia had passed off and both discs were pale. Wassermann test negative; X-ray of sella turcica showed no enlargement and no distortion of outline, but the depression appeared to be filled in with

Plate LXI.   DESCRIPTIONS OF PEDIGREE PLATES   407

something which gave a cellular or honeycomb-like shadow. I. 5 had good sight. I. 4, dead, was probably affected, she had two brothers who were so blind that they had to be taught in schools for the blind. I. 5 by his second wife had seven children, who saw well but were all young. No consanguinity recorded. Bibl. No. 108.

Fig. 845. *Fisher's Case.* Three cases of hereditary optic atrophy in two generations. The recorder suggests that the condition may be due to over activity, with enlargement, of the pituitary body associated with the period of adolescence or with the climacteric in women. II. 2, H. G., now aged 21 (1917), had good sight till August 1916, when it rapidly failed; in November he could barely count fingers at the distance of a foot with either eye; he saw better at night than in daylight; discs were pale; X-ray of sella turcica showed definite expansion with irregularity in definition and shape of the posterior clinoid process; no glycosuria; Wassermann test negative. II. 1, F. G., aged 22, saw well till about a year ago; now R. V. = L. V. = $\frac{1}{60}$; no error of refraction; an old patch of choroido-retinitis was noted in the right eye; optic discs were not obviously atrophic; fields were full; X-ray showed a normal sella turcica. A maternal uncle, I. 3, became affected at the age of 21. No consanguinity recorded. Bibl. No. 110.

Fig. 846. *Pollock's Case.* Two cases of Leber's disease in a brother and sister. II. 3, aged 11 (1915), had in October R. V. = L. V. = $\frac{6}{24}$; the discs were slightly congested; in December the discs were paler and vision became rapidly worse until, in September 1916, it was reduced to hand movements only; X-ray of sella turcica showed a shadow like a small bean in and a little below the centre of the fossa. The patient was then treated by organotherapy and improved; in February 1917, V. = $\frac{6}{60}$; this improvement ceased and vision deteriorated when the treatment was stopped for a month; discs were pale on the outer side, fundi were otherwise normal; central scotomata were noted, also a general contraction of the peripheral fields. II. 4, aged 8, gave a similar history with a similar X-ray picture. The mother, I. 2, had a divergent strabismus of the left eye and myopia of 30 D.; her fundus was normal apart from a myopic crescent; she had had two miscarriages and one still-born child before the birth of II. 3, also another miscarriage after the birth of her son; there was no history of blindness in her family; Wassermann test was negative for the mother and both children. The only brother and sister of I. 2 died of phthisis. I. 1 saw well. No consanguinity recorded. Bibl. No. 112.

Fig. 847. *Clemesha's Case.* Three cases of hereditary optic atrophy in a sibship of seven; the mother also was affected. II. 2, seen aged 6 months, had a typical optic atrophy with white discs and small arteries; media were clear. II. 3, seen aged 5 months, showed a similar condition. II. 1, aged 12 years, was affected to a lesser degree and was mentally dull; V. = $\frac{20}{200}$, discs were pale, vessels small; no central scotomata were present, but there was some imin ti n of the peripheral fields; colour vision was not affected. I. 1 had V. = $\frac{20}{70}$, with correction = $\frac{20}{40}$; she had some pallor of the optic discs with small vessels; no central scotomata were present but there was slight contraction of the peripheral fields; colour vision was intact. No other member of the mother's or father's family was affected. No consanguinity recorded. Bibl. No. 87.

Fig. 848. *Kauffmann's Case.* Hereditary optic atrophy in two brothers, vision commencing to fail in each at about the age of 12. The optic discs showed slight atrophy with smallness of vessels; central scotomata were present but no peripheral contraction of fields; both patients had nystagmus. These were the only two cases of the disease in a large sibship; the parents were healthy; no sign of syphilis; one patient had a posterior polar lens opacity. No consanguinity recorded. Bibl. No. 48.

Fig. 849. *Hormuth's Case.* Hereditary optic atrophy in Friedrich B., II. 3, and in three of his maternal first cousins; the age of onset of the disease is not given but is said to have been the same in each case. Two years after the onset of the disease II. 3 had R. V. = $\frac{20}{200}$, L. V. = finger counting at 11—12'; he had no contraction of the peripheral fields of vision but the right eye had a clearly defined central colour scotoma within which red appeared brown, rose was blue, green appeared whitish; discs were atrophic, the left being more so than the right; there was some narrowing of the vessels; injections of strychnine and electrical treatment led to no improvement; the patient had taken brandy regularly and smoked a good deal. A maternal aunt had two sons of whom one, II. 1, suffered from the same disease; another maternal aunt had three sons and a daughter of whom two sons were also affected.

II. 3 had been healthy up to the time of onset of his eye affection which progressed rapidly in the first three months; at the end of this time he could not see to read but was able to go about alone. No consanguinity recorded. Bibl. No. 64, p. 11.

Fig. 850. *Higgens's Case.* Optic atrophy in three siblings. I. 1, a compositor, had good health until he had rheumatic fever 14 years ago; he had varicose ulcers on his legs. Of his children II. 1, a son, was healthy; II. 2, a daughter, was rather delicate; II. 3 died aged 14 months; II. 4, Albert S., aged 15, said that his sight had failed suddenly three months before; he could count fingers using his lower fields of vision; discs were pale. After the birth of II. 4 his mother manifested evident signs of syphilis; she had cutaneous eruptions and sore throat, this was followed by four or five miscarriages. II. 6, Agnes S., seen aged 13, could then read 16 J. at six inches with each eye; her right eye had been failing gradually for 18 months; seven months later she could still find her way about but could not see to read; her discs were

52—2

dead white and the retinal blood supply was below normal. II. 7, female, was healthy. II. 8 died 24 hours after birth. II. 9, Frederick S., aged 10 (1881), could see well till within the last month; on returning to school after his holidays it was found that he could not see to read but was still able to find his way about; discs were quite white. The two youngest children of the family were said to be healthy.

None of the patients complained of headache or indeed of any symptom except loss of sight. No consanguinity recorded. Bibl. No. 16.

Fig. 851. *Story's Case.* Five cases of hereditary optic atrophy in a sibship of eight; no information is given of the parents or other members of the stock. II. 3, female, at the age of 40 reported that her left eye had been failing for about five weeks; her health had always been good until six months ago when the menopause had taken place; shortly after she suffered from acute pain in her right eye associated with loss of vision; there had been no pain in her left eye; the centre of the field was most affected and she saw better in twilight or on a dull day; R. V. = finger counting at ¾ m., L. V. = finger counting at 4 m.; could read 16 J.; tension was normal in both; pupils were dilated and slow to react; early cataracts were present in both lenses; right disc was atrophic; vessels were small and veins tortuous; the left disc was hazy with blurred margin and vessels as in right; some retinal haemorrhage in left; peripheral limits of fields were normal for white; colour vision was so defective that it was not possible to make charts of the colour fields; large central scotomata were present in each field, these were relative for white, absolute for colours. Four months later her vision was reduced to finger counting at 1 m.; the patient reported that her four brothers had all gone blind in exactly the same way, "from the brain."

II. 4 got sunstroke in India, also "ophthalmia"; he died, aged 23, from epileptic fits; he could only see in twilight and is reported to have had vision very similar to his sister's.

II. 5, a medical student, lost his sight at the age of 21; he used to drink to excess and became "excited" for a while; later he "settled down" and ultimately died "of decline."

II. 6 had a sudden fright at the death of his eldest brother and lost his sight either then or shortly after; he died in a lunatic asylum. II. 7 caught cold on a journey at the age of 30; after the cold he became unconscious but was "as well as ever" in a fortnight; about a month later he lost his sight and the specialist told him that he had a central scotoma; at the age of 45 his vision was reduced to finger counting at 1 m.; he had white atrophy of both discs and contracted retinal vessels; he was dull and sluggish in intelligence and had been sent to an asylum more than once.

Three sisters had good vision; one of them was examined and she, also the patient II. 3, were reported to be of highly excitable dispositions. No consanguinity recorded. Bibl. No. 24.

Fig. 852. *Mooren's Case.* Hereditary optic atrophy in three brothers in whom the onset of the disease was at the ages of 18, 19 and 21 years respectively. Their parents had always seen well; a married sister who was examined was normal. No consanguinity. Bibl. No. 17, p. 250.

Fig. 853. *Hormuth's Case.* Hereditary optic atrophy in two brothers. Heinrich D., II. 1, aged 39, complained that five or six months ago he had noticed a diminution in his vision which had gradually progressed; up to that time he had always seen well and been healthy; he was accustomed to take alcohol freely; now, it was found that R. V. = finger counting at 10', L. V. = finger counting at 8—10'; colour sense was not demonstrably disordered though he would sometimes confuse yellow and green; no central scotomata were detected and peripheral fields were not contracted; the right disc was hyperaemic with blurred margins and some exudate in the surrounding retina; the left disc was whitish with clearly defined margins; the arteries were narrowed, the veins dilated and tortuous. The patient received varied treatments but no improvement was shown and after four years vision was reduced to finger counting at 2'; after this time some temporary improvement followed the use of amyl nitrite.

II. 2, Ernest D., aged 26, was affected in the same way as his brother; in his case the onset was sudden, at the age of 18; eight years after the onset vision was reduced to finger counting at 8'; central scotomata were doubtful; peripheral fields of vision were not contracted; colour vision was defective, only blue and yellow were recognised; the discs were atrophied; vessels showed some narrowing; treatment had no effect upon the condition which remained stationary. No other case of optic nerve disease was known to have occurred in the family. No consanguinity recorded. Bibl. No. 64.

Fig. 854. *Hormuth's Case.* Hereditary optic atrophy in two brothers and a sister; two sisters and the parents saw well; no other case of eye disease was known to have occurred in the family. II. 3, aged 42, Frau von B., had a history of different nervous and hysterical complaints; she was in a highly irritable state, annoyed and excited by the slightest trifle; diminution in her vision had been noticed about ten weeks ago and was progressing; she had previously been examined but nothing abnormal ophthalmoscopically was then found and treatment with iron, baths and electricity had been of no avail; she took a good deal of alcohol. Now it was found that R. V. = L. V. = finger counting at 14'; fields of vision were full, colours were recognised in large samples only; ophthalmoscopic changes were slight but the papillae were pale and arteries were narrowed; retrobulbar neuritis was diagnosed, mercury and salt baths were prescribed and alcohol was to be reduced as much as possible. Five years later the visual acuity was reduced to finger counting at 4' in R. and at 7—8' in L.; she had for two years suffered from giddiness

PLATE LXI.   DESCRIPTIONS OF PEDIGREE PLATES   409

and occipital headaches. Two brothers, older than the patient, were similarly affected; the eldest became affected, II. 3 believed, at the age of 25, and the younger at 17; the affection was severe in both cases, the younger brother was in a hospital for the blind for some time but he was never completely blind. The two sisters, II. 4 and 5, saw well. No consanguinity recorded. Bibl. No. 64.

Fig. 855. *Hormuth's Case.* Hereditary optic atrophy in two brothers and their maternal uncle. II. 2, Friedrich S., suffered at the age of 9—10 years for about three months from severe rheumatism of his joints, since then he had only had slight recurrences lasting for a few days; he was a printer and had a history of repeated severe attacks of colic which ceased when, on account of his eyes, he had to give up his work (? lead colic). At the age of 20, II. 2 noticed that he could not read so well as he had done and then followed dimness of vision and giddiness and rapid progress of his disability; four months from the onset vision was reduced to finger counting at 5—6'; fields of vision were contracted; only blue and yellow colours were recognised; bilateral optic neuritis was present; treatments by means of inunction, pilocarpine, potassium iodide, strychnine and electricity were all without result; four weeks later the papillae were grey, margins blurred; arteries were narrowed; ten years later condition remained unchanged.

II. 1, Hermann S., first complained of his eyes at the age of 27; he had a severe "nervous fever" at the age of 10. Four months from the onset of his eye affection vision was reduced to hand movements in L., finger counting at 1' in R.; five months later defects in the fields were noted and colours were not recognised; papillae were pale, margins clear; arteries were narrowed; whilst the condition was progressing he had pain in his eyes, forehead and neck; treatment with inunction and potassium iodide was without result; the patient drank freely but smoked little. A brother of the mother also had suffered with his eyes and saw very badly; the onset in his case was at the age of 24 following a cold; he had treatment but no improvement followed. No consanguinity recorded. Bibl. No. 64.

Fig. 856. *Hormuth's Case.* Hereditary optic atrophy in two first cousins and in their maternal uncle. II. 1, aged 21, pianist in a café, reported that during five months he had noticed a diminution of vision and that after four weeks he was no longer able to see the notes of his music; he was still able to find his way about the streets; he had been treated by potassium iodide, mercury and strychnine with no improvement; he had a history of sexual indulgence and too much alcohol. Five months from the onset vision was reduced to finger counting in the right eye at 1—2', and in the left at 2'; fields of vision were full; of colours, only blue and yellow were known with any certainty; the right pupil was a trace wider than the left but reactions and eye movements were normal; post-neuritic white atrophy of the optic nerve was diagnosed; the arteries were slightly narrowed, the veins normal; sweating was tried but no improvement took place. The only sibling of II. 1, a sister, aged 16 years, saw well.

II. 3, aged 31, a shoemaker, reported that he had never been ill; he had had very good sight until nine months ago when, one morning, he noticed that he could not see the stitches in his work; on the following day he could not read his newspaper; during about three or four months his vision slowly diminished and since then had remained stationary; the patient gave no history of pain in his eyes or head, no giddiness or other cerebral symptoms; all his functions were normal. Nine months after the onset vision was reduced to finger counting in the right at 2—3', in the left at 3—4'; there was some contraction of fields; only blue and yellow colours were correctly named; green appeared whitish, red yellowish and rose bluish; post-neuritic atrophy of the nerve was diagnosed. II. 3 was seen at intervals during three years and vision remained unchanged; no central scotomata were demonstrated; the papillae became very white, the vessels remained normal; colour vision did not improve; electrical treatment and inunction were without result. II. 3 had a brother and sister who saw well.

The mothers of the two patients were sisters and saw well, but they had a brother, I. 5, who, whilst serving in the army, had taken a cold bath when he was overheated and had, following this, developed the same disease; no other relations were known to have suffered from eye disease. No consanguinity recorded. Bibl. No. 64.

Fig. 857. *Hormuth's Case.* Optic atrophy in two brothers. Theodor W., aged 24, reported that he had always seen well until six weeks ago when he had noticed a diminution in his vision which had become much worse the last ten days; he complained of headache, a sense of pressure in his eyes and cloudiness in his vision; in other respects he was healthy and showed no signs of syphilis; vision was reduced to finger counting at 6 m. in each eye; peripheral fields of vision were not contracted; the papillae were slightly hyperaemic but clearly outlined, veins were dilated; all possible treatments were tried without improvement; nine months later vision was reduced to finger counting at 2 m. in R. and at 3 m. in L.; small absolute central scotomata were present. An elder brother, aged 32, was unable to earn his living on account of disease of the optic nerve; no other cases of eye disease were known in the family. No consanguinity recorded. Bibl. No. 64.

Fig. 858. *Hormuth's Case.* Optic atrophy in two brothers. II. 2, Hermann H., aged 20, had noticed a gradual diminution of vision for four months; after three weeks the condition had progressed so far that he was unable to read; he was anaemic but otherwise healthy; vision was now reduced to finger counting at 12' in the R. and at 12—14' in the L.; bilateral central scotomata were present, peripheral fields were not contracted; red and green colours were not recognised; ophthalmoscopically there was little to note but there was some dilatation of the veins and after three weeks the papillae were paler. The patient had seven siblings of whom one, a brother, now aged about 40, had become affected with the same disease at the age of 18 when he was serving in the army. No consanguinity recorded. Bibl. No. 64.

Fig. 859. *Hormuth's Case.* Optic atrophy in two brothers; the onset in each case was at the age of 18. II. 1 was completely blind, he had been a baker but was obliged to give up his work. II. 2 was seen nine months after the onset of the disease; he was a joiner; his left eye became affected a few months before the right; R. V. = finger counting at 3 m., L. V. = finger counting at 3—4 m.; in the left field was a large central scotoma, the right visual field was contracted on the upper and outer sides; the patient was red-green blind; his left disc was markedly discoloured, its margins clear; arteries were narrowed and veins normal; the right disc was less uniformly pale, the temporal half being paler than the nasal, on this side also the arteries were narrowed; pupils reacted but were slightly dilated. The patient had been treated with inunction, bleeding and potassium iodide; some improvement was noted in the vision of the right eye. No consanguinity recorded. Bibl. No. 64.

Fig. 860. *Heinsberger's Case.* Optic atrophy in two brothers and in their two maternal uncles. I. 1 died, aged 70, of apoplexy; I. 2 died, aged 60, from dropsy; I. 3 and 5 became affected with some eye disease at the age of 20 and had weak sight up to their deaths; one of these affected brothers of I. 2 had a son who had "weak sight." II. 2 became affected at the age of about 27, the onset in his case being associated with occipital headache, lacrymation, cloudy vision, diminution of visual acuity and difficulty in recognising colours; and at the age of 41 he could count fingers with the right eye at 1·5 m. and with the left at 0·5 m.; he recognised red and green in large objects. II. 1 became affected at the age of 21; he appears to have been under treatment from that time until his present age of 47, but the condition had remained stationary since shortly after the onset; he had strabismus. Both brothers had had gonorrhoea at some date before the onset of the disease; neither had had syphilis. No consanguinity recorded. Bibl. No. 67.

Fig. 861. *Leber's Case.* (From Hormuth.) Optic atrophy in two brothers. II. 1, seen aged 51, had had trouble with his eyes and been under treatment for two and a half years; central vision in both eyes was wholly gone and absolute central scotomata were present; he was able to count fingers excentrically; there was some disturbance of colour sense for red and green; bilateral marked white discoloration of the papilla was noted, vessels showed some narrowing. A brother of the patient had developed the same disease at the age of 27; previous to his onset he had smoked much and drank whisky but he had since given up smoking and takes now only a moderate amount of alcohol. Parents had good eyes. No information is given of other siblings. No consanguinity recorded. Bibl. No. 64.

Fig. 862. *Nicolaï's Case.* I. 2 had three sons; the eldest, II. 1, was aged 32 when seen, he had atrophy of the optic nerve and his vision was reduced to $\frac{2}{60}$. II. 2, aged 29, also had white atrophy of the optic nerve, his vision was reduced to $\frac{5}{60}$ in right, $\frac{2}{60}$ in left; there was a central scotoma in the left; tension was normal, colour perception diminished; he had been under treatment for a long time without showing any improvement; II. 3, aged 25, had vision reduced to $\frac{6}{60}$ in each, ophthalmoscopic signs were those of optic neuritis. These three brothers had no other siblings. The mother's twin sister, I. 3, had a son and three daughters; the daughters saw well but the son at the age of 36 had vision reduced to $\frac{3}{60}$ in each, he had seen badly for thirteen years and had atrophy of the optic nerve. The mothers I. 2 and 3 had never complained of bad sight. No consanguinity recorded. Bibl. No. 34.

Fig. 863. *Hutchinson's Case.* Optic atrophy in a woman, her son and her nephew. I. 2 was aged 43 at the onset of the condition; she was seen six months later when she had white atrophy of the optic nerve in both eyes; she had never smoked and Hutchinson suggests that the exciting cause in her case was probably the cessation of menstruation. One of the sons of I. 2 had formerly been a patient of the recorder's for the same condition and a nephew was under the care of Mr Hulke; in each case it was found that the condition had been diagnosed as tobacco amaurosis. No consanguinity recorded. Bibl. No. 7.

Fig. 864. *Pufahl's Case.* Optic atrophy in three brothers and in their maternal uncle; three sisters had seen well but two of them were dead and one was aged 13. I. 3 became affected in his youth; at a later date his condition improved so that he was able to read and carry on his work. The condition in the three brothers was typical of the disease. No consanguinity recorded. Bibl. No. 12.

Fig. 865. *von Graefe's Case.* Optic atrophy in three brothers. II. 1, now aged 28, had at the age of 20 suffered from periodic acute headaches, giddiness and singing in his ears; at the same time a weakness in his sight developed which progressed so rapidly that the patient after 3 months could only go about with difficulty and could only read large print, such as the headlines of newspapers; at this stage the condition remained stationary for 1½ years. The patient then had a very energetic sweating treatment and, according to the statement of his brothers, became so much better that in four weeks he was able to read the smallest print without difficulty. II. 2, aged 23 (1858), became affected at the age of 20 with the same head symptoms and amblyopia as in the case of his brother; no improvement in vision had occurred three years later; fundus was normal. II. 3 became affected with headache and giddiness and was only able to read large

PLATE LXI.   DESCRIPTIONS OF PEDIGREE PLATES   411

print at the age of 19. All three brothers were healthy and had good vision up to the time of the onset of the disease. The father, I. 1, was short-sighted. No consanguinity recorded. Bibl. No. 3.

Fig. 866. *Leber's Case.* (From Hormuth.) Optic atrophy in a male and in his maternal uncle. II. 1, seen aged 37, reported that six years ago he had noticed a rapid diminution of vision; inunction, electricity, strychnine and potassium iodide were administered but the visual weakness progressed until now V. = finger counting at 1 m. A brother of the mother was blind from optic atrophy; no other member of the family was known to be affected. No consanguinity recorded. Bibl. No. 64.

Fig. 867. *Leber's Case.* (From Hormuth.) Optic atrophy in two brothers and their maternal uncle; the parents, grandparents, two uncles and one sister were short-sighted; other siblings saw well. II. 2 was seen aged 23; he had noticed a diminution in vision eight or nine months earlier and had been unable to read for five months; he had gonorrhoea five years ago; no syphilis and no excess in the use of alcohol or tobacco; vision in both eyes was now finger counting at 1⅓ m.; no central scotomata were demonstrated and no contraction of the peripheral fields; blue and yellow colours only were recognised; marked discoloration of the temporal halves of the discs was noted; some improvement followed treatment by potassium iodide. II. 1, aged 25, had seen badly for two years and was now unable to read. I. 3 had been unable to see to read for many years but could go about alone. No consanguinity recorded. Bibl. No. 64.

Fig. 868. *Nettleship's Case.* Blindness from birth with optic neuritis and large skull in three siblings; the parents were first cousins, they had eight children with no miscarriages. II. 1, 2, 6 and 7 all had good sight and health though one of them squinted; II. 4 died aged 7 weeks but could see. II. 3, female, was quite blind from birth; she was taken to Middlesex Hospital when a baby and the mother was then told that "the nerve was inflamed"; at the age of 7 pupils were motionless without a midriatic but dilated widely after its use; the left disc was seen with difficulty, it was hazy and one vein was decidedly enlarged but no swelling and no visible atrophy was reported; the right disc was not seen; cranium was rather large with a broad and prominent forehead; the patient spoke well and seemed intelligent. II. 5, male, died at 15 months, he was blind from birth, no particulars were available. II. 8, female, seen aged 7 months; she appeared to have no perception of light and her mother said she was certain the child had never seen; pupils were small, equal and motionless to light; irregular slow nystagmic movements and frequent strong convergence of eyes were noted; the discs were swollen and very hazy and veins were tortuous; head was large and square, fontanelle large, frontal eminences square, ribs slightly beaded, spleen 1½ inches below costal margin; the child had had no illness and no fits, she was breast fed but for the last two months had had some bread and oatmeal in addition; she was quite blind but screwed up her eyes in sunlight though she took no notice of lamplight. There was no history of blindness in the rest of the family except perhaps in a male, second cousin to one of the parents, who was said to have been blind all his life. The parents were healthy. Nettleship considered this was probably not a true case of Leber's disease. Consanguinity. Bibl. No. 85, p. clxxxiv.

Fig. 869. *Schlüter's Case.* Optic atrophy in five males and one female in two generations. II. 1, Minna R., aged 44, had suffered for five years from a bilateral diminution of vision; the condition had remained stationary during the last four years; eight years before the patient had had a difficult labour but had not been gravid since; menstruation had always been rather irregular and tiresome; vision was now reduced to finger counting at 3′ and was excentric, only a small part of the visual field functioning; colour vision was defective but blue in large objects was still recognised; the discs were atrophic with sharp contours, the vessels narrowed. II. 2, Friedrich M., aged 33, was healthy and robust but had had weak sight since the age of 12; the diminution of vision then noticed soon became stationary and had not progressed since that time; vision was now found to be finger counting in the right at 6′, in the left at 7′; central scotomata were present and colour vision defective; red and green were not recognised; peripheral fields were full. These siblings had two brothers, one of whom was normal, the other, II. 3, became amblyopic at the age of 25 and three years later developed Diabetes mellitus. A maternal uncle, I. 3, became amblyopic at the age of 20; two cousins, whose mother was sister to I. 2 and 3, also became amblyopic at the age of 20; none of the affected members were completely blind. No consanguinity recorded. Bibl. No. 19, pp. 50—51.

Fig. 870. *Schlüter's Case.* Optic atrophy in four males of two generations. II. 2, Albert B., aged 11, noticed six weeks ago some diminution in his visual acuity; he suffered from headaches and occasional vomiting; peripheral fields were full, absolute central scotomata were present; colour sense was very uncertain; discs were hyperaemic with blurred margins; arteries were slightly narrowed, veins dilated. Two maternal uncles of II. 2 also saw very badly; the onset of eye trouble in one of them was at the age of 20; the other was known to have seen well at one time. A cousin of the mother suffered from a similar defect of vision. II. 1, 3 and 4 saw well. No consanguinity recorded. Bibl. No. 19, p. 51.

Fig. 871. *Nettleship's Case.* (Habershon's Case II.) Optic atrophy in three brothers; no information of parents or other siblings is given. II. 1, aged 32, had been accustomed to smoke more than ½ oz. of the strongest and best shag daily; his vision began to fail in Dec. 1879, a month later he was unable to work; ten months later Nettleship found V. = about 12/50 and 14 J., hypermetropia ·5 D.; discs were rather pale all over; the defect was quite characteristic and well-marked colour scotomata were present. A similar history is given in the case of two brothers of the patient who also smoked much shag. No consanguinity recorded. Bibl. No. 29.

Fig. 872. *Nettleship's Case.* (Habershon's Case V.) *O*ptic atrophy in two brothers; a maternal uncle had had bad sight for many years. II. 2, J. C., aged 20, reported that his vision had failed six months ago and for six months before this he had almost constant frontal headaches and occasional faintness; his vision reached its worst in about a month and had remained unchanged since; he smoked $\frac{1}{2}$ oz. shag daily; no history of sexual excess; V. = $\frac{4}{200}$ about; temporal sides of discs were pale, nasal sides probably too red and oedematous; six years later vision was unchanged. II. 1, aged 22, reported that his sight had been failing for some time; R. V. = $\frac{10}{100}$, L. V. = $\frac{5}{200}$. No consanguinity recorded. Bibl. No. 29.

Fig. 873. *Posey's Case.* Optic atrophy in father and son; in each case the onset was in very early childhood; no other members of the family were affected. Vision in the father, aged 51, was about $\frac{6}{40}$; in the son, aged 16, V. = $\frac{5}{35}$. No consanguinity recorded. Bibl. No. 107.

Fig. 874. *Posey's Case.* Optic atrophy in father, son and maternal uncle; in all cases the onset of the disease was at the age of 25; the resultant vision in each case was about $\frac{5}{40}$; all patients smoked in moderation. No further information is given; it would be of interest to hear whether the parents I. 1 and 2, each of whom came of affected stocks, had any unaffected offspring. No consanguinity recorded. Bibl. No. 107.

Fig. 875. *Nettleship's Case.* Optic atrophy in two brothers and possibly in a sister. II. 2, aged 19, complained that his sight had been failing for four months; he was thrown from a cart six months before the onset of the disease when his left eye was closed for a week with swelling; he cannot now see to read or write nor can he distinguish colours; he had led a loose life for two years and admitted sexual excesses and that he was subject to nocturnal emissions; no history of syphilis; he was a moderate drinker and for two years had smoked two or three cigars each evening, five or six on Sunday. II. 1 was a soldier in India when at the age of 23 his sight failed; it was then said to be the effects of the sun and he was invalided home; he smoked a good deal and now at the age of 30 could not see to read or write. II. 3, another brother, saw well but died of phthisis. A sister, II. 4, had bad sight and wore spectacles always; she was not seen but was said to be always ailing and to be subject to fits (? epilepsy). Two other sisters saw well. The father, I. 1, had died of phthisis but had good sight; the mother was living. No consanguinity recorded. Bibl. Nos. 29 and 85, p. clxvi.

Fig. 876. *Browne's Case.* Optic atrophy in three brothers. II. 1, aged 40, was the eldest of a sibship of five; he had been seen at the age of 27 when his vision was failing and was then told that he was suffering from the use of tobacco; he had had splendid sight up to this age, had never been ill and had no headaches; he smoked $\frac{1}{2}$ oz. of twist daily and chewed about the same amount; his discs now showed a typical skim-milk white. II. 2, aged 33, had very good vision until five months ago when a gradual failure set in; he was accustomed to smoke 1 oz. of twist weekly and chewed indefinitely; he saw better in a dim light; general health was good; ophthalmoscopic appearances were those of recent atrophy of the discs. II. 3 said that his eyes had been uncomfortable for three months but his vision had only failed two weeks ago; he was a heavy smoker but took no alcohol; discs were pale; no scotomata were discovered. No other member of the sibship or collateral relative had suffered from an early failure of sight. No consanguinity recorded. Bibl. No. 28.

Fig. 877. *Snell's Case.* Optic atrophy in two brothers at the age of 17 years. In the case of II. 1 the onset was rapid; when he was first seen vision in the left eye was reduced to finger counting but the right eye still saw $\frac{6}{9}$; a month later R. V. = $\frac{6}{60}$; discs were pale; visual fields were contracted and central scotomata were present; this patient had had a blow on the head several months before his sight began to fail; he did not smoke. No cases of blindness were known to have occurred in other members of the family. No consanguinity. Bibl. No. 55.

Fig. 878. *Leber's Case.* (From Hormuth.) Optic atrophy in two brothers. II. 1, aged 47, had noticed a diminution in his vision for two months; right pupil was a trace wider than left; both pupils reacted normally; vision was reduced to finger counting at 5 m.; there was no contraction of visual fields but central scotomata for red and green were demonstrated; temporal halves of papillae were pale; in other respects the patient was healthy and complained only of headaches; syphilis was denied; he used tobacco and alcohol with moderation; treatment was followed by no improvement; five months later R .V. = finger counting at 1·5 m , L. V. = finger counting at 3 m.; green was no longer recognised, red was uncertain, yellow and blue were recognised. II. 2, aged 40, had been examined at the age of 14 when atrophy of the optic nerve was diagnosed; at this time R. V. = finger counting at 7—8′, L. V. = $\frac{20}{200-100}$. Twenty-six years later II. 2 reported that his vision had in the interval gradually diminished, it was now equal to finger counting in the R. at 1·5 m., in the L. at 4 m.; the papillae were white, vessels not narrowed; the smallest colour samples were correctly named. No other members of the family were affected. No consanguinity recorded. Bibl. No. 64.

PLATE LXI.   DESCRIPTIONS OF PEDIGREE PLATES   413

Fig. 879. *Leber's Case.* Optic atrophy in two brothers. II. 2, A. S., aged 18, had noticed for a year that objects were confused and appeared cloudy; he had also been subject to temporal headaches; fourteen days after this condition set in he could not see the pavements in the streets and could not tell at a short distance whether a man or a woman was in front of him; a year from the onset his vision was found to be finger counting in the R. at 1 m., in the L. at 1·5 m.; no definite scotoma was demonstrated; absolute red-green blindness was noted; the discs were greyish white with clear edges; vessels showed some narrowing; pupils reacted well. After five weeks' treatment with potassium iodide the vision remained unchanged; red and green were recognised in no part of the visual fields. No inheritable disease was known to exist in the family; the parents saw well. Of two siblings, a sister was healthy but an elder brother aged 27 had the same disease as the patient; his vision gradually became so bad that he no longer recognised people at a short distance, but later he improved and was now able to read the newspaper. No consanguinity recorded. Bibl. No. 64, pp. 154—5.

Fig. 880. *Pockley's Case.* Optic atrophy in two first cousins whose mothers were sisters; the onset in each case was at the age of 32 and when seen at the ages of 34 and 38 respectively the conditions found were almost identical in the two cases. II. 3 was a moderate smoker; he had never had syphilis though he had "risked it often enough"; about six weeks after the onset he had pains in his head and eyes and when his head ached he noticed "showers of sparks"; pupils reacted to accommodation but contracted sluggishly on exposure to light and on continued exposure dilated again and remained so; both discs were atrophic; colour-blindness to red and green was demonstrated all over the field; a central scotoma was present in each with normal peripheral limits of the field. There were apparent signs of trouble in the accessory nasal sinuses. II. 1 became almost blind in four or five weeks from the onset and condition had remained stationary since. No consanguinity recorded. Bibl. No. 106.

Fig. 881. *Norris's Case.* Fifteen cases of optic atrophy in four generations. IV. 9, aged fourteen (1883), complained that his sight had been gradually failing for the past year; both eyes were affected and he complained of frontal headaches and dizziness; R. V. = $\frac{3}{60}$, L. V. = $\frac{1}{60}$; the discs were atrophic; no changes were seen in the macular region; retinal vessels were contracted; the patient was colour-blind. No improvement followed treatment with strychnine. Examination was carried out on all the seven cases of this sibship, the age of onset for members from IV. 6 to IV. 12 being respectively 14, 19, 18, 14, 8, 8 and 7 years; the most prominent symptoms were frequent frontal headaches with gradual loss of central vision; the fields for form and for yellow, blue and red colours showed varying degrees of contraction; the loss of sight came on gradually except in one case where the ability to read ordinary type was lost in a week after the first signs of diminishing vision; two of the cases showed improvement whilst under observation, the others progressed or remained stationary.

The eyes of the parents of this sibship were examined and found to be normal. The mother had two brothers and a sister affected and one unaffected sister; the onset of the disease in the brothers was at the ages of 15 and 19 years respectively; the sister, III. 5, became affected at 35, the progress of the disease in her case was said to be rapid. II. 2 became affected at the age of 14; III. 3, the son of II. 2, became affected at 18 years. III. 5 had four children of whom two were affected. No consanguinity. Bibl. No. 23.

Fig. 882. *Despagnet's Case.* II. 3 was a heavy drinker and had had delirium tremens, he had good sight up to the time of his death at the age of 62; he was twice married; by his first wife he had two children, a daughter who died young, and a son III. 2, aged 48 at the time of observation, who had good sight but was subject to neuralgia and to nervous crises. By his second wife II. 3 had seven children, of whom two died young; III. 4, aged 41, had a sudden diminution of vision at the age of 20, the left eye was first affected and the right eye three months later; central scotoma were present; only blue and yellow were recognised; the onset of the disease was associated with headaches; the condition progressed for three months and then became stationary; fourteen years after the onset the discs were bluish white and the vessels normal. III. 4 had a son who became similarly affected at the age of 20 years; he had no central scotomata but there was some contraction of the peripheral fields. III. 5 became affected at the age of 31; central scotomata were present, peripheral fields were normal; the onset was associated with severe headaches and photophobia; the condition progressed for six months and then became stationary; six years later the discs were white with blurred margins and the vessels were narrowed. III. 6 became affected at the age of 32, the onset was associated with headaches and photophobia; central scotoma were present, also some concentric contraction of fields; one year from the onset R. V. = $\frac{1}{10}$, L. V. = $\frac{7}{10}$; discs were greyish white and vessels normal. III. 8 and III. 10 became affected at the age of 30 years.

The father of this sibship had normal parents and twelve normal siblings; the mother, II. 4, had normal parents and three siblings of whom two had good sight, but one brother at the age of 50 years had become weak-sighted. II. 6 and II. 8 had children who saw well. No consanguinity recorded. Bibl. No. 36.

Fig. 883. *Velhagen's Case.* Optic atrophy in two brothers, in their maternal uncle and in their mother's sister's son. IV. 3 and 4 both became affected at the age of 21; at the ages of 44 and 29 respectively the disease was seen to be typical in both; vision = $\frac{5}{10}$—$\frac{1}{10}$; there was pale bluish discoloration of the papillae; retinal vessels slightly narrowed; central scotomata were present, peripheral fields normal; vision for green was imperfect. A maternal uncle aged 50 and a cousin aged 27 both became affected at the age of 21. The maternal great-grandfather, I. 2, died insane; he had numerous other descendants who were normal. No consanguinity. Bibl. No. 69.

PLATE LXII. Fig. 884. *Mann's Case.* Hereditary optic atrophy in a brother and sister. No eye disease is known to have occurred in the parents or their siblings, or in the grandparents, but the maternal aunt, II. 6, married to a man in whose stock retinitis pigmentosa had occurred, had eight children of whom four had retinitis pigmentosa and four had pathological changes in the fundus indicative of retinitis pigmentosa. III. 5, aged 21, Ivy C., was examined by Dr J. C. Powell who reports that her sight failed about the age of 10 years; R. V. = L. V. = fingers at about 16 inches; pupils were large, equal and reacted sluggishly to light; fundi showed primary greyish atrophy of the optic nerves; retinal vessels were perhaps smaller than normal; central scotomata were present; colour perception was very defective, red only could be seen just at the central part of the right field; she could walk about fairly well alone in known localities; hereditary optic atrophy was diagnosed. III. 6, aged 19, had normal fundi and good vision; visual fields were full. III. 7, Herbert C., aged 18, was noted to have weak vision at the age of 8 years since when some improvement had occurred; now (1928) R. V. = $\frac{6}{18}$ with some letters of $\frac{6}{12}$ and $\frac{6}{9}$; L. V. = fingers at 1 m.; refraction of the right eye is $\frac{+1}{+0.25}$ cyl. ax. vert., but glasses do not improve vision; the left eye is convergent; the right fundus shows pallor of the optic disc with slightly tortuous vessels, not diminished in size; the periphery of the fundus presents the pigmented appearance known as "choroid tigra" which is probably not pathological; there is nothing suggestive of retinitis pigmentosa; in the left fundus the disc is quite white, the vessels are a fair size and "choroid tigra" is present as in the right eye; refraction of this eye is $\frac{-1}{+2}$ cyl. ax. hor., but glasses do not improve vision; the right field of vision is quite full, the left shows a central scotoma and also concentric contraction; an X-ray of the pituitary fossa showed no abnormality; the patient was alert and slightly above the average of his class in intelligence. III. 8 had healthy fundi and normal visual fields; she had mixed astigmatism in the right and hypermetropic astigmatism in the left eye; corrected vision was $\frac{6}{9}$ and $\frac{6}{9}$ respectively. III. 9, Ernest C., aged 13, had R. V. = L. V. = $\frac{6}{6}$; reactions of pupils were normal and visual fields full; examination of the fundi revealed a peppery appearance of the pigment which was, however, within physiological limits; in the right upper temporal quadrant a colloid body was apparent and there were two near the left macula; these are rare at so early an age but may be of no significance in this case.

The mother of this sibship was examined and appeared to have been always healthy and to show no sign of any eye abnormality. The father, II. 5, was separated from his wife and was not seen but his brothers state that his whole family are extremely healthy and long lived.

A full account of the early and fully developed cases of retinitis pigmentosa in the eight children of II. 6 is given in the original history. III. 21, Harry N., aged 30, a paternal first cousin to the siblings III. 10—17, had a typical history of retinitis pigmentosa and could not walk about at night though he could see to drive a van in a good light. III. 23 and 24, aged about 24, were reported to see badly at night. For further information see the original account. No consanguinity. Bibl. No. 152.

Fig. 885. *Fortunati and Mingazzini's Case.* Hereditary optic atrophy in two brothers. I. 1 and 2 had enjoyed good health and died in old age of some acute malady. II. 2, aged 50, neither drank nor smoked, he had never suffered from syphilis or any other venereal disease and had had no serious illness; ten years ago he had first noticed a lowering of his visual sensation, now vision was reduced to $\frac{1}{10}$ in each eye; peripheral limits of the fields of vision were practically normal; he had two little sons who were healthy. II. 3 became affected at about the same age as his brother; when first seen R. V. with correction of 6 D. for myopia = $\frac{2}{3}$, L. V. = $\frac{1}{30}$; a few months later R. V. = L. V. = $\frac{1}{40}$; peripheral limits of fields were normal; no syphilis, alcoholism or tuberculosis was known to have occurred in the antecedents or collaterals. No consanguinity recorded. Bibl. No. 78.

Fig. 886. *Hogg's Case.* Hereditary optic atrophy in a male and his two maternal uncles; his sister, parents and maternal grandparents saw well. No information is given of the cases. No consanguinity recorded. Bibl. No. 151.

Fig. 887. *Burroughs's Case.* Optic atrophy in father and son. II. 2, aged 40, was a non-smoker and was healthy though nervous; he had defective vision which was first noticed at about the age of 12 years; now R. V. = L. V. = $\frac{6}{60}$; he had slight myopic astigmatism but glasses did not improve his vision; discs were ivory white, lamina cribrosa was visible; visual fields showed central scotomata extending to about 10° from the fixation point, peripheral limits normal; Wassermann and von Pirquet reactions were normal; blood coagulation rate was normal. II. 2 had an uncle who had had "very bad sight" for the greater part of his life, he saw numerous specialists and glasses did not help him; this uncle was run over and killed in the street as a result of his defective vision.

II. 2 had two children, a little girl aged 7 who saw well and a boy aged 12, III. 1, who had noticed that his vision was bad 18 months before; the condition had progressed rapidly and now R. V. = L. V. = $\frac{6}{18}$;

Plate LXII.   DESCRIPTIONS OF PEDIGREE PLATES   415

he had slight hypermetropia but vision was not improved by glasses; pupils were large and equal and reacted to light and accommodation; he was healthy but nervous and became pale and agitated when the street doorbell rang; his discs showed a moderate degree of secondary optic atrophy, lamina cribrosa was visible; central scotomata extended to about 10° from the fixation point in each eye, there was also a definite temporal contraction of the peripheral limits of each field. The radiologist reported that "in my opinion there is no doubt that in the pictures of Mr L. and his son the pituitary fossae are not normal either in size or shape; they are larger and deeper than normal, moreover the rounded globular appearance is unusual." No consanguinity. Bibl. No. 129.

Fig. 888. *Lang's Case.* Hereditary optic atrophy in three siblings and in their nephew. III. 1, aged 18, noticed a diminution in his vision; R. V. = L. V. = $\frac{6}{10}$ on examination; central scotomata were present; a fortnight later paleness of the outer halves of the papillae was noted and visual acuity was now reduced to $\frac{3}{60}$. There was no history of eye disease in the father's stock, but the maternal grandmother suffered from some eye disease. The mother, II. 3, was healthy but one sister and two of her brothers were affected; in the sister, II. 4, the disease was unilateral, a central scotoma was present and V. = $\frac{6}{12}$; the condition was bilateral and much more severe in the brothers II. 5 and 6; one of them was examined and was noted to have complete optic atrophy with large central scotomata. No consanguinity recorded. Bibl. No. 133.

Fig. 889. *Holz's Case.* Optic atrophy in three members of a sibship of five; parents and grandparents saw well. III. 1, aged 28, saw well. III. 2, Anna P., aged 22, a dressmaker, noticed in 1884 that her vision was failing; six months later R. V. = finger counting at 2·5 m., L. V. = finger counting at 3·0 m.; discs were pale, especially on the temporal side, vessels were normal; there was some contraction of the visual fields. This patient was healthy in other respects; she menstruated normally from the age of 16. III. 3, Paul P., a shoemaker, aged 20, became affected at the age of 18 and was unable to carry on his work; R. V. = finger counting at 2·0 m., L. V. = finger counting at 3·5 m.; discs were pale and clearly outlined; vessels were a little narrowed; visual fields were contracted above; in other respects III. 3 was healthy; treatment was without effect. III. 4, aged 18, was normal. III. 5, Alwine P., aged $15\frac{3}{4}$, became affected; she had never before had trouble with her eyes; nine months after the onset R. V. = finger counting at 10·0 m., L. V. = finger counting at 7·0 m.; discs were pale, especially the temporal halves; there was some contraction of the visual fields. No consanguinity recorded. Bibl. No. 22.

Fig. 890. *Hansell's Case.* Hereditary optic atrophy in three brothers. II. 3, aged 56, reported that on the morning of the previous day he discovered on attempting to leave his bed that he was nearly blind, the night before he had been in his usual health and saw well, also he had had a good night's rest; there was no pain or headache and had been no injury; he had taken no medicine: there was no haemorrhage and no signs of disturbance in his general health; on ophthalmoscopic examination he was said to have a low grade of optic neuritis, veins were tortuous and distended, the arteries slightly contracted; the peripheral fields were not contracted but positive central scotomata were present; pupils were moderately dilated but responded to light and accommodation; R. V. = L. V. = $\frac{1}{100}$, excentric; no signs of syphilis or of nephritis; for years he had smoked one or two cigars daily; he drank very little or nothing. The patient had been subject to repeated exposure to cold during the six weeks preceding the attack.

The parents, I. 4 and 5, saw well up to old age but several maternal aunts and uncles became nearly blind in adult life; the eldest brother, II. 1, a physician, had sunstroke at the age of 35 and two years later was almost blind, he was now aged 60 and had a small amount of vision. II. 2, a farmer, lost his sight suddenly at 50 whilst working in a field. From his patient's account and also through a doctor's report the recorder concludes that all these members suffered from the same affection. No consanguinity recorded. Bibl. No. 62.

Fig. 891. *Gallemaerts's Case.* (Taken from Nettleship.) This case is so incompletely abstracted that all we can be sure of is that II. 1 and II. 2 became affected with optic atrophy at the ages of 21 and 17 years respectively. The age of onset for II. 3 is not given. I. 4 was not seen by the recorder, but was said to be affected in the same way as the cases described; Nettleship refers to "his" five children who were said to have "bad sight of the same kind," but enters the case as a female in the chart. No consanguinity recorded. Bibl. No. 65.

Fig. 892. *Pufahl's Case.* (Taken from Hormuth.) Hereditary optic atrophy in two brothers and in their three maternal uncles. II. 1, at the age of 19, had a bilateral diminution of vision which came on without any known cause; after five weeks he was unable to see to read; there was a central scotoma in the left eye, and six months later in the right eye also; the peripheral fields were not contracted; five weeks after the onset some signs of optic neuritis were present; the discs were reddish and slightly blurred and the veins were dilated; four months later partial atrophy of the discs was noted; the youth had been completely healthy up to the onset of the disease and there had been no abuse in the use of tobacco and alcohol; no improvement had occurred after six months' treatment. II. 2 became affected at the age of 17; in his case the peripheral fields were markedly contracted; no information is given of the presence of central scotomata; six years later he was able to go about alone in the streets. The parents, I. 5 and 6, had no visual defect but two brothers of I. 5 became so weak-sighted that they were unable to read at the age of 20 years; a third brother remained free from the disease in his youth, but he also became affected at the age of 57 years; he probably had central scotomata but it was thought that his peripheral fields of vision were not contracted. There was a history in this last case of excessive use of alcohol but the man did not smoke. No consanguinity recorded. Bibl. No. 14.

Fig. 893. *Magers's Case.* Hereditary optic atrophy in two twin brothers and probably in their maternal uncle. I. 1 died from tuberculosis. I. 2 died from puerperal fever. I. 3 became affected with some eye affection leading to loss of vision at about the age of 20 years. II. 2, Otto H., aged 16, complained that he had seen badly for about three months; at this time vision was much reduced, but excepting the veins, which were dilated and tortuous, the fundi were normal; the visual fields and colour perception were also normal; the condition, however, progressed and a year later the outer sides of the discs were pale, vision was further reduced and colour vision was defective; there was no peripheral contraction of the visual fields and no central scotomata could be demonstrated, though the patient appeared to use excentric vision on attempts to read test types. II. 3, Oskar H., became affected a year later than his brother; the onset in his case followed a blow in his right eye; a month later R. V. = finger counting at 1 m., L. V. = $\frac{6}{12}$; colour vision was normal; the discs were reddened and the veins dilated; at a later date the discs were pale, an absolute central scotoma was demonstrated in the right eye and a relative scotoma in the left; there was no peripheral contraction of the visual fields. These two affected brothers had eleven healthy unaffected living siblings. No consanguinity recorded. Bibl. No. 60.

Fig. 894. *Hensen's Case.* Optic atrophy in two brothers and in their maternal uncle. II. 1, Wilhelm T., had never been seriously ill and saw well until Dec. 1915 when, at the age of 34, he noticed that his vision was diminishing in both eyes; the condition progressed slowly and was associated with headaches; he never drank or smoked much and there was no history of infection; Wassermann test negative; the right pupil was wider than the left, reaction to light good; media clear; right temporal half of disc was pale with blurred margin, vessels normal; in the left, papillary margins were slightly blurred, veins hyperaemic; both fields showed large central scotomata and in the right the whole nasal half of the field was insensitive. II. 2 became affected in 1909 and now R. V. = L. V. = $\frac{1}{36}$ with excentric fixation; he had slight peripheral contraction of fields and large central absolute scotomata; discs were pale, temporal halves white; vessels normal; both brothers recognised colours fairly well. The age of II. 2 is not given. Both parents saw well, but a brother of the mother became amblyopic at the age of 30 years and has remained so. No consanguinity recorded. Bibl. No. 111.

Fig. 895. *Mooren's Case.* Hereditary optic atrophy in three brothers. No details of cases or family history are given. No consanguinity. Bibl. No. 17.

Fig. 896. *Rönne's Case.* Hereditary optic atrophy in a male aged 24 years (1910); the mother of the patient had a brother, a nephew and a niece who had experienced a sudden diminution of vision at about the age of 20 years, without other symptoms of eye disease; they had been under treatment and were diagnosed as cases of hereditary optic atrophy. II. 1 showed no symptoms of general nerve disease, he was a moderate smoker and denied any excess in the use of alcohol; in 1909 he noticed a diminution of vision in the right eye and a week later the left eye was in a similar state; the weakness progressed for 14 days, since when it had remained stationary; no other symptoms were complained of; now (1910) R. V. = finger counting at 1 m., L. V. = finger counting at 3 m.; central scotomata were present but the outer margins of the fields were normal; slight signs of optic neuritis were present and the temporal side of each disc was paler than normal. No consanguinity. Bibl. No. 91.

Fig. 897. *Beresinskaja's Case.* Hereditary optic atrophy in two brothers. II. 1, aged 32, noticed a sudden diminution of vision at the age of 18; the condition did not respond to treatment; absolute central scotomata were present; R. V. = 0·02, L. V. = 0·08; both optic nerves showed atrophic changes; general examination was negative. II. 2, aged 22, became affected with a diminution of vision at the age of 19; the condition improved markedly after a time and now (1924) R. V. = L. V. = 0·9; paleness of the temporal side of both discs was noted; relative central scotomata for green were present. The parents and siblings of the affected brothers were normal. No consanguinity recorded. Bibl. No. 128.

Fig. 898. *Climenko's Case.* Optic neuritis in two brothers. II. 2, aged 24, had a gradual diminution of vision at the age of about 15 years; he complained of giddiness at the time of the onset for a few weeks, but had had no similar trouble since, and no history of headaches or vomiting at any time; his vision was now reduced to finger counting in the lower and outer parts of the peripheral fields and to hand movements in the other regions; both discs were whitish especially on the temporal side. II. 1, aged 27, became affected about five years ago, first in the right eye and a few months later in the left; the onset was associated with temporal headaches; vision was now reduced to hand movements in the extreme periphery of each field only; discs were bluish white especially on the temporal side; mentality was normal. No other affected members were known in the family. No consanguinity recorded. Bibl. No. 88.

Fig. 899. *Rönne's Case.* Hereditary optic atrophy in two brothers each of whom became affected at the age of 21 years; no other relations were known to be affected. II. 1, examined six years after the onset of

PLATE LXII.   DESCRIPTIONS OF PEDIGREE PLATES   417

the disease, had R. V. = L. V. = $\frac{2}{60}$; absolute central scotomata were present but the fields showed no peripheral contraction; the patient had indulged in excess of alcohol but was a moderate smoker. No consanguinity recorded. Bibl. No. 91.

Fig. 900. *Barrett's Case.* Optic neuritis in two brothers. II. 1, aged 28 years, a country labourer, complained of failing sight for the past six weeks; he had had no illness, no headaches or sickness, and showed no signs of syphilis; he smoked two small plugs of tobacco a week; R. V. = finger counting at 2 feet, L. V. = $\frac{2}{60}$; the right field was a little contracted for white and had a large central scotoma; blue, red and green were not recognised; the left field was full for white but had a large central colour scotoma; red and green were not recognised; refraction was + 2 D. in both; the discs were pale and showed distinct traces of neuritis in tortuous vessels and organised exudation; treatment for six weeks with iodides, mercury and strychnine led to no change; the nervous system otherwise showed no abnormal symptoms. II. 2, aged 23, complained that his sight had been failing for three months; R. V. = $\frac{2}{60}$, L. V. = $\frac{4}{60}$; right field showed slight contraction for white and a large central scotoma for red; green was not recognised; left field was normal for white with a large relative scotoma for red; green was not recognised; the discs showed signs of a subsiding neuritis. II. 2 had never been ill, was not liable to headaches and showed no signs of syphilis; he smoked two plugs of tobacco a week; nervous system was normal in other respects. As far as could be discovered no other members of the family suffered from defective eyesight. No consanguinity recorded. Bibl. No. 43.

Fig. 901. *Crauell's Case.* "I know a marriage with seven children and only the oldest is with sight, the others being blind. They were born with sight, which they have gradually lost. I have examined their eyes, and I did not find opaqueness in them, but I believe that their blindness is due to atrophy and weakness of the optic nerves. The children are agile, they are not deranged and have great strength, with nothing abnormal. However, their parents suffer from uremy (? uraemia) and their sight is somewhat weak, for they cannot see further than 20 to 30 metres, lacking 80 centimetres necessary for normal sight." No consanguinity recorded. Bibl. No. 84, p. 34.

Fig. 902. *Bedell's Case.* Optic atrophy in three brothers and in their cousin; the three brothers were aged 19, 26 and 28 years respectively at the time of the record. Stereoscopic X-ray plates show a very prominent clinoid process with deep sella turcica in the three brothers; the plate of the cousin does not show these peculiarities. No consanguinity recorded. Bibl. No. 95.

Fig. 903. *Alsberg's Case.* Hereditary optic atrophy in a father and his son; each case had vision reduced to about $\frac{5}{60}$ in each eye; the discs of each were pale and sharply outlined, the paleness being more marked in the outer halves; no other fundus changes were present; Wassermann test was negative in each. No further case of the disease was known to have occurred in the family; the father, now aged 43, became affected at the age of 25; the son, aged 7 (1927), became affected three years ago; radiographs of the sella turcica showed no abnormality. This case is unusual both from the apparent transmission of the disease from father to son and from the very early age of onset in the son. No consanguinity recorded. Bibl. No. 139.

Fig. 904. *Suckling's Case.* Optic atrophy in a male who became affected at the age of 50; his mother became blind at 50, his sister and a female first cousin on his mother's side were also blind. II. 1 was seen at the age of 63 when he had double optic atrophy with complete blindness; he gradually lost his sight at the age of 50; pupils were small but reacted to light; no signs of syphilis or of other nerve disease were present. No consanguinity recorded. Bibl. No. 27.

Fig. 905. *Mügge's Case.* Optic atrophy in two brothers; the onset was at the age of 6 and 13 years respectively; the disease progressed slowly and became stationary whilst there was still fair vision; after some years the discs were seen to be pale; small relative central scotomata for green and yellow were demonstrated. No further cases of the disease had been known to occur in the family. No consanguinity recorded. Bibl. No. 90.

Fig. 906. *Lawson's Case.* Optic atrophy in mother and son. The mother, I. 1, seen at the age of 14, had then R. V. = $\frac{6}{12}$, L. V. = finger counting at 25 cm.; the left disc was pale and cupped in the temporal half; 17 years later, vision remained unchanged; the disc on the right side was normal, on the left it was pale especially the temporal half; peripheral fields were practically normal, there was a large central scotoma in the left eye only. II. 1, aged 10, had had defective vision since early infancy, now R. V. = $\frac{6}{60}$, L. V. = $\frac{6}{36}$; not improved by glasses; striking pallor of the temporal half of both discs was noted; central scotomata for colours were present, large in the left, small in the right eye; peripheral fields were normal. One other child of I. 1, a daughter, saw well at the time of observation. No consanguinity recorded. Bibl. No. 77.

Fig. 907. *Valude's Case.* Optic atrophy in a mother and her only child. I. 2 died of pneumonia. I. 1, now aged 46, had been long under treatment for optic atrophy; V. = $\frac{1}{10}$ in each eye; discs were uniformly white with clear contours, vessels somewhat diminished; no improvement followed treatment. II. 1, aged 14, became affected six months ago; the onset was associated with severe headaches, no vomiting; discs were pale with slightly blurred margins and vessels were tortuous; R. V. = finger counting at 20 cm., L. V. = finger counting at 50 cm.; various treatments were without result until ten months after the onset when injections of strychnine were followed by marked improvement; a year from the onset vision was almost normal in each; on stopping the injections the vision fell, but on resuming them recovery occurred and now R. V. = 1, L. V. = $\frac{2}{3}$; ophthalmoscopic appearances remain unchanged and the patient complains that he easily tires when reading. No consanguinity recorded. Bibl. No. 94.

Fig. 908. *Bickerton's Case.* Optic atrophy in two brothers. II. 1, aged 32, said that his sight began to fail at the age of 22; he had always been a heavy smoker but gave it up for six months and took strychnine; vision was now barely $\frac{1}{60}$ and J. 19; red and green were not recognised in 20 mm. test objects; there was a concentric contraction of the fields; discs were pale, vessels normal; no history of syphilis. II. 2, aged 35, a marine, was discharged for defective vision; his sight began to fail at 27; he gave up smoking for six months and took strychnine; now vision was barely $\frac{1}{60}$ and J. 19; discs were pale; fields were much contracted and had central scotomata; colours were scarcely recognised. The mother's brother, I. 3, had been invalided from the army in India owing to defective vision. No consanguinity recorded. Bibl. No. 71.

Fig. 909. *Wilbrand and Saenger's Case.* Hereditary optic atrophy in two brothers and in their maternal uncle. II. 1, aged 17, noticed suddenly that he saw badly during a voyage to China as steward; he had a shimmer before his eyes and could not see clearly what was in front of him; he was a moderate smoker and drinker; his father had died of some chest disease, his mother was still living; he was seen six months after the onset when he was fairly well nourished and his other organs were healthy; R. V. = L. V. = finger counting at 1 m.; discs were pale; there was peripheral contraction of fields, also central scotomata were present; he recognised no colours except blue. The patient thought his trouble was the result of getting his feet wet. He was seen again twelve years later when his condition remained unchanged; in the meantime a younger brother had developed the disease; he said that a maternal uncle also was similarly affected. No consanguinity recorded. Bibl. No. 101, p. 165.

Fig. 910. *Lundsgaard's Case.* Hereditary optic atrophy in nine males and two females of four generations; the disease in every case was transmitted by an unaffected female of the stock. The age of onset in I. 3 was at 30 years; II. 2 and II. 9 became affected at 25 and 30 years respectively; III. 2 became affected at 18 years, III. 3 at 27 years, III. 10 at 25 years, III. 15 at 8 years and III. 17 at 16 years; the ages of onset in IV. 3, 4 and 11 were 16, 12 and 6 years respectively. No consanguinity recorded. Bibl. No. 142.

Plate LXIII. Fig. 911. *Kawakami's Case.* Hereditary optic atrophy in nineteen males and twelve females of four generations. The pedigree has been very fully worked out and a large number of members of the stock have been examined; the age of onset of the disease in the affected members varies over a wide range of years, the youngest to be affected was aged 12 years and the oldest at the time of onset was aged 51 years. All generation V and many members of generation IV are still of an age at which the disease may develop. In generation I the only male, I. 3, was reported to have been affected; his three sisters appear to have been normal but to have transmitted the defect; thus probably all the children of I. 2 were affected, all the married daughters of I. 4 had affected sons, and all the married daughters of I. 6 were affected or had affected offspring. II. 1 died aged 65; he was reported to have been affected in his youth. II. 2 died aged 60; according to her nephew, III. 20, she became affected after her marriage but her daughter, III. 2, reported that she could see well; she had three affected children and seven affected grandchildren. II. 4 died aged 60; III. 20 reports that II. 4 also became affected after her marriage but there appears to have been some evidence that she had also suffered from trachoma; none of her children were affected but three of her grandchildren were affected and others had died young or were still of an age at which the disease might develop. II. 6, aged 70, was not seen but his wife and his sons report that he became affected at the age of 20 years; according to the statement of his sons he was able to see to read fairly small print; he married his first cousin, II. 7, and had four children of whom two sons became affected at the ages of 40 and 12 years respectively, one normal son was aged 25, one daughter was aged 18. II. 7, aged 61, was healthy and had normal fundi; R. V. = L. V. = 0·9. II. 8 had R. V. = L. V. = 0·1; fundi were normal, ?cataract; she had two sons of whom one, III. 25, was affected. II. 10 died aged 37. II. 11 and her husband died aged 50; they had two children of whom a son, III. 28, was affected. II. 13 died aged 37; his four children and twelve grandchildren were normal. II. 15, aged 78, had R. V. = 0·1, L. V. = perception of light; she had an immature cataract in the right eye, a mature cataract in the left; fundi could not be observed; she had seen well in her youth. II. 16 died aged 70; she became blind at 40 and it is reported that her eyes watered very much at that time; the recorder considers it is very doubtful whether this is definitely a case of Leber's disease; she had six children of whom three sons were affected. II. 18, aged 76, had R. V. = L. V. = 0·6; fundi normal; she had an affected son and three affected grandchildren.

III. 2, aged 67, was healthy, she became affected at the age of 50; now R. V. = L. V. = finger counting at 1·5 m.; papillae are pale, the retina somewhat degenerated, the macular region blurred; three of her six children were affected, her grandchildren were all below the age at which the disease is liable to develop. III. 3 is reported by III. 20 to be affected; her four children are normal, her grandchildren are still

PLATE LXIII.   DESCRIPTIONS OF PEDIGREE PLATES   419

young. III. 5 was normal up to the time of his death at 30. III. 6, aged 40, was affected, no details are given of his case. III. 7 died aged 31; four of her eight children were affected. III. 9 died aged 24; she was not affected and her three children aged 25, 20 and 18 respectively were unaffected. III. 12, aged 56, was reported by III. 20 to have had bad eyes; he had six children of whom IV. 27 died aged 12, the second son was aged 32, the third son aged 27 had R. V. = L. V. = 1·2, fundi normal; two daughters aged 23 and 20 respectively were normal; IV. 30 was aged 16 and not yet affected. III. 13, aged 50, was unaffected and had five children of whom IV. 31, aged 27, and IV. 32, aged 21, were normal, two sons died aged 10 and 7 years respectively. IV. 34 was only aged 8 years. III. 15, aged 46, had R. V. = L. V. = 1·0, fundi were normal; her husband aged 49 had R. V. = L. V. = 1·0, fundi were normal; he had a history of a transitory visual disturbance some years previously; they had seven children of whom three became affected rather early in life and two were still quite young, viz. 15 and 8 years of age respectively. III. 17 died aged 24; he had two children aged 18 and 10 respectively.

III. 20, aged 41, was an intelligent and healthy man; he had had no eye trouble until April 1923 when he was aged 40 and had noticed a sudden diminution of vision in both eyes; the condition progressed for five months since when it had remained stationary; the papillae were pale and yellowish, not clearly outlined, the macula and fovea were normal and there were no peripheral changes in the retina, the retinal vessels were normal; R. V. = L. V. = finger counting at 1 m.; refraction was emmetropic; large absolute central scotomata were present and there was some slight contraction of the outer limits of the visual fields; light sense was normal; colour sense was markedly affected, colours of large surfaces only being recognised; X-ray showed a normal base of skull. III. 19, aged 38, wife of III. 20, was examined, fundi were normal and R. V. = L. V. = 0·9. III. 21, aged 30, became affected at the early age of 12 years; he is able to carry on his work as an agricultural labourer; his papillae are very pale, outlines clear; R. V. = L. V. = finger counting at 1·5 m. III. 22, aged 25, was healthy, he had slight myopia; R. V. = L. V. = 0·9; there was some slight opacity of the left cornea. III. 23, aged 18, was healthy, fundi were normal and R. V. = L. V. = 1·5. III. 19 and 20 had three young children who were examined; the eldest, aged 15, had R. V. = 1·5, L. V. = 2·0, fundi normal; the second child, aged 11, had R. V. = 1·5, L. V. = 1·2, fundi normal; the youngest child, aged 3, had normal fundi. III. 25, aged 39, became affected at 27; papillae were very pale; R. V. = L. V. = finger counting at 0·5 m. III. 24, wife to III. 25, was normal; their three children were aged 12, 9 and 6 years respectively, all had normal fundi and saw well; III. 26, aged 36, had normal fundi and R. V. = L. V. = 1·5; his wife was tested and had normal vision; of his three children, aged 11, 7 and 2 years respectively, the eldest was examined and found to be normal. III. 28 became affected at about the age of 30 and died aged 36. The children of III. 31 were aged 30, 24, 22, 18 and 16 years respectively and were believed to be normal; two grandchildren, V. 22 and 23, were aged 7 and 2 years respectively. III. 32 was aged 47.

III. 39, aged 61, became affected at 51; R. V. = L. V. = finger counting at 1·0 m.; central scotomata were present, also definite peripheral contraction of fields; the papillae were atrophied and the foveal reflex was scarcely visible; the wife of III. 39 had normal vision and no cases of the disease had yet occurred in their children or grandchildren; the children were aged 41, 38, 35, 28, 26, 20, 16, 12 and 9 years respectively; one grandchild was aged 20, all the other grandchildren were less than 16 years of age. III. 41 died aged 45, he became affected at 30. III. 42 and 43 were examined and found to be normal; they had two normal children aged 26 and 22 respectively and two grandchildren aged 6 and 4 years respectively. III. 44, aged 51, became affected at the age of 29 and has seen badly since; R. V. = finger counting at 0·25 m., L. V. = finger counting at 1·0 m.; papillae were pale, foveal reflex scarcely visible. III. 45, aged 43, was believed to be normal; he had three children aged 21, 18 and 7 years respectively. III. 48, aged 51, became affected at 43; R. V. = L. V. = finger counting at 0·5 m.; bilateral central scotomata were present with slight contraction of the peripheral visual fields; papillae were pale, macular ring and foveal reflex were absent. III. 48 had seven children aged 29, 24, 24, 21, 19, 19 and 12 years respectively, none of whom were yet affected. III. 49 had eight children and R. V. = L. V. = 1·2; she had eight children of whom IV. 74, aged 31, was normal, IV. 75, aged 27, was reported by members of the family to have bad eyes, IV. 76, aged 24, had normal fundi and R. V. = 0·9, L. V. = 1·0; IV. 77, aged 22, became affected at 19, the condition became stationary after two months, since when R. V. = finger counting at 2·5 m., L. V. = finger counting at 2·0 m.; bilateral central scotomata are present; papillae are pale. IV. 78, aged 17, became affected at 17; after three months the condition became stationary and R. V. = L. V. = finger counting at 3 0 m.; papillae were pale, macular ring normal, foveal reflex scarcely visible. IV. 79, aged 17, and IV. 80 were not yet affected. III. 51, aged 37, had normal fundi and R. V. = L. V. = 1·2; he had four children aged 8, 6, 4 and 1 year respectively.

III. 54, aged 50, was normal and had nine children aged 26, 24, 21, 16, 14, 10, 1 9, 7 and 4 years respectively, none of whom were yet affected. III. 55 died aged 43, he was reported to have had bad eyes. III. 57, aged 28, was examined and was normal. The eldest son of II. 25, aged 26, was normal; his second son, aged 24, had R. V. = L. V. = 0·8; slight corneal opacities in both eyes are noted.

IV. 2, aged 42, had five living children aged 19, 17, 14, 11 and 8 years respectively and one son who died aged 11. IV. 3, aged 42, was in America; his mother said he saw well but III. 20 reports that he sees badly. IV. 4, aged 41, was unaffected. IV. 5, aged 37, had seen badly for twenty days; R. V. = L. V. = 0·4;

papillae were somewhat pale, there were no signs of inflammation in the fundi; she had five children of whom the eldest was aged 14, the youngest 2 years. IV. 7, aged 33, was examined and was normal; her two children were aged 6 and 1 year respectively. IV. 9, aged 26, saw badly at the age of 21; R. V. = finger counting at 3·0 m., L. V. = finger counting at 2·5 m.; papillae somewhat pale; her two children were aged 5 and 2 years respectively. IV. 12, aged 46, had four children aged 17, 13, 9 and 5 years respectively. IV. 14, aged 40, had six children aged 23, 18, 16, 11, 8 and 4 years respectively. IV. 15 were aged 30 and 27 years respectively. IV. 17 had two children aged 19 and 17 years respectively not yet affected. The elder of IV. 18, aged 37, was normal, the younger died aged 27, there was some doubt as to whether she had good vision. IV. 20, aged 32, became affected at 14; R. V. = finger counting at 0·5 m., L. V. = finger counting at 1·0 m.; papillae were pale and macular region blurred; her only child was aged 10. IV. 21, aged 30, and IV. 22 were reported to have had bad eyes. IV. 23 was normal. IV. 24 had R. V. = finger counting at 0·5 m., L. V. = finger counting at 1·0 m.; papillae were pale, macular ring invisible.

IV. 35, aged 28, became affected at 19; his family say that he saw worse than his two affected siblings. IV. 36, aged 26, was normal and had an infant son V. 21. IV. 39, aged 20, became affected at 16; the papillae were pale. IV. 40, aged 18, the onset was sudden and in both eyes; the condition progressed for three months and then became stationary; the papillae were pale yellowish not clearly outlined; the vessels and media were normal; oedematous changes were noted in the macular region; R. V. = L. V. = finger counting at 2·5 m.; relative central scotomata were present; X-ray showed a normal base of skull. Consanguinity. Bibl. No. 137.

Fig. 912. *Isiguro's Case I.* Hereditary optic atrophy in one male and three females of two generations. III. 3, aged 31, became affected at the age of 26; she had four children aged 15, 12, 6 and 3 years respectively, the eldest became affected at the age of 14 years. III. 4, aged 27, became affected at 17. Two sisters of III. 4 died young. The parents and grandparents of the sibship III. 3—5 saw well; the mother, II. 4, died aged 55; I. 3 and 4 died aged 71 and 60 years respectively; the brother of II. 4 had six children of whom III. 7, aged 34, became affected at the age of 21; III. 9—12 were aged 30, 25, 21 and 16 years respectively at the date of the record. No consanguinity recorded. Bibl. No. 137. (Abstracted by Kawakami from *Ganka Rinsho Iho,* 1923.)

Fig. 913. *T. Nakamura's Case.* Hereditary optic atrophy in three males and seven females of three generations; every member of generations II, III and IV was either affected or had died young or (two cases only) was of an age at which he may still become affected. I. 1 died aged 82, I. 2 died aged 60, I. 3 died aged 42; all these appear to have been normal. I. 1 and 2 had eight children of whom II. 1 died aged 47, and became affected at the age of 14. II. 2, aged 59, became affected at 25, she had two children who were both affected. II. 4 died aged 3 years. II. 5, aged 50, was affected and had an affected child. II. 7, aged 47, became affected at the age of 27. II. 9 died aged 4 and 2 years respectively. II. 10, aged 33, became affected at the age of 12. III. 1 became affected at 13; III. 2, aged 33, became affected at 18 and had an affected child. III. 4, aged 20, was not yet affected, his brother, III. 5, aged 15, became affected at the early age of 7 years; it is not clear to which sibship III. 4 and 5 belong but it would appear that they are possibly siblings of III. 6, aged 13, who became affected at the age of 8 years. III. 7 died young; III. 8 was aged 12 and not yet affected. IV. 1 died young; IV. 2, aged 12, had this year become affected. No consanguinity recorded. Bibl. No. 137. (Abstracted by Kawakami from *Nippon Ganka Gakkai Zassi,* 1909.)

Fig. 914. *Kako's Case.* Hereditary optic atrophy in three brothers and in their mother's first cousin once removed. IV. 1, aged 26, became affected at 19; IV. 2, aged 24, and IV. 3, aged 20, became affected at the age of 20 years; IV. 4 was aged 15; each case was examined and showed atrophy of the optic nerve; two of the brothers had central scotomata; all had some concentric contraction of the visual fields. The parents, aged 55 and 54, were normal and had normal siblings; the grandparents, II. 1—4, were also normal but the first cousin of II. 3 was reported to have been affected. No consanguinity recorded. Bibl. No. 137. (Abstracted by Kawakami from *Nippon Ganka Gakkai Zassi,* 1913.)

Fig. 915. *Takahasi's Case.* Hereditary optic atrophy in five males of three generations. I. 1 and 2 and their children were normal; one son, II. 1, married II. 7, whose brother now aged 76 became affected at the age of 20; II. 1 and 7 had seven children of whom III. 1 transmitted the defect to two of her sons, see later; III. 2, aged 55, became affected at 20 and III. 5, aged 37, became affected at the age of 20 years; III. 3, 6, 8 and 10 were normal and probably will remain so; we are not told the ages of their children so cannot be assured that they will remain free from the defect. III. 1 had six children of whom IV. 1, aged 32, and IV. 2, aged 28, were normal; the three children of IV. 2 were aged 8, 6 and 4 years respectively. IV. 4, aged 28, became affected at 25; IV. 5, aged 22, was not yet affected; IV. 6, aged 18, became affected at 17 and IV. 7 died aged 3 years. The father of this sibship, III. 13, appeared to come of a normal stock. No consanguinity recorded. Bibl. No. 137. (Abstracted by Kawakami from *Tohoku Igaku Zassi,* 1923.)

Fig. 916. *Yo-Kansyo's Case.* Hereditary optic atrophy in ten males and two females of four generations. I. 1 was known to have been affected, but no information is given with regard to the age of onset of the disease; he had seven children of whom II. 2 became affected at the age of 30, II. 8 became affected at 25; II. 1, 4, 5, 6 and 7 were normal and no information is given of their marriage. II. 2 and 8 were both

Plate LXIII.   DESCRIPTIONS OF PEDIGREE PLATES   421

married and had affected children; three of the five children of II. 2 were affected, III. 3 at the age of 30, III. 6 at the age of 23 years; the age of onset for the case of III. 2 is not given. Three of the six children of II. 8 were affected, III. 8 at the age of 40, III. 10 at 34, and III. 11 at the age of 33 years. III. 3 had four children of whom one, IV. 2, became affected at the age of 32. III. 8 had three children of whom one, IV. 5, became affected at 29. III. 11 had two children of whom one, IV. 9, became affected at the age of 28. IV. 9 had four children whose ages are not given, we cannot assume that they will remain free from the disease though none of them are yet (1923) affected. No consanguinity recorded. Bibl. No. 137. (Abstracted by Kawakami from *Ganka Rinsho Iho*, 1923.)

Fig. 917. *Nisizaki's Case*. Hereditary optic atrophy in three males and three females of two generations. I. 1 and 2, and their five children, aged 51, 45, 36, 31 and 26 years respectively, saw well. I. 3 and 4 were free from the disease but three of their six children were affected. II. 7, aged 44, became affected at the age of 21 years; she was married to II. 1 and had three children, of whom III. 5, aged 24, was affected at 19; III. 6, aged 20, was affected at 19; III. 7 was aged 7 years. II. 8 was unaffected and had two young children aged 8 and 4 years respectively. II. 10, aged 38, was unaffected. II. 11, aged 35, became affected at 30; she had four young children aged 14, 9, 4 and 2 years respectively, of whom the second child aged 9 years was already affected. II. 13, aged 30, was affected; no information is given of his age at the onset of the disease. II. 14, aged 22, was unaffected. III. 1 was aged 3; III. 2—4 were aged 14, 10 and 7 years respectively. No consanguinity recorded. Bibl. No. 137. (Abstracted by Kawakami from *Nippon Ganka Gakkai Zassi*, 1909.)

Fig. 918. *Fuzihira's Case*. Hereditary optic atrophy in three males of two generations. I. 1 and 2 had two children, a son, II. 3, aged 51 (1914), who became affected with the disease at the age of 36, and a daughter, II. 2, who was herself normal but had two affected sons. III. 1, aged 22, became affected at the age of 18; III. 5, aged 15, became affected at 14 years; III. 2 was unaffected; four other siblings died young. II. 3 had four children of whom III. 8 died aged 19, III. 9—11 were aged 29, 27 and 20 years respectively. No consanguinity recorded. Bibl. No. 137. (Abstracted by Kawakami from *Nippon Ganka Gakkai Zassi*, 1914.)

Fig. 919. *Kusunoki's Case*. Hereditary optic atrophy in three males and one female of a sibship of six; the mother's brother was also affected. II. 4 was aged 23; the age of onset in his case was 18. No further information is given. No consanguinity recorded. Bibl. No. 137. (Abstracted by Kawakami from *Ganka Rinsho Iho*, 1924.)

Fig. 920. *Okazaki's Case*. Hereditary optic atrophy in three males and one female of a sibship of nine; other members were below the age at which liability to develop the disease occurs. II. 1, aged 24, became affected at 15; II. 2, aged 21, became affected at 18; for II. 3, aged 20, the age of onset was 16; II. 4, aged 18, was unaffected; II. 5, aged 16, became affected at 15; other members of the sibship were aged 13, 10, 8 and 1 year respectively. No consanguinity recorded. Bibl. No. 137. (Abstracted by Kawakami from *Chuo Ganka Iho*, 1920.)

Fig. 921. *Isiguro's Case II*. Hereditary optic atrophy in five males and two females of three sibships. I. 1 and 2 were normal and lived to the ages of 75 and 72 years respectively; they had three children of whom II. 2, aged 49, had optic atrophy at the age of 23, and II. 4 had an affected son, III. 11. II. 2 had ten children of whom five were affected and probably three others were still of an age at which liability to develop the disease is present. III. 1, aged 26, and III. 5, aged 18, became affected at the age of 13; III. 4, aged 21, was affected at 14; III. 2, 6, 7 and 8 were aged 25, 17, 15 and 13 years respectively; the age of onset for III. 6 and 7 is not given. III. 11 was aged 20, no information is given of his age at onset of the disease, or of the ages of his five still unaffected brothers. No consanguinity recorded. Bibl. No. 137. (Abstracted by Kawakami from *Ganka Rinsho Iho*, 1923.)

Fig. 922. *Inouye's Case*. Hereditary optic atrophy in five members of a sibship of six; their mother and maternal grandmother were also affected. The age of onset for these cases is as follows: I. 1, II. 1 and III. 3 became affected at 15; III. 1 and 2 became affected at 19; III. 4 became affected at 13, and III. 5 at 14. The ages of members of the sibship III. 1—6 at the time the case was reported were 34, 31, 28, 22 and 19 years. The age of III. 6 is not given, but as he appears to be the youngest member of the sibship he was still of an age at which the disease may develop. No consanguinity recorded. Bibl. No. 137. (Abstracted by Kawakami from *Nippon Ganka Gakkai Zassi*, 1919.)

Fig. 923. *Kuwahara's Case*. Hereditary optic atrophy in five males and one female of three generations. I. 1 was affected but the age at which the disease developed in him is not given; he had three children of whom one daughter transmitted the disease, which had already affected three of her nine children, and the two sons became themselves affected; the onset in II. 3, now (1918) aged 45, was at 28 years; II. 4, aged 38, became affected at the age of 35. III. 4, aged 22, had become affected this year; III. 5, aged 18, became affected at 15; III. 6, aged 11, had this year become affected. III. 7, 8 and 9 were probably too young to be definitely regarded as free from the disease. No consanguinity recorded. Bibl. No. 137. (Abstracted by Kawakami from *Chuo Ganka Iho*, 1918.)

Fig. 924. *Kisi's Case I.* Hereditary optic atrophy in two males and one female of a sibship of nine; parents and grandparents were unaffected. III. 1 died aged 2 years. III. 2, aged 22, became affected at 21; III. 3, aged 20, became affected at 14; the onset in III. 4, aged 17, was at the age of 11 years. All other members of this sibship were of an age at which the disease may still develop, thus III. 5 and 6 were aged 13, III. 7 aged 11, III. 8 aged 8, and III. 9 was aged 6 years. No consanguinity recorded. Bibl. No. 137. (Abstracted by Kawakami from *Nippon Ganka Gakkai Zassi*, 1910.)

Fig. 925. *Kozaki's Case.* Hereditary optic atrophy in two sisters aged 23 and 15 years respectively; the onset in the former case was at 16 years, in the latter case at 15 years of age; the parents and their siblings, also grandparents, were normal. The affected sisters had three siblings of whom the two younger were aged 7 and 5 years respectively. No consanguinity recorded. Bibl. No. 137. (Abstracted by Kawakami from *Chuo Ganka Iho*, 1923.)

Fig. 926. *Fuzii's Case I.* Hereditary optic atrophy in three males and five females of three generations. I. 1 became affected at the age of 20, she was married and had five children of whom four were affected. II. 2 and II. 4 became affected at 27, II. 3 at the age of 19, and II. 6 at the age of 18 years. II. 2 was married and had four children of whom III. 1 became affected at 22, III. 3 and 4 became affected at the age of 12. We suspect that this is the same case as the one published by Fuzita two years before at which time III. 1 had not yet become affected. No consanguinity recorded. Bibl. No. 137. (Abstracted by Kawakami from *Okayama Igakukai Zassi*, 1922.)

Fig. 927. *Fuzii's Case II.* Hereditary optic atrophy in two males and one female of a sibship of seven, and in their maternal grandfather; the onset of the disease occurred in III. 4 at fifteen years, in III. 6 at 21 years and in III. 7 at 18 years. No consanguinity recorded. Bibl. No. 137. (Abstracted by Kawakami from *Okayama Igakukai Zassi*, 1922.)

Fig. 928. *B. Nakamura's Case.* Hereditary optic atrophy in three males and three females of a sibship of nine; the three unaffected siblings were still below the age at which the disease may develop. The ages of III. 1—9 at the time the history was reported were 29, 27, 24, 22, 20, 18, 15, 13 and 9 years respectively; the age of onset of the disease in the affected members was as follows: 20 years for III. 1, 14 for III. 2, 18 for III. 3, 16 years for III. 4 and III. 5, and 14 years for III. 7. The parents and grandparents were unaffected. No consanguinity recorded. Bibl. No. 137. (Abstracted by Kawakami from *Nippon Ganka Gakkai Zassi*, 1918.)

Fig. 929. *Fuzihira's Case.* Hereditary optic atrophy in two males and one female of a sibship of six; the mother and the maternal grandmother were also affected; we are not given the age of onset in any case, but present ages of III. 1 and 2 are given as 22 and 20 years respectively. No consanguinity recorded. Bibl. No. 137. (Abstracted by Kawakami from *Nippon Ganka Gakkai Zassi*, 1914.)

Fig. 930. *Kisi's Case II.* Hereditary optic atrophy in two sisters and in the two sons of one of them. II. 3, aged 44, became affected at 21; we are not told the age of onset for her affected sister II. 4. III. 1, aged 25, and III. 2, aged 20, became affected at 19. III. 3 was only aged 7 years at the time the case was reported. The father, II. 2, of the affected brothers was aged 50; he and the grandparents, I. 1—4, appear to have been normal. No consanguinity recorded. Bibl. No. 137. (Abstracted by Kawakami from *Nippon Ganka Gakkai Zassi*, 1910.)

Fig. 931. *Oguchi's Case.* Hereditary optic atrophy in two males and one female of a sibship of seven; the affected members were aged 37, 27 and 22 respectively, but we are not told in the abstract of this case at what age the onset occurred; of the normal siblings II. 1 was aged 42, II. 2 died aged 35, II. 4 was aged 35, II. 5 was aged 30; the parents were apparently normal, the father died aged 60. No consanguinity recorded. Bibl. No. 137. (Abstracted by Kawakami from *Nippon Ganka Gakkai Zassi*, 1909.)

Fig. 932. *Imamura and Ichikawa's Case.* Optic atrophy in a brother and sister. I. 1, aged 56, and I. 2, aged 53, were well and had good vision; there had been no amblyopia in their antecedents, direct or collateral, so far as could be discovered. II. 1, aged 28, noticed some defect in his vision at the age of 18, since then he had had xanthopsia and myiodesopsia; his vision progressively diminished for five months and had since been stationary; now V. = finger counting at 30 cm. in the right and at 50 cm. in the left; media were normal, pupils reacted briskly to light; the papillae were clearly outlined and were pale over their whole area; some narrowing of vessels was noted; only blue and yellow colours were recognised; central absolute scotomata were present with no contraction of the peripheral fields. II. 2, aged 25, noticed a diminution of vision at the age of 24; she had at this time and since some headaches which were not very severe; now pupils reacted normally, media were clear; discs were hyperaemic, contours a little blurred; vessels dilated; V. = finger counting at 3 m. in the right eye and at 4 m. in the left; colour vision was not perceptibly defective; central scotomata were present with no peripheral contraction of fields. II. 2 also showed signs of mental weakness, slowness in intellectual operations with feeble memory; she had tremors of lips, eyelids, protruded tongue and of extended fingers; rigidity of limbs was noted and defective movements of fine coordination; Romberg's sign was negative. II. 3 and 4, aged 23 and 21, saw well. II. 5

PLATE LXIII.   DESCRIPTIONS OF PEDIGREE PLATES   423

died aged 4 years. II. 6 and 7, aged 15 and 13 years respectively, showed no signs of defect at the time of the record. No consanguinity. Bibl. No. 115.

Fig. 933. *Kusunoki's Case.* Optic atrophy in two brothers one of whom became affected at the age of 9 years. No consanguinity recorded. Bibl. No. 137. (Abstracted by Kawakami from *Ganka Rinsho Iho*, 1924.)

Fig. 934. *Komoto's Case.* Hereditary optic atrophy in two males and in their maternal aunt. II. 1 was aged 20; II. 2, aged 17, became affected at the age of 13; II. 3, aged 14, became affected at this age; II. 4 was aged 8 years; II. 5 died young. No consanguinity recorded. Bibl. No. 137. (Abstracted by Kawakami from *Nippon Ganka Gakkai Zassi*, 1909.)

Fig. 935. *Masuda's Case.* Hereditary optic atrophy in a male aged 14 and in three of his mother's siblings. The age of onset in II. 7 was 14; we are not given the ages of his six siblings so have no idea whether they should or should not be regarded as definitely free from the disease; the parents I. 1 and 2 were apparently normal; the age of onset for I. 3, 4 and 5 is not given. No consanguinity recorded. Bibl. No. 137. (Abstracted by Kawakami from *Nippon Ganka Gakkai Zassi*, 1911.)

Fig. 936. *Fuzita's Case.* Hereditary optic atrophy in two males of a sibship of three; the mother's brother was also affected. II. 1, aged 26, became affected at the age of 14; the onset for II. 3 was at the age of 16; I. 3 was aged 25, but we are not told how long he had suffered from the disease. I. 1 died aged 56 years. No consanguinity recorded. Bibl. No. 137. (Abstracted by Kawakami from *Ganka Rinsho Iho*, 1920.)

Fig. 937. *Onisi's Case.* Hereditary optic atrophy in two males and two females of two related sibships. II. 1 was aged 33 (1913), the age of onset of the disease in her case is not given; II. 2, aged 15, became affected at the age of 14. The age of onset of the disease in II. 5 and 6 was 14 years; they were now aged 16 and 14 respectively. The father of II. 1 and 2 was related to one of the parents of II. 5 and 6. No consanguinity recorded. Bibl. No. 137. (Abstracted by Kawakami from *Nippon Ganka Gakkai Zassi*, 1913.)

Fig. 938. *Kakutani's Case.* Hereditary optic atrophy in a mother and in two of her three daughters; the onset for the mother was at the age of 33 years; both daughters became affected at the age of 23. No further information is given. No consanguinity recorded. Bibl. No. 137. (Abstracted by Kawakami from *Chuo Ganka Iho*, 1920.)

Fig. 939. *Takagi's Case.* Hereditary optic atrophy in a female and in her maternal aunt and uncle. II. 1, aged 15, had just become affected; I. 3 became affected at 18; I. 4 became affected at 19 years. No consanguinity recorded. Bibl. No. 137. (Abstracted by Kawakami from *Nippon Ganka Gakkai Zassi*, 1922.)

Fig. 940. *Kawabata's Case I.* Optic atrophy in a brother and sister. II. 1, aged 22, became affected at 21. II. 2, aged 17, became affected at 16. No consanguinity recorded. Bibl. No. 137. (Abstracted by Kawakami from *Chuo Ganka Iho*, 1918.)

Fig. 941. *Kawabata's Case II.* Optic atrophy in a brother and sister. II. 1, aged 28, became affected at 18. II. 2, aged 25, became affected at the age of 24 years. No consanguinity recorded. Bibl. No. 137. (Abstracted by Kawakami from *Chuo Ganka Iho*, 1918.)

ADDENDUM

Since completing my introduction to this memoir a brief preliminary notice of the first anatomical examination of a case of Leber's Disease has been published. This communication is of so great an interest that I reproduce it here. A full account of the case is to be published in *von Graefes Archiv.*

Rehsteiner, K.: Die erste anatomische Untersuchung eines Falles von Leberscher Krankheit. *Klinische Monatsblätter f. Augenheilkunde*, Bd. LXXXV, S. 280. Stuttgart, 1930.

Bulbi und Sehnerven eines an typischer hereditär-geschlechtsgebundener Sehnervenatrophie leidenden und 7 Jahre nach Beginn des Leidens gestorbenen Mannes. Ganglienzellschicht und Nervenfaserschicht der Retina stark atrophisch, sonst nichts Abnormes an den Bulbi. Atrophie der Nervenfasern im Sehnerven sehr ungleich, neben partiell und ganz atrophischen auch wieder normale Nervenfaserbündel. Gliafasern in den atrophischen Bezirken vermehrt, sekundäre Bindegewebssepten atrophisch, auf dem Querschnitt statt eines zarten Maschenwerks von Septen nur noch plumpe Bindegewebsinseln an den ehemaligen Knotenpunkten der Septen zu sehen. Atrophie dicht hinter dem Bulbus am stärksten temporal, weiter hinten gegen die Mitte rückend. Sie schloss also stets das papillomakuläre Bündel ein, war aber viel grösser als dasselbe. Damit stimmt überein, dass in vivo ein Zentralskotom bestanden hatte, das aber nicht nur den Fixierpunkt, sondern auch grosse Teile des angrenzenden Gesichtsfeldes umfasste.

Der vorliegende Fall wies keine Befunde auf, die für eine Entzündung sprechen. Da es sich aber um ein Spätstadium handelt, in dem eventuelle frühere entzündliche Zeichen wieder verschwunden sind, wurde eine Parallele gezogen zu einigen toxischen Degenerationen (Atoxyl, Diabetes), die als nicht entzündliche Degenerationen bekannt sind und die im Spätstadium aussehen wie unser Fall (im Gegensatz zu postneuritischer Atrophie nicht Verdickung, sondern Schwund der feineren Septen!). Wir fassen daher auch unsern Fall als primäre Atrophie auf, ohne indessen Toxine für diese verantwortlich zu machen. Die Lebersche Krankheit ist eine hereditäre, durch das Keimplasma bedingte, nicht entzündliche Degeneration des Sehnerven.

ON SOME STRUCTURAL ANOMALIES OF THE EYE AND ON THE INHERITANCE OF GLAUCOMA

In this section of the *Treasury* I propose to consider: A. Anomalies in size of the eye—Anophthalmos, Microphthalmos, Megalocornea, Buphthalmos—and to include with this group Glaucoma. B. Some Anomalies in the development of the iris—Aniridia, Coloboma iridis. C. Ectopia lentis. It has been decreed that the Nettleship volume can hold no more and must now be closed; the omission from it of a section on Hereditary Nystagmus is to be regretted, for this subject is of wide interest and is one to which Nettleship made valuable contributions; it is hoped, however, that the condition may one day find a place in another volume of *The Treasury of Human Inheritance*.

The selection of subjects for inclusion in this section may appear slightly arbitrary; it was influenced, to some extent, by the consideration as to which anomalies appear to have a tendency to be associated in the same individual, or in different members of the same family; such associations may well provide valuable hints regarding the source of the defects and carry considerable aetiological significance. It was intended to include in this part hereditary opacity of the cornea, but this has had to be excluded owing to lack of space. A number of anomalies of which hereditary examples are very rare have been omitted, because the great labour of an exhaustive examination of the literature concerning them is hardly justifiable if the fruits are likely to be too meagre.

A. ANOMALIES IN SIZE OF THE EYE.

Under this heading I propose to include microphthalmos and megalocornea. The extreme difficulty of the undertaking becomes at once apparent, for we have no criteria as to what does or does not constitute either condition.

That an eye may be of a size to constitute an anomaly has long been recognised; thus Guillemeau, in a delightful little volume, published in 1585[1], writes under *Ensemble de l'œil petit dict œil du couchon et en Grec Microphthalmos*—"or le microphthalmos est quand des la premiere conformation la personne à les yeux petits et peu fendus, n'estant enfoncez en l'orbite plus qu'il ne faut : et comme chose nee avec la personne ne se peut amender, nestant besoin d'y mettre aucun remede." Or again under *Ensemble de l'œil de bœuf, ou gros œil*—"telle affection est quelquefois naturelle, comme l'on void a ceux qui ont les yeux gros et a i ceux n'est besoin d'y mettre la main."[2] Bartisch, in 1583, in a large folio volume[3], gives full-page illustrations—"von unnatürlichen kleinen und engen Augen," and "von unnatürlichen grossen weiten Augen." These drawings are not very convincing, but they do call attention to the fact that the conditions they purport to represent are "unnatural" or anomalous.

All will agree that an eye the size of a pea is microphthalmic, but are we to call

---

[1] *Bibl.* No. 3.   [2] Spelling and accenting of original preserved.   [3] *Bibl.* No. 2.

a small eye in a small orbit in a small skull microphthalmic? If we are to rely upon general impressions, an eye which is deeply sunken in a large orbit may well pass as microphthalmic, when it would be regarded as normal if judged with regard to size alone; or, again, a narrow palpebral opening may be the determining factor in a personal judgment. Similar difficulties arise in the consideration as to what constitutes megalocornea. Moreover, is the size of the cornea, in these cases, a measure of the size of the eyeball? Or, if the anomaly in megalocornea consists in an abnormally large cornea relatively to the size of the eye—which is urged by some authorities—how can we be sure that any particular case, diagnosed as megalocornea, belongs to this category, in the absence of measurements on the eyeball as well as on the cornea? Yet recorders have been content to measure corneae, and state that all eyes having a corneal diameter above a certain fixed value are to be classified as megalocornic; the difficulty is complicated by the fact that this fixed limiting value differs from one observer to another. Thus, eyes regarded as anomalous by one observer would be classified as normal by another, and corneal measurements, which should perhaps be regarded as anomalous in a rather small eye, would be classified as normal in a larger eye. The observer who takes measurements on the cornea, and makes praiseworthy efforts to establish criteria, does not go far enough and indeed may be more commonly in error than his fellow who judges from general impressions alone[1]. It is unfortunately impossible to measure the size of the eyeball in the living person. If it is a fact that the *relative* size of the cornea is what constitutes the anomaly in megalocornea, then we may of course have megalocornea in a microphthalmic eye, and it is idle to regard a megalocornic eye as a large eye determined by measurements exceeding a certain limiting value in the corneal diameter. There is indeed some reason for supposing that the microphthalmic eye, viewed as a possibly immature or ill-developed eye, may be not unlikely to have a relatively large cornea, in as far as the cornea is normally precocious in development relatively to the rest of the eye, and is disproportionately large in the embryo.

Again, I wonder whether similar standards with regard to these matters can be taken to hold for both sexes. Are we justified in assuming that the size of the cornea relatively to the size of the eyeball is the same for the two sexes? It is unquestionable that both these anomalous eyes do occur; families in which they occur are fully alive to the condition and have usually little hesitation in asserting which are the affected individuals, but I am not prepared to define the anomalies within their limits, nor can I encourage my readers to accept every case designated anomalous or normal, with regard to size, in the pedigrees below, as certainly belonging to the categories in which they are placed.

Efforts have been made, from time to time, to determine between what limits the size of the normal cornea may lie; notable amongst these are the investigations of Priestley Smith[2] in 1891 and of Peter[3] in 1925; the former measured the corneal

---

[1] We are told by Kayser that the "Calwer" eyes of his cases and by Gronholm that the "kuppelformige" eyes of his cases were recognised by the laity of the neighbourhood and by the parents at the birth of the affected children.　　　[2] *Bibl.* No. 107.　　　[3] *Bibl.* No. 262.

diameter in 1000 eyes (in 250 males and 250 females); the latter took a similar measurement in 1024 eyes of 245 males and 267 females; the two series are unfortunately not readily comparable, and Peter alone gives detailed measurements in a form suitable for analysis; both these authors agree that their material shows no demonstrable increase in the size of the cornea after the age of 5 years. Priestley Smith finds some slight shrinkage late in life. Peter's measurements provide the following distribution and enable statistical constants to be calculated.

Corneal Diameter in mm.	Males	Females	Males and Females
10·25	—	2	2
10·50	—	4	4
10·75	2	10	12
11·00	24	38	62
11·25	56	91	147
11·50	105	142	247
11·75	129	122	251
12·00	90	86	176
12·25	59	29	88
12·50	22	8	30
12·75	3	2	5
Totals	490	534	1024

Corneal Diameter in mm. (Peter's Data.)

	No.	Mean Value	Standard Deviation	Coefficient of Variation
Males	490	11·74 ± ·01	0·376 ± ·008	3·20 ± ·07
Females	534	11·59 ± ·01	0·380 ± ·008	3·28 ± ·07
Males and Females	1024	11·67 ± ·01	0·385 ± ·006	3·30 ± ·05

It would appear that the female cornea tends to be slightly smaller than that of the male on the average, but the frequencies combined for the two sexes provide a distribution which fits the normal curve given by $y = \dfrac{1024}{\sqrt{2\pi} \times \cdot 3854}\, e^{-\frac{x^2}{\cdot 2970}}$ so closely that I think we are fully justified in examining this curve with a view to the consideration of what constitutes an anomaly in the size of the cornea for both sexes.

The accompanying diagram shows the histogram for Peter's male + female distribution with the best-fitting normal curve; the χ^2 for the determination of the measure of fit is 8·95 and the corresponding value of $P = \cdot 53$. The curve then may be regarded as a very fair representation of the range and frequencies of corneal measurements in the general population, and on the basis of it I would suggest that any cornea which measures 10·0 mm. or less is probably anomalous, any cornea which measures 13·0 mm. or more is likely to be anomalous; corneae measuring 12·0 to 12·75 mm. are only justifiably described as megalocornic if this anomaly includes corneae which are large relatively to the size of the eyeball, or if such corneae are

55—2

more bulging and prominent than normal; it is of significance with regard to these
points that the anterior chamber in megalocornea is very commonly said to be deep.

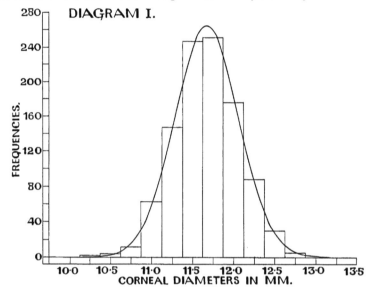

Hereditary Microphthalmos.

Published cases which fall into this category are for the most part of an extremely
anomalous character, and my warning here would lie not in any hesitation regarding
the acceptance of the cases designated microphthalmic, but rather in some caution
regarding the normality of other members of the affected stocks. The cases described
mostly show gross defect, quite apart from the question of size of the eyeball, and it
is, perhaps, not unlikely that a member of the family who saw well, and showed no
demonstrable departure from the normal in development, would escape having his eyes
classified as anomalous owing merely to the smallness of the eyeball; yet surely some
reduction in size of the eyeball should not be incompatible with good vision and a
serviceable eye; just as there is a considerable overlap at the end of the normal range of
size in the cases described as megalocornic, so also, if the pedigrees were fully investigated, an overlap should reasonably be looked for at the microphthalmic end of
the normal range.

Only 81 eyes of 43 individuals belonging to my collected series of cases of
microphthalmos have been measured; the grade of defect was generally closely
similar for the two eyes. It will be seen, from the table given below, that the range
of measurements of the corneal diameter varies from 2 mm. to 10·5 mm.; it might

appear from the distribution that eyes with a corneal diameter exceeding 10·5 mm.
were no longer classed as microphthalmic and that perhaps it has been judged that
eyes showing larger measurements than this should be regarded as normal with
regard to size. On the other hand, it is evident from an examination of the histories
appended, that not alone microphthalmos, but also the grade of microphthalmos tends
to be inherited; and the fact that multiple anomalies are so commonly associated

Some Analysis of 191 *Cases of Hereditary Microphthalmos (or Anophthalmos),*
indicating the very high grade of defect throughout the series.

(1) Least Corneal Diameter in mm.	(2) No. of Eyes	(3) Description of Eyes; no measurement given	(4) No. of Cases	(5) No description of Eyes or measurement given	(6) No. of Cases
2, 2·5	2	Bilateral Anophthalmos	9	Born blind	26
3, 3·5	1	Unilateral Anophthalmos	8†	Blind or nearly blind	6
4, 4·5	2	{Eyes rudimentary, diminutive}	38	Vision very bad	7
5, 5·5	9	{ or very small }		Good sight at one time	4
6, 6·5	3	Eyes smaller than normal	14‡	{Nystagmus and other anomalies} { noted }	6
7, 7·5	12			Other anomalies noted	13
8, 8·5	12			Other defects probable	2
9, 9·5	18			Probably no other defect	3
10, 10·5	22			No mention of other defect	12§
Totals	81*	.	69		79

* Measurements taken on the affected eyes of 43 individuals.
† Seven of these cases had an extreme grade of microphthalmos in one eye.
‡ Nine of these cases exhibited other anomalies; four cases were not examined.
§ Three of these cases were unilateral; nine of the cases came of stocks exhibiting other anomalies.

with the defect in size points to the conclusion that we are probably justified
in accepting the accuracy of the, pedigrees, and may regard them as illustrative examples of a severe grade of hereditary microphthalmos. Nevertheless, it would
be of great interest to have corneal measurements taken on the "normal" members
of these defective stocks. It may well be that a human eye with a corneal diameter
less than 10 mm. is almost sure to be an imperfectly developed or malformed eye, but
that pedigrees would be readily found, if sought for, exhibiting the inheritance of
eyes a little larger than this, and presenting no associated structural anomalies and
allowing of good vision. I could in fact put my hand on a few such pedigrees, but in
the absence of any criteria as to what constitutes a microphthalmic eye I have not
included them here; they could not with certainty be described as anomalous and
were evidently not homogeneous with my material illustrative of high grade cases.

Columns (3) and (4) of the table above refer to cases on which no corneal measurements were taken, but some idea of the degree of abnormality with regard to size of
the eyes of 69 individuals is there given; in the majority of these cases the eyes were
evidently very anomalous, described as "rudimentary," of the size of very small
green peas with diminutive or undifferentiated corneae, and so on; it is unlikely that
more than very few of these 69 cases had corneae measuring more than 5 or 6 mm.

Seventy-nine cases, for which no measurements were taken and no description is given to indicate the size of the eyes, are analysed in columns (5) and (6); it will be seen at once from what a severe grade of defect many of these individuals suffered; indeed an examination of this table as a whole amply supports my statements regarding the high grade of defect to which cases described in the literature under hereditary microphthalmos belong; these cases go to the ophthalmologist because of the severity of their symptoms and are subsequently described by him; the material in fact tends to be selected because of its high grade defect, and is probably by no means a random sample of material which might reasonably be included under our title.

On Defects associated with Hereditary Microphthalmos. The table on the following page gives some analysis of the defects found in association with microphthalmos in my collected cases; the list includes some mention of associated defects in 119 individuals; in addition to these the records include eight cases of bilateral anophthalmos; in ten further cases the eyes were diminutive and associated defects were probably too gross for analysis; 27 cases were blind at birth or very early in life and thus certainly had associated defects of which no mention is made. In a few cases, nearly all of which were not examined, no associated anomaly is described; most of these cases came of stocks in which multiple anomalies were known to have occurred. I think we may readily agree that it is rare to find a case of high-grade hereditary microphthalmos unaccompanied by other gross developmental defect; on the other hand, if we can trust our records, the associated defect is very generally confined to the eyeball, and it is surprising to find so little evidence of the occurrence of such abnormalities as hare-lip and cleft palate, or digital anomalies, in association with microphthalmos. It is true that the cases of my series are generally described by an ophthalmologist, who may well have failed to consider the question of associated bodily deformities, but he would be unlikely to pass over so gross a deformity as hare-lip or cleft palate without notice if such were present, yet in the whole series of cases I find only one example of an associated hare-lip and no single recorded case of cleft palate. Turning to the section on Hare-lip and Cleft Palate in *The Treasury of Human Inheritance*, Vol. I, I find no fewer than 12 microphthalmic individuals amongst 122 isolated cases of hare-lip and cleft palate; the number of cases presented here in which a highly arched palate[1] is described and in which some anomaly of the teeth is noted, suggest some developmental instability in these regions which might well lead us to look for references to cleft palate, but I think it is clear that in hereditary microphthalmos there is no evidence of an associated liability to this defect.

With regard to anomaly in the dental system, White Cooper wrote[2]: "In every case of double microphthalmos which has fallen under my notice, there has been imperfect dental development....The teeth, in such cases, are small, jagged, discoloured and soon decay: the cause which impedes the due development of the

---

[1] I do not know what constitutes a highly arched palate or according to what standards the common references to its existence in medical literature are based.

[2] *Bibl.* No. 40.

Associated Defects *	No. of individuals		
	♂	♀	♂
Unilateral anophthalmos with gross defects in the other microphthalmic or rudimentary eye	4	5	—
Cataract	7	10	6
,, with aniridia	1	—	—
,, ,, aniridia and defective teeth	1	2	—
,, ,, aniridia and corneal defects	2	—	—
,, ,, aniridia and strabismus	1	—	—
,, ,, aniridia, ptosis, high arched palate	1	—	—
,, ,, aniridia, ptosis, ectopia lentis, high arched palate, defective dentine	—	1	—
,, ,, aniridia, ectopia lentis, high arched palate, defective dentine	—	1	—
,, ,, colobomata of iris or choroid	2	1	—
,, ,, colobomata and high arched palate	1	—	—
,, ,, colobomata of iris and lens	1	—	—
,, ,, colobomata, strabismus, retinitis pigmentosa, high arched palate	—	1	—
,, ,, corectopia and high myopia	1	—	—
,, ,, corectopia and ptosis	—	1	—
,, ,, corectopia, high myopia, choroidal atrophy, strabismus	1	—	—
,, ,, corectopia, high myopia, choroidal atrophy, ectopia lentis	—	1	—
,, ,, corectopia, myopia, choroidal atrophy, tremulous iris	1	—	—
,, ,, corectopia, ill-developed iris, strabismus	—	1	—
,, ,, corectopia, strabismus, persistent pupillary membrane	—	1	—
,, ,, corectopia, strabismus, ill-developed iris, high arched palate, badly placed teeth, mental weakness	—	1	—
,, ,, colobomata, no central fixation, anomalous skull	—	1	—
,, ,, oval pupil, gerontoxon, anomalous skull	1	—	—
,, ,, glaucoma, high hypermetropia, defective teeth	—	1	—
,, ,, high myopia	—	1	—
,, ,, strabismus	—	1	—
,, ,, strabismus and mental defect	1	—	—
,, ,, anomaly in skull	1	—	—
Aniridia	—	4	—
,, with ectopia lentis	—	1	—
,, ,, aphakia	—	1	—
,, ,, deaf-mutism	—	1	—
Colobomata of iris or choroid	1	3	—
,, with corectopia	—	1	—
,, ,, strabismus	—	2	—
,, ,, opaque nerve fibres	—	1	—
,, ,, high arched palate	—	2	—
,, ,, hare-lip	1	—	—
,, ,, deaf-mutism, talipes equinus, etc.	1	—	—
Corectopia	—	1	—
,, with atrophic irides	—	2	—
,, ,, choroidal atrophy	—	1	—
,, ,, high myopia and albinism	—	1	—
,, ,, high myopia and choroidal atrophy	—	1	—
,, ,, high myopia, choroidal atrophy, ptosis, high arched palate	1	—	—
,, ,, myopia and conical cornea	—	2	—
,, ,, ptosis	—	1	—
,, ,, aphakia	—	1	—
,, ,, blue sclerotics	1	—	—
High myopia with strabismus and aphakia	2	—	—
High hypermetropia	2	2	—
,, with epicanthus	2	—	—
,, ,, strabismus and defect in macula	—	1	—
,, ,, remains of hyaloid artery	—	1	—
,, ,, dental anomalies	1	—	—
,, ,, mental defect	—	1	—
Glaucoma	1	1	—
Epicanthus	2	—	—
,, with persistent pupillary membrane	—	1	—
Corneal opacities	1	3	—
Ptosis	1	—	—
Strabismus	—	1	—
Deformity of skull	—	1	—
Deafness, with nystagmus and very bad vision	1	—	—
	45	68	6

* ... reciation of the si ... d th ... h an examination

globe of the eye...influences the growth of the teeth;...many of these children are stunted in stature, bow-legged or knock-kneed, of wayward, irritable temper, and not infrequently obtuse in intellect." We do not know how many cases of double microphthalmos this author had seen, but the condition is rare and the observation may be of limited significance; he describes four cases in his paper, three of whom were siblings. I can only add that among my 119 analysed cases, dental anomalies are described in two males and six females belonging to four families. Usher made a special examination of the teeth in four members of the family described under Fig. 982, and found no anomalies in the dental system; but I have no reason to believe that more than very few cases of my series have been demonstrated to have normal teeth; I suspect that, if looked for, dental anomalies would be found to occur with considerable frequency in the general population. With the possible exception of dental or palatal anomalies, mental defect, deaf-mutism or other anomalies outside the eyeball do not occur in association with microphthalmos with any significant frequency, as far as can be judged from the published accounts of cases.

Ou consideration of the associated defects in the eyeball it is at once evident that the defect is rarely purely quantitative. The microphthalmic eye of our series is not merely a small eye, but is usually an ill-developed eye showing multiple qualitative defects, or indeed may be so completely disorganised as to render the identification of parts difficult or impossible. The most commonly described associated defects in the eyeball, when analysis is possible, concern the lens and the iris, the former exhibiting some type of cataract, which may be congenital or occur early in life; capsular cataract is often described; in a few cases the senile type of cataract is suggested; some defect of the lens, with or without other anomalies, is described in no fewer than 58 of our 119 analysed cases of microphthalmos. Again, 57 cases show some associated defect in the development of the iris which may vary from complete aniridia through various degrees of colobomata to a simple corectopia; of the 21 cases of corectopia, the displacement was upwards and inwards in nine cases, inwards in seven cases, and was generally of a very noticeable character. The association of microphthalmos with anomalies of the iris, when it exists, is an extremely intimate one, and it is often immaterial whether the pedigree is classed under the heading of the particular iridal defect or under microphthalmos, so closely are the two conditions linked[1] (see for example Fig. 942 under microphthalmos, Fig. 1106 or Fig. 1116 under aniridia, or Fig. 1158 under coloboma iridis). Other anomalies found in the eyeball in association with microphthalmos include strabismus in 14 cases, ptosis in six cases, corneal defects in eight cases; anomalies in refraction are common, but high hypermetropia or high myopia occur with a similar frequency; there is some evidence that high refractive errors of either type tend to be linked with the microphthalmic condition in pedigrees in which they occur; Usher's pedigree showing microphthalmos with myopia and corectopia is the best example showing linkage of these three conditions; this author considers the source of the myopia in his cases,

---

[1] I have adopted the policy in such cases of publishing the pedigree under the heading to which it is relegated by its recorder.

concluding that it is axial in character and not resulting from corneal or lenticular anomalies.

It is not within the scope of this work to investigate the pathogenesis of congenital anomalies, but undoubtedly the examination of the microphthalmic eye with its multiple associated anomalies presents an intensely interesting study from this point of view; in particular one observation seems to me to be of significance: it is the total absence from my series of cases of any description of an associated orbital cyst. Usher definitely notes the absence of cyst formation in his cases of Fig. 982; further, in no case in the literature, to my knowledge, in which cyst formation is described in connection with a microphthalmic eye, is a hereditary history given; I think it probable that the microphthalmic eye with cyst formation is not a hereditary condition and has a totally different etiological significance from the cases of my series.

Another observation, which seems to me to be of great interest, is the rarity with which glaucoma occurs in individuals with microphthalmos of hereditary origin; if the small eye predisposes to glaucoma, as Priestley Smith's investigations give reason to suppose[1], it would appear that the association is not due to smallness of the eye, but perhaps to a disproportion of parts constituting the eye. May we deduce that the microphthalmic eye of our cases is, for all its many failings, a better proportioned eye than the small eye which develops glaucoma? I shall return again to this point in the section below dealing with hereditary glaucoma.

There may be seen at the Royal College of Surgeons a beautiful skeleton of Caroline Crachami[2], an ateleiotic dwarf, aged 9 years, of stature 19·5 inches; this child must have had a truly microphthalmic eye, for the orbits are in proportion to the skeleton. I have sought in vain for accounts of defective vision or anomalies in the eyeball in such cases; one is repeatedly driven to the conclusion that our cases belong to a small group, exhibiting an extreme grade of defect, which are inadequately described under so general a title as microphthalmos.

To sum up the chief points of interest concerning the question of associated anomalies in the microphthalmic eye, I would emphasise:

(a) The great number of cases showing some intimately linked defect in the development of the iris.

(b) The large proportion of cases exhibiting defect in the lens.

(c) The lack of uniformity in the high associated errors of refraction from one pedigree to another, though the same type of error tends to occur within the family.

(d) The absence of orbital cysts.

(e) The rarity of the occurrence of glaucoma.

(f) A profound interference with the development of the eyeball would appear to be compatible with perfect development of the rest of the body, and has rarely been demonstrated, so far as can be judged from published records, to be associated with any other severe grade of deformity, in cases which have survived to be described.

[1] *Bibl.* No. 107.

[2] A photograph of this skeleton appeared in *The Treasury of Human Inheritance*, Vol. i, Plate Z.

Symmetry in Microphthalmos. There is no doubt that in hereditary microphthalmos, as in the normal-sized eye, symmetry is generally a striking feature, extending to all grades of the defect. In anophthalmos both eyes are commonly absent; both eyes may be rudimentary; both eyes may be blind at birth; both eyes are like very small green peas in size; both corneae may be pear-shaped and present identical small measurements; or the grade of defect may be slight in each eye; the associated anomalies too are very commonly bilateral. Cases however are not rare in which a marked asymmetry is presented, and when this occurs it is frequently noted in more than one member of the affected family; such cases are described in 15 females and nine males belonging to 11 families of my series, which provides a by no means negligible percentage from only 190 individuals. Some analysis of these cases is given in the following table. A striking feature of this table is the frequency of

Examples of Asymmetry in Hereditary Microphthalmos.

No.	Fig.	Case	Sex	Right Eye	Left Eye	Remarks
1	961	I. 1	♂	Anophthalmos	Normal, good vision	Grandfather to No. 2
2	,,	III. 1	♀	Anophthalmos	Rudimentary	See No. 1
3	957	II. 2	♀	Rudimentary	Normal size, nystagmus	Son with bilateral anophthalmos
4	973	I. 1	♀	Normal size	Deeply sunken, very reduced globe	Mother to Nos. 5 and 6
5	,,	II. 2	♀	Rudimentary	Anophthalmos	See Nos. 4 and 6
6	,,	II. 3	♀	Rudimentary	Anophthalmos	See Nos. 4 and 5
7	980	II. 1	♂	Size of a pea, blind	Anophthalmos	Brother to No. 8
8	,,	II. 2	♀	Size of a pea, blind	Anophthalmos	See No. 7
9	1170	II. 2	♀	Normal size, opaque nerve fibres	Microphthalmos, coloboma iridis	Sister to No. 10
10	,,	II. 3	♀	Slight microphthalmos with colobomata and cataract; vision always bad	Rudimentary	See No. 9
11	1158	II. 2	♂	Normal size, good vision	Microphthalmos, coloboma iridis, cataract	Uncle to No. 12
12	,,	III. 3	♀	Microphthalmos, colobomata, strabismus	Normal size, colobomata	See No. 11
13	1161	III. 5	♀	Normal size, good vision	Microphthalmos, colobomata, etc.	Aunt to No. 14
14	,,	IV. 2	♀	Normal size, saw well	Microphthalmos, colobomata	See No. 13
15	958	II. 2	♀	No anomaly	Microphthalmos, coloboma iridis, corectopia	Mother to No. 16
16	,,	III. 2	♂	Microphthalmos	Normal size	See No. 15
17	974	I. 1	♀	Microphthalmos, colobomata	Normal size	Mother to No. 18
18	,,	II. 1	♂	Microphthalmos, colobomata	Normal size	See No. 17
19	982	VI. 28	♀	Very small, undeveloped, and blind	Small, coloboma iridis, $V. = \frac{6}{18}$	Sister to Nos. 20—22.
20	,,	VI. 29	♂	Anophthalmos	Small, undeveloped, and blind	A sister with bilateral anophthalmos. See Nos. 19, 21, 22
21	,,	VI. 30	♂	Size of a large pea, undeveloped, blind	Anophthalmos	See Nos. 19, 20, 22
22	,,	VI. 31	♀	Small, undeveloped, and blind	$V. = \frac{6}{12}$	See Nos. 19, 20, 21
23 & 24	978	I. 1 & II. 1	♂ ♂	Unilateral microphthalmos in father and son		

anophthalmos and of very high grade defect in cases which exhibit asymmetry; the severity of the anomaly may affect both eyes and merely differ in degree, or one eye may be entirely normal. It will be noted that in only one case is the asymmetry confined to a single member of the affected family.

The most striking and valuable illustration of asymmetry is provided by Usher's family of Fig. 982 and Plate B; the asymmetry is conspicuous in all cases except in that of the youngest affected child, VI. 36, with bilateral anophthalmos; this child was too restless to be measured, but the photograph suggests symmetry in the two eyes. Usher took rough measurements on the palpebral fissures and orbits of the other affected members of the family. It is not possible from any data known to me to determine within what limits measurements of the orbit *in children* may be regarded as normal with regard to size, but the right orbit of VI. 29, aged 14, is undoubtedly very anomalous with a vertical diameter of only 10 mm. and a horizontal diameter of 14 mm.; in each child the more grossly undeveloped eye is associated with a smaller size of orbit and the difference in the orbital measurements on the two sides is very significant, as will be seen in the table given below. Dr Morant estimates that a difference greater than 3 mm. between the right and left orbital heights or breadths in the same individual would probably not be found more frequently than about once in a normal sample of 1000 skulls.

Orbital measurements.

Case	Sex	Age	Height in mm.			Breadth in mm.			Remarks
			Right	Left	Difference	Right	Left	Difference	
VI. 29	♂	14	10	14	4 mm.	14	24	10 mm.	
VI. 30	♂	13	22	18	4 mm.	33	27	6 mm.	Cases of
VI. 28	♀	16	25	28	3 mm.	28	28	0 mm.	Fig. 982
VI. 31	♀	12	20	24	4 mm.	24	26	2 mm.	

English Adults (a) Spitalfields (Biometrika, Vol. XXIII),
(b) Farringdon Street (Biometrika, Vol. XVIII).

Sex	Height in mm.			Breadth in mm.		
	No.	Mean	Minimum	No.	Mean	Minimum
♂ (a)	(124)	32·6	27·6	(109)	42·5	37·7
♂ (b)	(83)	34·3	27·5	(81)	42·3	38·8
♀ (a)	(32)	31·5	28·1	(32)	40·2	36·1
♀ (b)	(78)	33·7	29·2	(75)	40·3	36·0

It is difficult to suggest that the very undersized orbit of VI. 29, aged 14, has any direct bearing on the accompanying anophthalmos, when the grossly undeveloped right eye of his elder sister, VI. 28, has an orbit probably within normal limits with regard to size. I would call attention to the fact that the two boys of this family, with the most asymmetric orbits, are mentally defective. VI. 29 is an imbecile, VI. 30 shows a less severe grade of mental defect. Judging from the photograph, the small orbits of VI. 29 are small relatively to the size of the skull and are not part of a general microcephaly. The stock from which these children came carries mental defect on both sides of the family, and it will be seen from Usher's widely spread enquiries that no fewer than 39 cases of mental defect or epilepsy are noted in the pedigree. The parents of the affected sibship are normal and of the 66 members of the stock examined by Usher no further case of anomaly of the eyes was discovered or heard of. Thus it is difficult to know what is the source of the serious eye affection confined to the single sibship VI. 28—37, or whether it bears any relation to the mental defect of the pedigree. This pedigree is of very great value, not alone for the careful examination of all members of the affected sibship and the photographs of each individual, but also for the unique opportunity provided to study the nature of the ancestry at the back of so defective a single family.

Vision in Cases of Hereditary Microphthalmos. It is quite clear that the vision in this condition is in the great majority of cases extremely bad throughout life. In many cases no definite statement regarding vision is provided, but in some of these the deformity is severe and no doubt the visual defect is correspondingly high grade; in other cases no examination has been made, or the affected individual is too young to test; 26 cases, in which no statement regarding vision is given, suffered from cataract with or without other anomalies and certainly had grave visual inefficiency. I have no reason to regard the cases for which no information is given as selected in any way, or likely to present worse or better vision on the average than the cases of which we have some definite knowledge, which are analysed under broad categories in the table below. In addition to the cases included in this table, five individuals with unilateral microphthalmos had good vision in the unaffected eye; nine members with bilateral anophthalmos were of course without vision.

Vision in Cases of Microphthalmos.

	♂	♀	♂	Totals	Remarks
Blind from birth	17	7	9	33	5 with unilateral anophthalmos
Blind or nearly blind	11	14	—	25	Includes V. = p.l., V. = $\frac{6}{60}$ or less
Blind in one eye	2	6	—	8	In the eye V. = $\frac{6}{12}$, $\frac{4}{12}$, $\frac{6}{12}$, $\frac{12}{12}$, $\frac{6}{30}$, $\frac{6}{30}$, $\frac{not}{36}$, $\frac{6r}{36}$, "always bad"
Vision "very bad" or "always bad"	6	4	—	10	—
Vision good early in life	—	4	—	4	Cataract later in all
Vision = $\frac{6}{9}$—$\frac{6}{30}$ in each eye	3	4	—	7	Cataract in one case
Vision good	3	1	—	4	All members of one family
	42	40	9	91	

Surely few other hereditary eye anomalies lead to so much visual incapacity as this, but we must always remember that defective vision need not follow from smallness of the eye, except in extreme cases; it is the mal-developed eye with its multiple anomalies rather than the microphthalmic eye which is responsible for the high grade functional incapacity exhibited in the table above.

Sex incidence and the Inheritance of Microphthalmos. Of 164 examples of hereditary microphthalmos for which the sex is known, 74 are males, 90 are females, giving a male sex-incidence of $45 \cdot 1 \pm 2 \cdot 6 \, °/_o$. Thus we have some actual excess of females in this short series, which however cannot be regarded as demonstrating an increased incidence amongst females in general, having regard to the probable error; we can however state that microphthalmos is not one of the conditions to which the male sex is predominantly exposed. On considering the sex responsibility for the transmission of the defect, I find some actual excess of cases transmitted by females, but the numbers are so few that it would be unwise to generalise from them; I would prefer to leave it that either sex may readily transmit to their offspring. The figures on which these statements are based are as follows, but they must be regarded as provisional only:

	♂	♀	♂	Totals
Mother affected	16	19	5	40
Father affected	8	19	3	30
Transmission probably through unaffected Mother	12	7	2	21
,, ,, ,, Father	5	9	—	14
Source indeterminate	32	36	16	84

Usher's history to five generations, Fig. 942, provides the most fully worked out pedigree yet published showing transmission of the defect; in this case each affected member has an affected parent and no unaffected member has transmitted the defect; moreover each of the five married microphthalmic members has affected offspring. These facts do not always hold; Fig. 943, by Cunier, and Fig. 950, by Ash, provide examples showing the transmission through normal females of affected stocks; Fig. 947, due to Martin, presents an affected member who has only normal offspring in a history extending through three generations; such examples however are very infrequent. Occasionally the affection appears to be confined to a single sibship, as seen in Usher's case (Fig. 982), in Wolff's case in the offspring of two unaffected first cousins (Fig. 949), or in Stuelp's case (Fig. 944); the father in the latter case was alcoholic and there was some suspicion of syphilis, eight of the 14 members of the affected sibship died young, but there was no history of miscarriage on the mother's part; the collateral history was not investigated in either Wolff's or Stuelp's cases, but in each of these families affected individuals were married and had only normal offspring. A further analysis of pedigrees is provided in the following table:

Parentage	No. of Sibships	Offspring			Average Size of Family
		Affected	Normal	Percentage Affected	
One Parent affected	29	64	59	$52 \cdot 0 \pm 3 \cdot 0$	4·2
Neither Parent affected	33	79	82	$49 \cdot 1 \pm 2 \cdot 7$	4·9
Mother or Mother's stock affected	32	62	63	$49 \cdot 6 \pm 3 \cdot 0$	3·9
Father or Father's stock affected	15	35	37	$48 \cdot 6 \pm 4 \cdot 0$	4·8

Such tentative conclusions as may be deduced from these figures suggest that roughly $50 \, °/_o$ of the sibship is affected *on the average*, and that this percentage in the general population of affected families is not significantly increased when one parent is affected; nor does the mother appear to transmit the defect to a higher proportion of her offspring than does the father. I would however emphasise the need for an examination of the individual pedigrees and for the realisation that in certain cases all members of a sibship may be affected, or again only one of a large family may show the defect; the proportion of affected in particular cases may, and indeed does, vary between very wide limits.

Hereditary Megalocornea.

If it is difficult to write more than tentatively regarding the inheritance of microphthalmos, it is so much more difficult to write at all on megalocornea that I would prefer not to include any consideration of the condition in this volume. Several interesting pedigrees however have been worked out with great care, under this title, and ophthalmologists appear to be agreed upon the existence of the anomaly, and its distinction from buphthalmos. Whether the anomaly depends upon the absolute size of the cornea, or on the large size of the cornea relatively to the eyeball, it is one which may very reasonably be expected to occur, and it is evident that in the large majority of published cases the absolute size of the cornea is large, whatever the relative size may be. My chief anxiety is concerned with the fact that if the true anomaly consists in the *relatively* large cornea, then measurements on the cornea alone are not adequate criteria on which to base a diagnosis, and a number of individuals, who are classified as "normal" in the accompanying pedigrees, may not with accuracy be placed in this category. I propose then to present the few published pedigrees known to me, but do not claim to have made an exhaustive search in the literature for histories. The condition is evidently very rare, but I think the small amount of material collected is of considerable interest from the comparison it provides with cases of hereditary buphthalmos, and in the sharply contrasting pictures presented by the too small and the too large eyes, not only from the point of view of their mode of inheritance but with regard to the frequency of associated defect and disability.

It would be of interest to have orbital measurements on some of the more striking cases of megalocornea, for exophthalmos is rarely described, and the size of the orbit would perhaps provide some indication as to whether or no the whole eyeball takes part in the enlargement. In favour of the view that perhaps the eye is a malproportioned eye, characterised by an anomalous overgrowth of the cornea, is the fact that in cases of removal of the lens for cataract operation no enlargement of the lens has been found; further, the common description of a tremulous iris is evidence that the lens is not in a position to support the iris as in the normal eye.

Earlier writers appear to have regarded the rare cases of this anomaly as healed examples of congenital buphthalmos; this is not to be wondered at when isolated cases are under consideration, but on the accumulation of records it became evident that the two conditions were markedly differentiated and presented little in common. In 1889 Horner[1] writes:

[1] *Bibl.* No. 102.

"Die reine Cornea globosa, deren scharfe Abgrenzung und absolute Durchsichtigkeit durch mehrfache Beobachtung festgestellt ist, kann sich durchs ganze Leben als eine blosse Vergrösserung der Basis der Cornea sowohl beiderseits als auf einem Augen, häufig bei mehreren Gliedern derselben Familie, forterhalten und einzig durch die Veränderung der Refraction und im spätern Leben sich äussernde Disposition zu Cataract, und zwar leicht bewegliche Cataract für die Leistungsfähigkeit'des Auges bedeutsam werden."

More recently Seefelder and Kestenbaum have enumerated the criteria which differentiate the two conditions; Seefelder in 1916[1] gives ten characteristics by which megalocornea differs from buphthalmos: (1) the absence of corneal opacities or tears in Descemet's membrane; (2) the absence of widening of the limbus, in spite of the enlargement of the anterior part of the eye; (3) the sharp definition of the corneoscleral margin; (4) the normal appearance of the sclera in the region of the anterior chamber; (5) the absence of any excavation of the optic nerve; (6) the absence of functional disturbance; (7) the relatively high astigmatism not against the rule as in hydrophthalmos; (8) the radius of curvature of the cornea is rather shortened than increased; (9) the tension of the eyeball is normal; (10) the symmetry in the proportions of the two eyes.

Kestenbaum, in 1919[2], published the following table:

	Megalocornea	Hydrophthalmos*
a	Nearly always in males	Males : Females = 5 : 3
b	Nearly always bilateral	35 °/₀ unilateral
c	Nearly always symmetrical	The two eyes usually differ
d	Corneal curvature usually normal	Corneal curvature markedly diminished
e	Frequent embryontoxon †	No embryontoxon
f	Largely hereditary	Rarely hereditary
g	Megalocornea occurs in widely-spread family histories without a single case developing into hydrophthalmos	

* More commonly described as Buphthalmos in this country.
† A congenital opacity of the cornea similar in appearance to *arcus senilis*.

I would further call attention here to the marked contrast shown by the few pedigrees of the two conditions given on Plates LXVI and LXVII; it seems evident that cases of buphthalmos are commonly confined to a single sibship. This apparent difference in the mode of inheritance can only, within limits, be accepted as a differentiating criterion, as the reader will agree, in consideration of the difference shown in, for example, pedigrees of congenital stationary night-blindness of the two types or in those of hereditary optic atrophy in Europe and Japan. Moreover, buphthalmos is often associated with extreme disability and disfigurement,. which must influence the marriage incidence amongst its population; I have few records of cases in which buphthalmic people with affected siblings have married and had offspring, and have not a single case of a family history of the disease really fully investigated; we have no knowledge of the nature of the stocks in which these isolated families, showing multiple cases of buphthalmos, occur. Speaking generally, the sex-incidence and hereditary characters of a disease are not trustworthy guides as differentiating criteria with regard to its pathological or anomalous nature.

[1] *Bibl.* No. 221.   [2] *Bibl.* No. 230.

On examination of the ten pedigrees of megalocornea appended, it will be seen that the cases described as affected include 53 males and six females, giving a male sex-incidence of 89·8 °/$_o$. A percentage based on such small numbers can only be regarded as provisional, but the value provided is in keeping with the sex-incidence found for other conditions generally described as sex-limited, and in particular closely resembles that given for colour-blindness in Part II of this volume. It is of significance that all the six affected females have an affected parent, and that two of the cases, V. 25 and 26 of Fig. 985, have an affected father and a mother of affected stock: this again strikingly recalls the case of colour-blindness in which condition an affected father with a mother of affected stock so generally, but not invariably, led to the occurrence of the relatively rare cases of colour-blindness in women.

Corneal measurements were taken on 63 eyes of 32 affected members of the pedigrees; they vary between a minimum value of 12·0 mm. to a maximum diameter of 18·0 mm.; 54 of the measurements were 13·0 mm., or greater than this, and it will be seen from an examination of Peter's measurements on 1024 eyes that no single case of his series had a corneal diameter as great as 13·0 mm.; the measurements do for the most part suggest that the absolute size of the cornea is anomalous but I have no means of judging what its size relative to the eyeball may be. Grönholm definitely states that there was no exophthalmos in his cases of Fig. 985, and that the enlargement belonged to the corneae and not to the globe of the eye, whereas Bondi notes of his two cases belonging to Fig. 990 that the whole eyeball was enlarged. It is interesting that of the two most extreme cases, in which the corneal diameters measured 18·0 mm., one case, II. 1, of Fig. 986, had at the age of 16 R.V. $= \frac{6}{12}$, L.V. $= \frac{6}{9}$; the other extreme case, II. 1, of Fig. 989, aged 44, had seen well up to the age of 34, after which cataract developed and the left eye became phthisical following operation.

Some Characteristics of the Megalocornic Eye in 66 Cases.

Corneal Diameter in mm.	No. of eyes	Depth of Anterior Chamber	No. of Cases	Vision	No. of Cases
12·0—12·75	9	"Very deep"	5	No complaints of sight	1
13·0—13·75	29	"Deep"	10	Blind in old age	2
14·0—14·75	14	5·5 mm.	2	Perception of light	1*
15·0—15·75	1	5·0 mm.	5	Saw well till age 34	1†
16·0—16·75	4	4·5 mm.	3	Good	3‡
17·0—17·75	2	3·0 mm.	1	$\frac{6}{5}$—$\frac{6}{9}$	12
18·0—18·75	4	No statement	40	$\frac{6}{12}$, $\frac{5}{18}$	18
				No statement	28

    * Glaucoma.   † Cataract.   ‡ Young children.

The corneal enlargement in these cases, so far as can be judged from the histories, is entirely consistent with the criteria enumerated by Seefelder; in no single case is any corneal opacity, or thinning of the sclera, or stretching of the limbus noted. With regard to the depth of the anterior chamber, no statement is made in the majority of cases, but I think it may be accepted that the chamber is deeper than normal in cases of megalocornea; it is difficult to see from a consideration of simple proportions how it can be otherwise, for a cornea with enlarged base and a normal or not increased radius of curvature must in the absence of other abnormalities have a deeper anterior chamber, if absolute measures be considered. Parsons, in his *Text Book of Ophthalmology*, gives 2·5 mm. as the average depth of this chamber, presumably measured from the posterior surface of the cornea. Donders[1] gives 3·6 mm. as the average distance between the middle of the anterior surface of the cornea and the anterior surface of the lens.

The vision in megalocornea is evidently not uncommonly a little below normal, though an extreme grade of the anomaly is not incompatible with good vision; the source of the frequent deviation from perfect vision is not clear; the common note of a tremulous iris, in these cases, suggests some misfit in the proportions of the eye, and that the lens is not providing the normal support to the iris, but I do not know that this fact has any significant bearing on the reduction of visual acuity. In twelve of our cases the irides are said to be tremulous, in four cases—of the same pedigree, Fig. 983—no tremor could be detected; these figures provide no measure of the frequency of the occurrence, for in other cases no statement assuredly cannot be taken to indicate no tremor.

The apparent freedom from associated defects in the megalocornic eye is no less striking a feature than their variety and frequency in the microphthalmic eye; no single defect, apart from the iris tremor, which indicates malproportion, can be pointed to with any significant frequency. It is true that four cases of cataract have been noted, of which three occur in one pedigree, Fig. 983, and two cases of zonular cataract are described, in brothers aged 6 and 7 years respectively, of Fig. 985, but in view of the iris tremor with presumably some lack of instability in the position of the lens, it is only surprising that more instances of lens defect are not noted. Treacher Collins has made some most interesting observations on the growth of the cornea[2]; he writes, "The cornea in man's eye is smaller relatively to the size of the globe than in any other mammal. In all mammals below man the diameter of the cornea measures more than half the antero-posterior diameter of the globe; in the chimpanzee it is about half; in man alone is it considerably less than half." Or again "From the sixth month of foetal life, when the anterior chamber is first formed, to the end of the second year, the growth of the cornea is rapid; during that time it doubles its size; at the sixth month of foetal life the diameter is 5·5 to 6 mm.....During the whole of foetal life, and at birth, the diameters of the cornea measure more than half those of the eyeball whilst in the fully developed eye they are less than half." Treacher Collins suggests that the increase in the size of the cornea of the megalocornic eye might be due to excessive growth during the normal time of its expansion, or to a prolongation of the usual period of growth; the latter suggestion is discountenanced by the fact that the condition is marked at the birth of the affected individuals. Of great interest too is Usher's description of enlarged corneae in goldfish[3]; he tells us that enlarged and bulging

---

[1] *Accommodation and Refraction of the Eye*, p. 38. London, 1864.
[2] *Bibl.* No. 234. [3] *Bibl.* No. 236.

corneae in fish are not uncommon and may arise from environmental conditions; it is not clear whether the enlarged corneae in his five goldfish from the same tank are or are not analogous to cases of megalocornea in man.

With regard to the inheritance of megalocornea, it is not possible to draw any general conclusions from the few pedigrees available, though some individual pedigrees are of great interest and suggestiveness; a few facts of significance, however, may be

Analysis of Parentage in 59 Cases of Megalocornea.

Parentage	♂	♀	♂	Remarks
Mother affected	5	1	—	All cases of one sibship in Fig. 984
Father affected	8	5	1	5 ♂ and 2 ♀ of Fig. 984
Mother's Stock affected, Parents normal	24	—	—	In 9 cases Maternal Grand-fathers were affected
Both Parents normal, no knowledge of Stock	9	—	6	

pointed out. It will be seen from the table given here that all the six affected females had an affected parent; it may be added that two of them with an affected father also had an affected maternal grandfather; three of the affected females are from one stock, in which five affected parents (Fig. 984) transmit the defect to thirteen of the fourteen affected members of the pedigree; in one case the parentage was unknown. The last pedigree by Gredig was most carefully investigated; it provides a marked contrast, regarding the mode of inheritance, to the extensive histories described by Kayser in Fig. 983 and by Grönholm in Fig. 985. It would appear from the latter two pedigrees that the hereditary characters in certain stocks conform to those commonly noted in colour-blindness. Megalocornea, then, like congenital stationary night-blindness, presents pedigrees in which all affected members are of affected parentage and also typical relatively sex-limited pedigrees, in which the defect is transmitted for the most part through unaffected females to their sons; this defect differs from congenital stationary night-blindness in that in pedigrees where affected members directly transmit to their offspring, the anomaly is predominantly exhibited in males, if we may judge from Gredig's case.

The pedigrees on Plate LXVI undoubtedly suggest that megalocornea is an anomaly and that cases do not merely belong to the extreme end, with regard to size, of the normal range of corneal measurements. It seems likely that we have here a foetal type of eye in which the cornea has retained its large size relatively to the eyeball; perhaps the extreme rarity of cases and large absolute size of cornea are apparent characteristics due to the fact that it is the large cornea which attracts attention to the case and determines its recognition. The freedom from associated anomalies is of interest, though a number of authors have called attention to the common occurrence of embryontoxon, and a few cases of persistent pupillary membrane with megalocornea have been noted.

The megalocornic eye should rarely, if ever, be confused with a case of arrested buphthalmos, provided examination has been made, the history of the case given, and the pedigree observed. The contrast between the two conditions will be further emphasised in the next part of this memoir.

Hereditary Buphthalmos.

"Œil de bœuf ($\beta o\hat{v}s$ $o\phi\theta a\lambda\mu os$) est une maladie d'œil quand il est gros et éminent, sortant hors la teste, comme on voit les bœufs les avoir." Thus writes Ambroise Paré (1517–1590) in the sixteenth century, providing an early reference to a malady of the eye characterised by enlargement of the eyeball and proptosis, which suggests a recognition of buphthalmos and perhaps its differentiation from exophthalmos, without enlargement of the eyeball, and from megalocornea, which is no malady of the eye but an anomaly, unaccompanied by proptosis. Saint-Yves[1], however, in 1722, in an interesting chapter entitled *De la grosseur démesurée du Globe de l'Œil*, definitely distinguishes between (*a*) the naturally large eye, (*b*) exophthalmos due to causes other than increase in the size of the globe, and (*c*) an increase in the size of the globe, when he says there may be found too great an abundance of the aqueous humour constituting an hydropsy of the globe; Saint-Yves thus provides the first undoubted reference to buphthalmos within my reading, though the great people of early days—Hippocrates, Galen, Celsus and other writers—describe conditions rather vaguely, which may or may not indicate that they were familiar with the disease. Again, more than a century elapsed before the ophthalmoscope was invented and the discovery was made that these cases were also accompanied by an excavation of the optic nerve similar to that noted in glaucoma as the result of raised intra-ocular pressure; from this time it was recognised that the chief criteria of the disease included (1) Distension of the globe and of the cornea. (2) Increased intra-ocular tension. (3) Excavation of the optic nerve. The suggestion was then made by Mauthner[2] and Dufour[2], that the condition was analogous to glaucoma, occurring at an early age when the tunics of the eyeball are still supple and capable of stretching under the influence of raised ocular tension; the disease then is generally regarded as the glaucoma of infancy. I may briefly enumerate other characteristics of the disease: they include (*a*) Opacities in the cornea with widening of the limbus and tears in Descemet's membrane. (*b*) Bluish coloration of the sclerotic in the region of the limbus owing to its thinning under the influence of tension. (*c*) Deepening of the anterior chamber. (*d*) Flattening of the cornea. (*e*) A tremulous iris. (*f*) Asymmetry in the shape of the cornea and in the appearance of the two eyes. (*g*) Gross defects in the visual function, with optic atrophy and limitation of the fields of vision[3]. In 1836, Grellois, in his *Dissertation sur l'Hydrophthalmie*, writes[4]:

"C'est ici le lieu d'aborder une question qui n'a été soulevée par aucun auteur: je veux parler de l'hérédité. Je n'ai point de faits assez concluants pour me prononcer sur l'influence de cette prédisposition, cependant l'observation permet d'émettre les deux propositions suivantes: (1) Chez les hydrophthalmiques étudiés à Alger, il est rare que le père et les enfans ne soient point atteints du même mal; (2) il ne frappe jamais l'Européen, le soldat, quelles que soient les circonstances défavorables où le jettent les chances de la guerre. De là ne pourrait-on point conclure à la transmissibilité héréditaire de l'hydrophthalmie, puisque d'une part elle attaque ordinairement plusieurs lignées d'une même famille, et que d'une autre, elle épargne les étrangers qui sont à l'abri de l'influence héréditaire, quelles que soient les circonstances dans lesquelles ils se trouvent placés?"

---

[1] *Bibl.* No. 8, pp. 166—172.　　　　　[2] *Bibl.* No. 131, p. 9.

[3] For a very full and interesting study of the general features of the disease I would recommend the French thesis by Gros, *Bibl.* No. 131.　　　　[4] *Bibl.* No. 25.

Grellois recognises that the fact of hereditary transmission has not been established but is only suggested by his observation; he refers to the disease depending on a fault in the equilibrium between the secretory and excretory mechanisms of the eye, and makes suggestions regarding the influence of climate upon it; we are told that the condition is common in some parts of Scotland, Holland and North America, also that it is very common on the coast of Barbary; it is a sad spectacle, he says, to see in the narrow streets of Algiers files of six to eight blind people following one another, almost all blind from hydrophthalmos[1]. I have found no further reference to a special liability to the disease in certain countries, but if the disease be hereditary and intermarriage freely occurs amongst the blind of the district, this fact rather than the climate may determine an increased local incidence of the disease. Many writers now stress the importance of heredity as an etiological factor in the causation of the disease, but I am not sure that they have adequate grounds for doing so, for published histories are very rare and scanty; indeed, the only justification for including any consideration of buphthalmos in a memoir, the primary function of which is the elucidation of factors bearing upon heredity in man, is to exhibit the contrasting picture provided by multiple cases occurring in the same family with the also rare but widely spread histories of megalocornea, and with those of glaucoma. If buphthalmos is indeed to be regarded as the glaucoma of infancy, the comparative study of pedigrees of each condition should be of value and of considerable interest. Here, however, I would note that in long series of recorded cases heredity can commonly be demonstrated in only a few examples; in particular Seefelder, in his investigation of 47 cases, finds evidence of heredity in no single case; a similar statement holds with regard to the glaucoma of later years.

The enlargement of the eye, consequent upon buphthalmos, may occur at any time up to the age at which the sclerotic has become rigid and unable to yield to a raised intra-ocular pressure; it rarely occurs later than the age of 7 years, but the large proportion of cases becomes noticeable at birth or in the first years of life, as will be seen from the following table; the cases, however, said to be congenital present a variety

| Author | No. of Cases | Onset of the Disease | | Totals | % Congenital or 1st Year |
		Congenital	In 1st Year		
Seefelder	47	9	24	33	70·2
Zahn	57	24	28	52	91·2
Gros	45	27	6	33	73·3
Golomb	27	14	11	25	92·6
Totals	176	74	69	143	81·3
Hereditary Cases	39	24	8	32	82·1

of appearances at birth according to the phase of the disease, which may be already far advanced. Buphthalmos may affect either sex but occurs more commonly among males than females; the sex incidence for purely hereditary cases does not differ significantly from that calculated from 304 cases due to all causes, which is of interest, in view of the

---

[1] We have no guarantee that these were not cases of secondary buphthalmos.

fact that hereditary disease does on the whole tend to become manifest in men more frequently than in women, and we might have expected our group of cases to show a rather higher percentage of males than other cases.

Amongst my collected records of hereditary buphthalmos, definite unilateral defect occurs so rarely that I came to regard asymmetry in this respect as exceptional; of 58 cases, for which information on this point is suggested, I find only 6 cases in which

Author	No. of Cases	Males	Females	Male Sex Incidence
Gros	116	71	45	61·2
Zahn	73	43	30	58·9
Kunzmann	37	26	11	70·3
Seefelder	46	31	15	67·4
Golomb	32	24	8	75·0
Totals	304	195	109	64·1 ± 1·86
Hereditary Cases	83	51	32	61·4 ± 3·60

unilateral affection is probable; of these six, two cases had not a normal unaffected eye—one had cataract and a luxated lens in the eye free from buphthalmos, the other had normal vision but an enlarged cornea in the unaffected eye. It was then a surprise to find a relatively high percentage of unilateral cases from the not essentially hereditary group of cases. Some figures are given below. The difference in the percentages

Author	No. of Cases	Bilateral	Unilateral	Percentage Bilateral
Gros	116	74	42	63·8
Zahn	73*	51	22	69·9
Seefelder	47*	32	15	68·1
Golomb	32*	17	15	53·1
Totals	268	174	94	64·9 ± 2·0
Hereditary Cases	58	52	6	89·7 ± 2·7

* Zahn's cases include 14 of hereditary origin; Seefelder could find no evidence of heredity in his cases; Golomb includes four hereditary cases.

for the hereditary and for all cases is certainly significant; the only explanation I can offer for it is that primary inherent affection which is the rule in my series is more likely to be bilateral than is secondary affection arising as a result of infection or local injury of which many cases may be included in the other groups; the percentage of 90 for bilateral cases of my series would probably be raised if knowledge were available of all the 85 hereditary cases of the pedigrees appended, for unilateral affection tends to be noted when it occurs in a condition which is generally bilateral, so that no knowledge is more likely to refer to bilateral than to unilateral affection. It is not however any difference that may be noted in the two comparative series which is matter for surprise, but it is difficult to see why common characteristics with regard to sex-incidence and age of onset should hold for a disease due to the accumulation of fluid within the eyeball, whether it be the result of some developmental anomaly or be due to inflammatory products and adhesions interfering with the processes of filtration. Thus I think we can deduce little indication, from an examination of comparative material, as to how far isolated cases diagnosed as buphthalmos tend to be primary affections or secondary to other causes. If hereditary buphthalmos tends to symmetry in as far as the affection is usually bilateral, there is often very marked asymmetry in the condition of the two eyes; sometimes this would appear to follow from the effect of varied treatments, but the onset is not always simultaneous in the two eyes and the progress and ultimate interference with function may differ markedly.

I have too few definite observations on the eyes of affected individuals to make any statements regarding them, but have condensed in the following table such descriptions as are available, to give some general idea of the size of the eye in these cases and of the severe grade of the resulting disability. It is of interest to compare the facts given here with those of the corresponding table for the megalocornic eye given on p. 440.

Some Observations on Buphthalmic Eyes.

Corneal diameters in mm.	Anterior Chamber	Vision
12·5—13·5 in 3 eyes 14·5—15·5 ,, 7 ,, 16·5—17·5 ,, 4 ,, 19 ,, 1 ,, ——————————— 5 eyes "Voluminous" 7 ,, Excised 5 ,, Ruptured or Atrophied	Very deep in 6 eyes Deep in 1 eye Normal in 4 eyes Rather shallow in 2 eyes Very shallow in 2 eyes	Blind in both eyes or p.l. 19 cases Blind in one eye* ,, 6 cases Other measurements of Vision include: V. = $\frac{1}{3}$, $\frac{1}{20}$, $\frac{1}{2}$, $\frac{4}{5}$, $\frac{5}{6}$ Finger counting at 1 m. "Saw well after operation"

* The other eye, of these cases, counts fingers in four individuals; one was a case of unilateral defect with good vision in the other eye; the sixth case had a good result from operation in the other eye.

Most writers on buphthalmos refer to a deep anterior chamber as an almost invariable characteristic. Elliot, however, writes[1]:—"the anterior chamber is greatly deepened in buphthalmos...it remains to mention, however, that in certain cases of this affection the anterior chamber, instead of being deepened, is narrowed or even obliterated. It is probable that these cases do not belong to the same aetiologic class as the commoner ones, which are to be attributed...to defects in the development of the parts concerned in excretion." It is of interest then to find examples of deep and shallow anterior chambers amongst our examples of hereditary buphthalmos; I have no reason to suspect that the cases of hereditary buphthalmos of my records are not homogeneous from the aetiological standpoint.

With regard to the inheritance of the disease, the material is so poor that I can only ask the reader to examine the pedigrees—Plates LXVI, LXVII. Figs. 993—1021—and note the need for fully worked out histories; it seems likely, however, that the disease is commonly confined to a single sibship, for the disease is of so serious and disabling a nature that any family would probably be aware of cases occurring amongst near relatives. Yet I would call attention to the fact that of the four histories in which the disease was not confined to a single sibship—Figs. 993, 997, 998 and 1001—

[1] *Bibl.* No. 247, p. 407.

(excluding the cases in which a parent was affected) three were provided by the same author, Zahn, whose main purpose was to enquire into the hereditary factor; it cannot therefore be accepted as proven in any way that the disease is limited to one sibship as generally as the available pedigrees appear to suggest. The only case within my personal knowledge—that of Fig. 1000—certainly appeared to be confined to a single sibship so far as the parents could discover. There are certainly very striking distinctions in the modes of inheritance of the three conditions—megalocornea, buphthalmos and glaucoma—which provide such different series of pedigrees as those illustrated on Plates LXVI—LXIX, scanty and imperfect though each series admittedly is.

We must not lose sight however of the possible influence of the varying clinical aspect of the three diseases on the hereditary picture; the megalocornic individual, well and free from all disabling or disfiguring symptoms, has a very different outlook with regard to marriage and parentage from that of the unhappy child, described in such moving terms by Elliot—"Buphthalmic children are naturally backward and diffident. If the corneae are exposed, pain frequently makes them fractious and irritable. The limitations in the excursions of the eyeballs necessitate constant turning movements of the head, which impart a characteristic staring look and a somewhat stilted attitude to the patient. The proptosis renders the eyes very liable to damage and the children consequently shun the rough companionship of their fellows. Taken all round, the lot of these little people is a very hard one[1]." The sufferer from glaucoma generally becomes affected at a relatively late age, when marriage may already have occurred and children be born; up to the time of his affection, he has probably appeared to be an entirely normal member of the community, such as the buphthalmic child has never been. It is difficult to estimate the extent to which apparent differences in the mechanism of heredity are really inherent, or may be modified by such adventitious secondary considerations. The very interesting, though limited, observation of hereditary buphthalmos in rabbits by Vogt[2] might well make us pause before insisting on any inherent distinction between the modes of inheritance of this disease and of glaucoma.

It is evident that in most cases of buphthalmos both parents are free from manifest defect, but we have no reason to doubt the observations of Argyll Robertson, Fig. 1013, of Venneman, Fig. 1021, and of von Ammon, Fig. 1004, who noted the direct transmission from mother to offspring in their cases. Cases of buphthalmos come before the ophthalmologist for treatment in infancy or early in life; by the time the patient has reached adult life there can as a rule be no question of further treatment, and I can find no hint as to what is the ultimate history of these afflicted individuals—how many of them reach adult life, or marry and have children. The available material provides no guide as to whether the marriage of a man or woman who has an arrested buphthalmos is justified, or whether such a parentage carries grave menace to the offspring.

If buphthalmos and glaucoma of hereditary source are essentially the same disease with the same underlying pathogenesis, it seems incredible that cases of the former variety should not arise commonly amongst the offspring of glaucomatous patients, but

[1] *Bibl.* No. 247, p. 412. [2] *Bibl.* No. 232. See Fig. 1022, Plate LXVII.

I have little evidence that such a sequence is liable to occur[1]. Is there then some inherent difference in the conditions determining the very early onset in buphthalmos, or have we another example of the hereditary factor including and controlling to some extent the age of onset with the other characteristics of the disease, so that a family exhibiting glaucoma later in life would be unlikely to provide examples of congenital affection? We know that microscopic sections of eyes affected with primary congenital buphthalmos have shown that the iris angle is blocked by tissue at the root of the iris which has not separated off from the back of the cornea during development. Is the source of hereditary glaucoma of the same nature, differing in degree only, so that in one case the individual is born with the affection, in the other case with a predisposition to the disease?

If hereditary buphthalmos is due to a developmental anomaly concerned with the secretory or excretory mechanism of the eye, leading to the accumulation of fluid within the eye and thus to raised tension and subsequent distension, we might look for other associated developmental anomalies in the structure of the eye. I find, however, no evidence of any associated liability, except such as might be expected to follow from the disturbance caused by the disease itself; further there is no evidence that cases of hereditary buphthalmos tend to arise in degenerate stocks or in stocks carrying any liability to developmental errors—I do not know whether such evidence could be found if information were complete. Glaucoma and buphthalmos certainly both arise as a result of raised intra-ocular tension, and both diseases may exhibit hereditary tendencies; the eyeball is no longer supple and capable of expansion in glaucoma, so that the clinical signs of the two diseases differ markedly. If the underlying cause of the raised tension in the two cases is the same, and if buphthalmos is truly the glaucoma of infancy, we should look more suitably for hints of the link in pedigrees of glaucoma, referring to an adult population and tending to cover a wider field of investigation. Some further consideration of this question will be given in the following section of this memoir dealing with glaucoma.

Hereditary Glaucoma.

The growth of knowledge regarding glaucoma, and the definition of the disease, has been progressing since the time of Hippocrates and Galen, when the term was used freely to indicate a number of conditions which were at a later date not included under this title; the history of this growth has been fully investigated by several authors, whose contributions may be found in readily accessible works: the most notable of these is that due to Schmidt-Rimpler[2] in 1908, based to some extent on an admirable thesis by Pamard[3] in 1861. Progress in recent years has been largely characterised by advances in operative technique, and by researches of a physio-chemical nature[4], which may well lead to a new epoch in the history of the disease. The hereditary character of glaucoma was apparently long unrecognised, the earliest reference known to me

---

[1] A case of buphthalmos occurs in association with glaucoma in Figs. 1077 and 1080 of Plate LXIX.
[2] *Bibl.* No. 186.   [3] *Bibl.* No. 45.   [4] See below, p. 450.

being that due to Benedict[1] in 1842; this late recognition may, or may not, have a bearing on the frequency or infrequency of heredity as a factor in the aetiology of the disease; certainly relatively few good pedigrees of the condition have ever been published. The literature of glaucoma is enormous. Schmidt-Rimpler gives a very valuable bibliography, up to 1907, including about two thousand references to books or papers on the subject; the number has continued to accumulate steadily since that date.

The following quotation, from Elliot, indicates the fundamental nature of conditions which may be included under glaucoma, and reveals something of the difficulties which such cases present:

"The term 'glaucoma' is not the title of any one single disease. It is rather a convenient clinical label for a large group of pathologic conditions, the distinctive feature common to all of which is a rise in the intra-ocular pressure. The causes of these conditions are many and varied, the pathological findings are most diverse, and the difference in the symptoms presented is so extraordinary that very careful study is required to detect the bond which serves to unite these very dissimilar manifestations of disease in a common category. When we speak of the hardness of a glaucomatous eye, or of its rise in tension, we are referring to the outward manifestations of an increase of the fluid pressure within the globe. To this increase all the causes of glaucoma lead up; on it every sign and symptom of the condition depend. If the rise in pressure can be traced to the action of some antecedent local disease, we speak of the glaucomatous condition as *secondary*, failing this we term it *primary*[2]."

The purpose of this section is to present all available material bearing on hereditary primary glaucoma; to endeavour to determine whether such cases are homogeneous, i.e. due to a common cause; to glean any information that can throw light on that common cause, if such there be, and thus to indicate what is the hereditary factor in these cases. It is obvious that multiple cases of glaucoma in the same family may be noted which are outside the scope of this investigation, if some other hereditary disease be of such a character as to predispose to glaucoma; one might, for example, expect to find multiple cases of glaucoma occurring in family histories of cataract or of ectopia lentis, though I can present little evidence that they do so with any significant frequency, but such cases indicate a secondary glaucoma, due to disturbances within the eyeball which may have no concern with the hereditary factors, and is probably not homogeneous with the material to be discussed in this memoir. I would, however, suggest that in face of the great number of cases of, say cataract, which are never followed by glaucoma, there is some significance to be attached to multiple cases of glaucoma, as such, following cataract in the same family, indicating perhaps, though not necessarily, an inherent predisposition to the onset of glaucoma which would perhaps never have been manifested without the strain put upon the physiological processes of the eyeball by the existence of the cataract.

If then a rise in the intra-ocular pressure is the one essential criterion in the determination of glaucoma, we may ask ourselves what are the possible causes of this rise. There are three main divisions into which possibilities fall. (1) The secretory mechanism of the eye may be over active, so that the fluid contents of the eyeball increase at a greater rate than they can be excreted or absorbed; the fibrous sclerotic

[1] *Bibl.* No. 27.   [2] *Bibl.* No. 247, pp. 1—2.

tunic of the eye is incapable of stretching to accommodate a greater volume of contents and thus tension is raised. (2) The excretory mechanism may be defective, so that secretory products tend to be retained in the eye. (3) The structure of the eye may be at fault or malproportioned, so that excretion is interfered with by, say, too large a lens impeding the exit of fluid, or some defect in the canal of Schlemm, or in the region of the angle of the eye, the patency of which is of fundamental importance for drainage purposes. All these possibilities are related and interact upon one another; for example, if the excretory mechanism tends to break down, the immediate effect must be one of irritation likely to lead to increased secretion and to congestion of tissues which will in their turn further tend to obstruct the excretory tracts.

It will be seen how extremely complicated the situation becomes and a little consideration will reveal the great number of factors concerned in the stability of circulation within the eye, and thus of the varied conditions which may give rise to the common symptom indicative of glaucoma. It is not within the scope of this memoir to consider any of these factors and their various modes of operation in detail; the literature concerning them is very extensive and often of so high a standard that only a specialist with wide personal experience of cases and the problems which arise therefrom is in a position to add to it. Moreover Elliot's book on the subject is readily accessible, giving a most thorough and scientific discussion of the many possibilities concerned in the aetiology of glaucoma. I have made no reference to the more recent extremely valuable investigation of Duke-Elder into the physio-chemical aspect of the circulation of the eye and its bearing on the questions of the regulation of intra-ocular pressure, and thus on glaucoma, nor to his work on the vascular responses of the eye, which to use his own cautious words "may form a factor in the aetiology of certain cases of glaucoma" (*Proc. R.S.* Vol. 109 B, p. 28, London, 1931), but would recommend the study of these far-reaching researches at first hand[1].

My preliminary remarks, quoted from Elliot, refer to the extraordinary difference in the symptoms presented by patients suffering from glaucoma; this is to be expected in a disease which may result from many different causes; the character of the onset also colours to a large extent the picture presented by the patient; if the onset be sudden and acute, congestive signs and pain predominate, irreparable damage to the eye may occur in a few hours if treatment be not immediate; the fall in vision may be very rapid and the patient is in dire distress for which there is all too much reason. On the other hand the onset may be slow and insidious, accompanied by no pain or signs of congestion and no diminution of vision over a long period; the only complaint may be that of occasional mistiness in vision, with perhaps coloured haloes seen round a light, for which some explanation is demanded. I think ophthalmologists would agree that the ultimate fate of any case of glaucoma, whatever the mode of onset or the causal factor, is the same, namely blindness and disorganisation of all the structures of the eye, if treatment be neglected and no preventive measures be put into operation.

[1] Duke-Elder, W. S.: "On the Clinical Application of the Newer Conceptions in the Physiology of the Eye" (*Lancet*, Vol. 1 for 1930, pp. 4—9, London, 1930) provides a most delightful introduction to this author's highly specialised line of work.

Once the equilibrium of the circulatory mechanism in the eyeball is disturbed, and tension is raised sufficiently to produce symptoms which attract the attention of the patient, the vicious circle is set in operation, and anatomical changes resulting from the raised tension tend always to lead to a further rise and the progress of symptoms. Yet the tension of the eye is not invariable; it may be raised within limits without the production of symptoms and without any ill effects; the safe limits almost certainly vary from person to person as well as at different periods of life. It is not improbable that exceptional circumstances may lead to an isolated case of glaucoma in a person whose limits are normal—just as they do in secondary glaucoma where the circumstances are demonstrable—but that relatively narrow limits are the source of the glaucoma in members of our pedigrees. For obvious reasons it is impossible to measure the limits of safety in individuals, nor can we obtain any idea of the number of people who may have occasional mistiness in vision and see haloes round lights, without consciously recognising the phenomena or attaching any importance to them. Some ophthalmologists take the view that probably all cases of glaucoma have an insidious onset with prodromal symptoms, such as those described, which sometimes remain unnoticed by the patient until an acute attack overtakes him.

Until recent times glaucoma was regarded as incurable and the patient doomed to blindness from the outset; now the prospect, though always precarious, is far less gloomy, provided always that treatment leading to the relief of tension is timely and adequate. I would put down here a few names among the pioneers who have brought this about. In 1830 Mackenzie[1] wrote: "As a superabundance of dissolved vitreous humour appears to form an essential part of the morbid changes which take place in the glaucomatous eye, it is not unreasonable to conclude that occasionally puncturing the sclerotica and choroid might prove serviceable, by relieving the pressure of the accumulated fluid on the retina. The puncture should be made..." and thus inaugurated the fundamental basis of all modern operative treatment in the artificial relief of pressure. Von Graefe again proved one of the benefactors to mankind in his discovery of the value of iridectomy as an aid to the filtration of the eye in certain cases and his observations regarding the need for *early* operation. Amongst many others of more recent years I would refer primarily to Elliot who has become famed through the success of his technique in the trephine operation for the relief of glaucoma. It is not however alone operation which constitutes the whole of treatment in glaucoma; other measures, such as the use of drugs to contract the pupil and the avoidance of prevocative factors in the daily regime, have their value and place in different stages of the disease and in special cases.

The outlook is always apt to be at its worst in hereditary disease, when the cause is inherent, and the trouble is not due to accidental transitory disturbance which may never recur—this is where the responsibilities of parentage should be considered. The sufferers from non-hereditary glaucoma may take a measure of comfort if the fate of the large majority of hereditary cases seems still to be very hard.

It is difficult to obtain any idea as to how commonly primary glaucoma is hereditary;

[1] Mackenzie, W.: *A Treatise on Diseases of the Eye*, p. 710. London, 1830.

opinions of ophthalmologists on the point are varied; several men of wide experience have expressed the opinion that the disease may very generally be traced to hereditary influence, if such causation be sought for; the disease however is relatively common whilst published pedigrees are few and mostly scanty. Nettleship, in 1909, refers to the urgent need for the collection of much more material relating to the heredity of glaucoma, but the material has accumulated slowly and is still quite inadequate for the purposes of a statistical inquiry. I have little doubt that if glaucoma were as commonly hereditary as is, say, retinitis pigmentosa, cataract or haemophilia, fully worked out family histories would be in our hands from Nettleship, Usher and others to whom we are so greatly indebted for their investigations in heredity; it is surely of some significance that we have only three small pedigrees of primary glaucoma due to Nettleship and a single case from Usher. It is true that glaucoma is for the most part a disease of declining years and the difficulty in tracing any evidence of heredity is enhanced by the death of many individuals who might have developed the disease had they lived longer.

Primary glaucoma is widespread in its incidence, affecting all races. The following table provides some idea of the relative incidence amongst patients suffering from eye disease in various countries, the figures given there are certainly in some cases influenced

Author and Country	No. of Patients	No. of Cases of Glaucoma	Percentage of Glaucoma Cases
Kagoshima (Japan)[1]	21,455	42	[0·20]
Schmidt-Rimpler (Goettingen)[2]	134,000	536	0·40
Schüssele and Neuffer (Tubingen)[3]	154,390	1052	0·68
Förster[2]	11,000	93	0·84
Magni (Pisa)[2]	64,729	615	0·95
Coppez (Belgium)[2]	148,000	1511	1·02
de Wecker (Paris)[4]	40,000	421	1·05
Lange (St Petersburg)[5]	74,244	847	1·14
Markow (Charkow)[6]	106,609	1329	1·25
Vienna (Univ. Clinic)[2]	8,451	107	1·26
Wiesbaden (Hospital)[2]	14,619	217	1·48
Cykulenko (Russia)[7]	60,977	939	1·54
Wagner (Gentiles in Odessa)[8]	9,622	155	1·61
Krukow (St Petersburg)[9]	79,440	1430	1·80
de Wecker (Constantinople)[4]	20,000	386	1·93
von Graefe's Clinic, 1859—1863[2]	12,076	269	2·23
Wagner (Jews in Odessa)[8]	9,903	255	2·57
Bossalino (Pisa)[2]	10,072	275	2·73

[1] Bibl. No. 215. [2] Bibl. No. 186, p. 122. [3] Bibl. Nos. 145, 211.
[4] Bibl. No. 152. [5] Bibl. No. 104. [6] Bibl. No. 137.
[7] Bibl. No. 282. [8] Bibl. No. 82. [9] Bibl. No. 103.

by special conditions and I cannot be sure of the significance to be attached to the varying frequency of the disease in the different clinics. The Japanese cases were private patients of Kagoshima; I do not know whether his figures can be taken as characteristic of Japan but am seeking further information on this point* as his small

* I am much indebted to Professor Kawakami of Tokyo for some explanation of Kagoshima's figures. He writes that, in Japan, patients tend to seek help at a public hospital for serious conditions such as glaucoma, and that private cases tend to be selected from amongst those suffering from less grave disease;

percentage of cases is entirely at variance with the statement commonly made that there is a high incidence of glaucoma amongst Eastern peoples. Elliot[1] writes that his experience in South India would lead him to think that glaucoma is a very common disease there and that the cause of this prevalence has a distinct connection with a want of development of the globes which is very common in India. It is likely that glaucoma patients would seek out Elliot and thus perhaps influence his views of their prevalence, but others have also noted the high incidence in India and the proportion of cases at the Madras Ophthalmic Hospital has continued to be high since Elliot's time there; he considers it impossible to say whether Europeans in India tend to develop glaucoma more readily than at home.

The high proportion of cases in von Graefe's clinic are almost surely due to the fame he had won by his treatment of glaucoma, and I can only conclude that patients in Pisa tended to go to Bossalino for a similar reason, for Magni in the same town saw relatively few cases of the disease. De Wecker compared cases in Paris and in Constantinople; he thought there was no doubt of the much greater prevalence of the disease in Constantinople. A special liability to glaucoma amongst the Jews has been repeatedly noted and possibly influences some of the figures of my table; recently however a Jew, writing in America, denies this liability and says that glaucoma is no more common amongst Jews than amongst Gentiles—"every Jew with glaucoma is registered at several hospitals and several private consultation rooms. Gentiles ask for advice of one person only. Jews pour into hospital in Vienna whereas Gentiles tend to stay at home, perhaps be looked after by a private physician, or perhaps just go blind[2]." The nervousness of the Jew, thus depicted by one of themselves, may well in itself tend to precipitate an attack of glaucoma in any subject with a predisposition to the disease. We learn from Wagner[3] that in Odessa amongst a population of 193,513, there were 140,809 Gentiles and 52,517 Jews; of these people 19,525 suffered from eye disease and attended at the hospital; the patients consisted of 9622 Gentiles, 155 of whom had glaucoma, and 9903 Jews of whom 255 had glaucoma; considering then the incidence of glaucoma in the hospital clinic relatively to the proportion of the races in the town as a whole, it would appear that the Jews of this city were about four times as liable as the Gentiles. I have no evidence that glaucoma tends to occur in individuals of poor physique, but would note here that the Russian and Polish Jewish children in this country have been found, from very detailed investigations, to fall on the whole considerably below Gentile children in physique, and to have bad sight as compared with English and Scottish children; evidence was given indicating that these defects were

he gives me comparative figures from other ophthalmologists in Japan varying from 2·1 °/₀ of all eye patients suffering from glaucoma to 0·5 °/₀, bringing the relative incidence amongst eye cases in Japan well within the range provided by European countries. Professor Kawakami does me the further service of explaining that the high incidence of trachoma in Japan reduces the relative frequency of other eye diseases. Thus are we warned that the table given here has only a limited significance but, bearing this in mind, it is not without interest.

[1] *Bibl.* No. 247, p. 134.
[2] *Bibl.* No. 288.
[3] *Bibl.* No. 82.

racial characteristics and not produced by the poverty and bad home environments of many of the immigrant families *.

(a) *Sex Incidence in Glaucoma.* The sex incidence in glaucoma varies to some extent for the different types of the disease commonly classified under such headings as "acute glaucoma," "chronic inflammatory glaucoma," "glaucoma simplex" or "glaucoma haemorrhagicum," there being apparently an excess of females exhibiting the acute and inflammatory types; this may follow from a supposed vaso-motor instability in women at certain periods of life leading to a flare up of an incipient but not yet recognised disease; or there may be a tendency amongst women to neglect minor symptoms and only seek advice when an acute attack overtakes them. The various types of the disease are of vital importance from the point of view of treatment, and the contrasting picture provided by them must be ever before the clinician's eye, but it is outside the scope of

Determination of the Male Sex Incidence in Primary Glaucoma.

Author and Country	♂	♀	Totals	Male Sex Incidence
Rydel (Vienna)[1]	46	33	79	58·2 ± 3·7
Markow (Charkow)[2]	845	660	1505[11]	56·1 ± 0·9
Vienna (Univ. Clinic, 1869)[1]	32	27	59	54·2 ± 4·4
de Wecker (Constantinople)[3]	207	179	386	53·6 ± 1·7
Schmidt-Rimpler (Goettingen)[1]	280	256	536	52·5 ± 1·5
de Wecker (Paris)[3]	214	207	421	50·8 ± 1·6
Lange (St Petersburg)[4]	399	448	847	47·1 ± 1·2
Schussele and Neuffer (Tübingen)[5]	473	579	1052	45·0 ± 1·0
Neuburger (Germany)[6]	120	152	272	44·1 ± 2·0
Priestley Smith (England)[7]	431	569	1000	43·1 ± 1·1
Haffmans[8] (Germany)	39	56	95	41·1 ± 3·4
Arlt[1] (Bohemia)	45	65	110	40·9 ± 3·2
Wagner (Odessa)[1]	476	750	1226	38·8 ± 0·9
Kagoshima (Japan)[9]	16	26	42	38·1 ± 5·1 [12]
Cykulenko (Russia)[10]	348	591	939	37·1 ± 1·1
Totals	3971	4598	8569	46·3 ± 0·4
Hereditary Cases	145	134	279	52·0 ± 2·8

[1] *Bibl.* No. 186, p. 123.   [2] *Bibl.* No. 137.   [3] *Bibl.* No. 152.
[4] *Bibl.* No. 104.   [5] *Bibl.* Nos. 145, 211.   [6] *Bibl.* No. 118.
[7] *Bibl.* No. 107, p. 167.   [8] *Bibl.* No. 43.   [9] *Bibl.* No. 215.
[10] *Bibl.* No. 282.   [11] These numbers include 176 cases of secondary glaucoma.
[12] Professor Kawakami sends me a number of determinations of the male sex incidence in primary glaucoma in Japan, dependent upon the experience of seven observers, varying from 47·5 to 30·1; he does not tell me on what number of cases the latter very low figure depends.

this memoir to consider the different types in any detail; all types are exhibited in hereditary cases. De Wecker pointed out that (a) Simple glaucoma frequently passes into the congestive form. (b) In the same patient we may meet with simple glaucoma on the one side and congestive glaucoma on the other. (c) In the same family, especially among the Jews, we may find some members suffering from simple and others from

* Pearson, K. and Moul, M.: "The Problem of Alien Immigration into Great Britain, illustrated by an examination of Russian and Polish Jewish children." *Annals of Eugenics*, Vol. I, pp. 5—127, Vol. II, pp. 290—317, Vol. III, pp. 1—76.

congestive glaucoma. (d) The operation of sympathectomy will sometimes cause a simple chronic glaucoma to assume a congestive course[1]. Elliot further insists that the distinction between congestive and non-congestive glaucoma is not a radical one[2].

The sex incidence varies between wide limits as we pass from one observer to another or from one country to another, as will be seen from the table on p. 454; it is difficult to explain such differences as are presented without an intimate knowledge of the type of population to which the statistics refer. Such conditions as follow revolution, war and famine are bound to be reflected in the incidence of a disease which may be precipitated in the predisposed by nervous crises, circulatory strain, or by the quality of the blood, and the sex incidence may well be changed by such causes; the markedly different sex indices provided by Markow's pre-revolution figures in Russia and by Cykulenko's recently published statistics may at any rate be partly due to the changed character of the population in the interval and to the nature of the selective action to which the Russian people has been subjected. Clearly the sex incidence in hereditary glaucoma provides no distinctive feature as compared with that for glaucoma in general.

(b) *The Age of Onset in Glaucoma.* We are indebted to Priestley Smith[3] and to Schmidt-Rimpler[4] for valuable statistics referring to the age of onset in primary glaucoma. Schmidt-Rimpler's records include his own cases and those reported by Bossalino, Wagner, Rydel and Haffmans, thus representing examples of the disease from Germany, Austria, Italy and Russia, giving the age of onset in 871 males and 1150 females. Priestley Smith's records on the other hand, concerning 431 males and 569 females, are drawn entirely from his own cases and from those of other English ophthalmologists, who responded to his request that schedules on the subject should be filled in, and returned to him. The close agreement of the two series is of great interest and

The Age of Onset in Primary Glaucoma.

Age of Onset	Continental		English			Means	Standard Deviation
	♂	♀	♂	♀			
10—19	7	3	2	3			
20—29	31	41	12	11	English Males	55·79 ± 0·41	12·50 ± 0·29
30—39	62	102	39	53	„ Females	54·63 ± 0·33	11·82 ± 0·24
40—49	156	272	75	126	Continental Males	55·59 ± 0·29	12·55 ± 0·20
50—59	259	369	125	168	„ Females	53·62 ± 0·24	11·87 ± 0·17
60—69	264	280	127	163			
70—79	88	77	49	42	All Males	55·65 ± 0·23	12·53 ± 0·17
80—89	4	6	2	3	„ Females	53·95 ± 0·19	11·86 ± 0·14
Totals	871	1150	431	569			

suggests a degree of uniformity regarding this feature of the disease amongst widely differing populations indicative of the slight part that racial and temperamental differences play in the manifestation of the disease at the appointed time, in the predisposed, under ordinary conditions of life[5].

[1] *Bibl.* No. 247, p. 466.   [2] *Bibl.* No. 247, p. 154.
[3] *Bibl.* No. 107, p. 123.   [4] *Bibl.* No. 186, p. 167.
[5] On applying the test to see whether the English and Continental series (♂ + ♀) provide random samples of the same population it is found that $\chi^2 = 7·12$, $P = 0·417$, indicating a close agreement between the two series.

It would appear that for glaucoma in general women tend to become affected a little earlier than men and to exhibit slightly less variation in the age of onset. The difference between the sexes is further illustrated by the following diagram calculated from Priestley Smith's data, showing the relative liability[1] to glaucoma

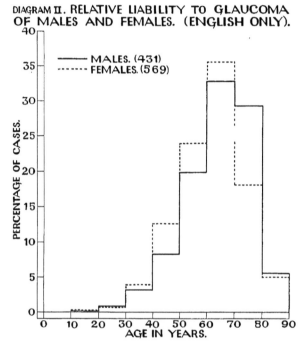

DIAGRAM II. RELATIVE LIABILITY TO GLAUCOMA OF MALES AND FEMALES. (ENGLISH ONLY).

of males and females at each period of life; the maximum liability for each sex falls within the same age group, 60—69 years, but females show a greater liability than males at ages before this period and males show a greater liability at more advanced ages. These curves must be taken to represent the results of experience in the medical profession rather than the true liability curves for the population as a whole. Priestley Smith made some investigation into the reality of the steep fall in liability after the age of 70 years and concluded that this was to some extent contributed to by the unwillingness of old people whose sight fails to attend at hospital or seek treatment; he estimated that the true liability continued to rise steeply until the age of about 70—80 and then fell. This fall may perhaps be interpreted as due to some selection in the death rate tending to the elimination of old people predisposed to glaucoma.

---

[1] Percentage of cases at each age group relatively to the size of the population at the corresponding age, as given by the English Census, 1911.

The ages of onset in recorded hereditary cases of primary glaucoma present a marked contrast from those of series which include all cases which arise; the actual figures for Priestley Smith's English cases, for Schmidt-Rimpler's Continental cases and for the hereditary cases of my collected records are given in the table below.

Age of Onset	Hereditary Cases			English Cases	Continental Cases	English and Continental
	$\male$	$\female$	$\male + \female$	$\male + \female$	$\male + \female$	$\male + \female$
10—19	24	29	53	5	10	15
20—29	23	26	49	23	72	95
30—39	14	7	21	92	164	256
40—49	17	17	34	201	428	629
50—59	10	7	17	293	628	921
60—69	6	8	14	290	544	834
70—79	4	2	6	91	165	256
80—89	1	1	2	5	10	15
Totals	99	97	196	1000	2021	3021

		Means	Standard Deviation
Hereditary Cases	$\male$	$35 \cdot 51 \pm 1 \cdot 22$	$17 \cdot 94 \pm 0 \cdot 86$
,,	,, $\female$	$33 \cdot 35 \pm 1 \cdot 23$	$17 \cdot 97 \pm 0 \cdot 87$
,,	,, $\male + \female$	$34 \cdot 44 \pm 0 \cdot 87$	$17 \cdot 99 \pm 0 \cdot 61$
English and Continental $\male + \female$		$54 \cdot 69 \pm 0 \cdot 15$	$12 \cdot 19 \pm 0 \cdot 11$

It will be seen that the mean age of onset in definitely hereditary cases is 20 years earlier than that for the general series of cases; the standard deviation is also much increased. Again, no fewer than 52·0 °/ₒ of the 196 hereditary cases occur before the age of 30 years, whilst only 3·6 °/ₒ of the 3021 general cases occur before the age of 30; these differences are surely too great to be explained by the possibly earlier recognition of symptoms in a family, whose members have previously suffered from experience of the disease, and suggest some very fundamental difference in the determining factors of the two groups of cases. It would appear that hereditary cases cannot be regarded as a random sample drawn from the larger population; I would, however, repeat that the number of cases known to be hereditary are few, and remind the reader that we have no knowledge as to what proportion of cases of the general series are free from genetic potentialities.

These very marked differences between the two series are further brought out by the graphs[1] shown in Diagrams III and IV (p. 458), which illustrate the close agreement between the English and Continental series, with the contrasting curves defining the age of onset in hereditary glaucoma[2], and the relative liability to the disease at different ages respectively. The curves in all cases start at the age group 10—19 years; this is a rather arbitrary proceeding, but cases arising at an earlier age

[1] I have combined the figures for both sexes in these graphs because of the small numbers of the hereditary series; the sexual differences in no way modify the general arguments though they should not be lost sight of. The graphs have been used instead of the customary histogram in order to aid the ready differentiation of three curves in one diagram.

[2] [It is possible that the contrast between the hereditary and non-hereditary cases may be largely ascribed to the fact that incomplete pedigrees have been used in the former case.—ED.]

B. T.

DIAGRAM III. AGE OF ONSET IN GLAUCOMA.
(MALES AND FEMALES).

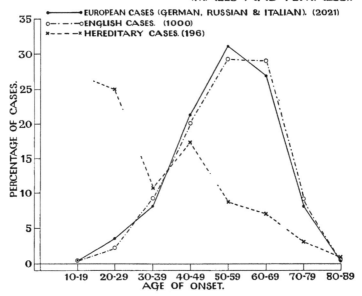

DIAGRAM IV. RELATIVE LIABILITY TO GLAUCOMA AT DIFFERENT AGE PERIODS. (MALES AND FEMALES).

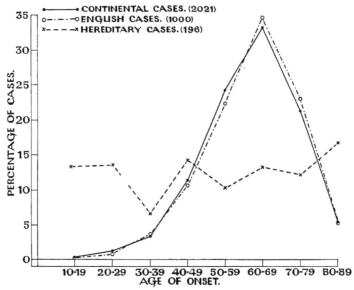

fall into the buphthalmic group, and though belonging to the same broad category of cases, due to the rise of intra-ocular pressure, there is a sharp discontinuity between the curve describing the ages of onset in this group and that for glaucoma cases of either series; over 80 °/₀ of cases of buphthalmos are congenital or become manifest in the first year of life, and the curves of Diagrams III and IV would fall almost to the zero line and rise again very steeply if any attempt were made to combine the cases. These facts lead to the conclusion that the determining factors in buphthalmos, in hereditary glaucoma and in non-hereditary glaucoma are by no means identical, though their effects are common to all the conditions in so far as they disturb the balance between secretion and excretion within the eyeball.

The relative liability curves shown in Diagram IV are of great suggestive interest, showing the almost steady or very slight increase of liability to hereditary glaucoma throughout life, and the contrasting steep rise to a maximum liability at 60—69 years for the disease in general[1]. The drop in the incidence of hereditary cases at the age of 30—39 years is difficult to explain; the fall is more marked in the case of females than for males, but it would be unwise to emphasise the point or indeed to attempt any explanation of the details of this curve based on so few cases.

I have endeavoured to obtain some estimate of the degree of uniformity in the age of onset of glaucoma within the family and have formed the correlation tables on p. 460 to determine the degree of association between the age of onset in parent and offspring, and in pairs of siblings; the results are extremely interesting so far as they go, but the numbers are so small that the conclusions to be drawn from them can only be regarded as tentative, pending the accumulation of more material. The correlation coefficient in each case is extremely high, suggesting that the age of onset in the parents closely determines the period of life at which predisposed offspring will show signs of the disease; members of a sibship evidently tend to become liable at the same age. It is of particular interest to compare these correlations with those for the age of onset in pairs of siblings affected with hereditary optic atrophy; the parent in that disease was rarely affected; the correlation coefficient for pairs of siblings was found to be about 0·5, calculated upon much more ample material. It looks as if the mechanism of heredity, which provides for manifestation of the disease in the parent who transmits, determines the character of the transmission more closely than under conditions of latency.

Further points I would call attention to in these correlation tables are: (a) the mean age of onset in the offspring is some ten years earlier than the mean age in the parent; (b) the standard deviation is greater for parents than for their offspring. I think no inherent significance can be attached to these observations without further confirmation; the onset of glaucoma early in life is likely to prejudice the marriage and parenthood of the individual, so that we see relatively few parents who developed the disease before the age of 30 years; further, the unaffected offspring of the affected parents have many of them not yet reached advanced years at which they may develop the disease; these facts would influence the relative mean ages provided

[1] The true maximum probably occurs at a later age as explained by Priestley Smith above.

by the table, also perhaps the lessened variation in the younger incomplete generation. In particular, the reduced age of onset in the younger generation must not be taken as proof of a general tendency to antedating on the transmission of the disease. This question of antedating is of such great practical importance that I much regret my inability to make any definite statement regarding it; the pedigrees available are too few and much too scanty to be able to demonstrate whether the phenomenon does or does not hold; such information as I have is in favour of some liability to antedate

Glaucoma in Parent and Offspring.

Age of Onset of Glaucoma in Parent

		10—19	20—29	30—39	40—49	50—59	60—69	70—79	80—89	Totals	
Age of Onset of Glaucoma in Offspring	10—19	14	11	5	6	1				37	Mean Age of Parent 42·080 ± 1·191 Standard Deviation 18·766 ± 0·842
	20—29	1	9	10	9		1			30	
	30—39	1	1	3	4	2	3			14	Mean Age of Offspring 30·664 ± 0·959 Standard Deviation 15·120 ± 0·678
	40—49				2		6	6		14	
	50—59				1	2	10			13	
	60—69						4		1	5	Correlation Coefficient + ·813 ± ·022
	Totals	16	21	18	22	5	24	6	1	113	

Glaucoma in Pairs of Siblings.

Age of Onset of 1st Sibling

		10—19	20—29	30—39	40—49	50—59	60—69	70—79	Totals	
Age of Onset of 2nd Sibling	10—19	48	21	4					73	
	20—29	21	26	7	2				56	
	30—39	4	7	2	5	6			24	Mean Age of Siblings 34·375 ± 0·718
	40—49		2	5	26	13			46	Standard Deviation 17·021 ± 0·507
	50—59			6	13	14	4		37	Correlation Coefficient + ·897 ± ·008
	60—69					4	10		14	
	70—79							6	6	
	Totals	73	56	24	46	37	14	6	256	

following the transmission of the disease, and I would ask the reader to note the few cases of the table in which the onset of the disease in the offspring was at a later date than its occurrence in the parent. The problem is complicated by the late age at which the onset of glaucoma may occur and by the common lack of information regarding the age, or age at death, of unaffected members of the pedigrees. I have been unable to demonstrate from my material that antedating does not take place[1].

[1] [For the determination of coefficients of inheritance and for the problem of antedating only *completed* pedigrees can possibly be used. The author has apparently used incomplete pedigrees.—ED.]

On the Size of the Eye in Glaucoma. Priestley Smith writes[1]: "Every operator must sometimes have been struck when performing an iridectomy for primary glaucoma, by the unusual smallness of the cornea." Elliot writes[2] that he has "constantly made the observation in Madras that the eyes which come on the operating table for hypertension are decidedly below the average in size"; and again, "Anyone who has a large surgical practice cannot fail to be struck with the difference between the glaucomatous globe and an average non-glaucomatous organ...the glaucomatous eye gives one the impression that whatever may be its length antero-posteriorly, it is smaller than natural in its other diameters, and is in fact too small for its socket." This view is repeatedly stated in the literature of glaucoma. The growth of the eye is precocious in that it reaches its maximum size in early childhood, whereas the lens continues slowly to increase in size throughout life; it is thus obvious that the increasing liability to glaucoma as age advances might well be associated with these facts. We are indebted to Priestley Smith for an investigation into the matter. He measured the size of the cornea on 1000 healthy eyes of 500 persons, and on 216 eyes of 112 persons with primary glaucoma; he found that the average horizontal diameter of the cornea in healthy eyes was 11·6 mm., that of the glaucomatous patients was 11·2 mm.; further, whereas 22·7 $°/_\circ$ of the corneae of the glaucomatous measured 10·5 or 10 mm., only 1·7 $°/_\circ$ of healthy eyes had corneae of so small a size. Thus the corneae of the greater number of glaucomatous eyes were within normal limits, but there were found to be a very unusual number of small eyes amongst them.

Priestley Smith further measured a large number of lenses—156 from the eyes of 91 persons—and provided the following extremely interesting table. He notes

Mean Value of Measurements on the Crystalline Lens[3].

Age	No. of Eyes	Weight (mgr.)	Volume (cub. mm.)	Specific Gravity	Transverse Diameter (mm.)
20—29	21	174	163	1067	8·67
30—39	22	192	177	1085	8·96
40—49	23	204	188	1085	9·09
50—59	21	221	205	1078	9·44
60—69	23	240	225	1067	9·49
70—79	12	[245]	[227]	[1079]	[9·64]
80—89	6	[266]	[244]	[1090]	[9·62]

of six eyes, blinded from glaucoma, which had been enucleated, that some or all of them were characterised by "A small globe; a disproportionately large lens; a shallow anterior chamber; a closed filtration angle; an atrophied ciliary body; an excavated optic nerve." These facts certainly suggest a possible source for glaucoma of hereditary origin, for size of globe and of lens are surely inherited, and thus a malproportioned eye with a tendency to obstruction in the filtration area might readily be expected to occur in family histories of glaucoma. I have, however, no evidence that such is

[1] *Bibl.* No. 107, p. 96.   [2] *Bibl.* No. 247, pp. 134, 222.

[3] No measurements included if there was any trace of opacity in the lens; few quite clear lenses were available after the age of 70. Great care and labour were expended on this investigation, as will be seen on examination of the original description by Priestley Smith.

a common source of hereditary glaucoma; some evidence indeed tells against the hypothesis. The cornea has been measured, or its size indicated, in only 25 eyes of my series of cases; of these only two can be described as small.

The Cornea in Cases of Hereditary Glaucoma.

Corneal Diameter	No. of Eyes	Age of Onset
14 mm.	3	23, 18, 15
12·5	1	47
12·0	4	55, 47, 29, 13
R. 12·0, L. 11·5	2	13, 13
11·5	3	17, 16, 10
11·0	8	33, 30, 19, 19, 15, 15, 15, 12
10·5	1	42
10·0	2	28, 19
Macrocornea	4	20—24
Cornea "full"	1	21

No detailed discussion of the clinical details of hereditary cases as compared with non-hereditary cases is possible with so short a series as I can present, for many of which no clinical description is given; so far as one can judge, however, the same types of cases running a similar course occur in hereditary or in non-hereditary glaucoma and there would appear to be a similar proportion of acute, chronic congestive and non-congestive cases in the two groups. One point however I may mention; it refers to the depth of the anterior chamber. In the great majority of recorded hereditary cases no statement is made regarding the depth of the chamber; it may be that no statement commonly means a shallow chamber, but I have no means of judging whether or no this is so; of the 32 cases for which information is given, no fewer than 21 are said to have deep or very deep anterior chambers; in 13 of these 21 cases the onset of the disease was at an age earlier than 19 years; four cases had a normal or (in one case) *rather* deep chamber; six cases had a shallow chamber, in one case the chamber was obliterated; five of the latter group of cases were of the acute or congestive type of the disease. I put these facts on record, but can make no general statement regarding the character of the anterior chamber in hereditary glaucoma.

Parsons writes[1]:

"Two great classes of cases of glaucoma can be distinguished, viz. (1) those in which the tension is usually only moderately increased, in which the anterior chamber is deep, and in which there are more or less definite signs of inflammation of the ciliary body; (2) those in which all grades of increased tension are met with, in which the anterior chamber is shallow, and in which, while there may be very evident signs of congestion and irritation, any definite signs of ciliary inflammation are either absent or secondary in onset. It is well to keep these two groups quite separate, since their pathogenesis is different and the differences in clinical history and treatment are marked. The term *glaucoma* should be limited to the second group...."

These statements have haunted my mind whilst writing this introduction. I can

---

[1] *Bibl.* No. 175, Vol. III, p. 1073.

only conclude that the deep anterior chambers of my records have a similar source to those of buphthalmos and perhaps bear some relation to the early age of onset in hereditary cases. All writers are agreed upon the shallow anterior chambers of glaucoma in general. Elliot writes[1]: "A shallowing of the anterior chambers of the eye is an anatomical feature which is met with, sooner or later, in the vast majority of cases of glaucoma"; he quotes further from Priestley Smith: "In primary glaucoma the anterior chamber is usually shallow. In the main this is a pre-existing and predisposing condition—a cause rather than a consequence—...." It is much to be regretted that a note of the depth of the chamber is made in so few of the available records of hereditary glaucoma.

With regard to the ultimate vision in hereditary glaucoma I would ask the reader to seek information from the records appended; if the number of reports of blindness appal him, he should remember that these records cover a long period during which the technique of operation and the possibilities of treatment have progressed so far as entirely to change the outlook for the patient; nevertheless a case of glaucoma must always be an anxious business for surgeon and patient. Let us then see what are its hereditary characters and learn whether it may not be prevented in perhaps a small proportion of cases.

(c) *The Inheritance of Glaucoma.* Such material as I have on which to base my conclusions regarding the inheritance of glaucoma covers 295 cases of the disease in so poor a collection of pedigrees[2] that only very tentative suggestions can be made from them; of 85 cases no knowledge of the antecedents is available; information concerning the parentage of other cases is given in the table below.

Parentage		Affected Offspring			Totals
		♂	♀	♂	
Mother Affected (43 sibships)		41	42	2	85
Father Affected (42 sibships)		37	41	6	84
Neither Parent yet Affected	Mother's Stock Affected	10	1	1	12
	Father's "	2	3	—	5
	— "	11	10	3	24

Two conclusions can be drawn from this table: (a) either parent is equally potent as a transmitter of the disease; (b) the parent who transmits the disease is usually himself affected; my pedigrees show manifest affection, at the time of observation, in the parentage of an affected individual in 80 % of 210 cases. Of the remaining cases information was mostly incomplete; in some cases the parent may have died before the age of maximum liability, in other cases the affected offspring was young at the date of the record and the parent, if living, was well within the age at which the disease is likely to become manifest. It is extremely difficult to declare that any member of a family afflicted with hereditary glaucoma is free of the affection so long as he lives. There is no doubt that members already affected at an early age should abstain from parentage, indeed there is probably grave risk to the offspring of any

. [1] *Bibl.* No. 247, pp. 115, 116.   [2] Plates LXVII—LXIX, Figs. 1023—1090.

member of an affected sibship belonging to a stock definitely known to carry the disease in a hereditary form.

So far as I can judge cases of hereditary glaucoma appear in otherwise healthy stocks and very few examples of associated hereditary diseases or anomalies are found amongst the affected individuals; it is true that many cases included in my records are very incompletely described from the clinical point of view, some are not described at all, but I find no evidence of associated defects in the circulatory or central nervous systems, and very little associated defect in the structure of the eye so far as it can be observed. With regard to refraction, I have too few records amongst my notes on which to base any general statement. Only examinations of excised eyes could reveal the true hereditary factor which leads to glaucoma; even this is apt to mislead from the reason that an excised eye is a grossly diseased eye and may be completely disorganised by acute inflammatory reactions to which it has been subjected. Priestley Smith's extremely valuable work, pointing to a small eye with a disproportionately large lens leading to glaucoma as the lens further increases in size with age, undoubtedly explains the source of glaucoma in many cases of later years; an ill-developed or absent canal of Schlemm has often been demonstrated in excised eyes from buphthalmic patients, a defect of this character, however, is not very likely to remain unsuspected and lead to no symptoms until the age at which hereditary glaucoma commonly develops. My material provides no evidence of the source of glaucoma in hereditary cases.

B. CONGENITAL ANOMALIES OF THE IRIS. (a) ANIRIDIA, (b) COLOBOMA IRIDIS.

I propose to limit this section almost entirely to a presentation of the hereditary characters of the conditions included under (a) and (b), and to some analysis of the associated defects in each case; any discussion of the pathogenesis and pathology of the conditions belongs primarily to the skilled embryologist and a memoir on this aspect of the subject is at the present time being prepared elsewhere; it is hoped that the material here collected may be of some value to that investigation, but I should like to suggest that samples of material confined to hereditary examples of a disease do not alone provide a satisfactory foundation for a description of what occurs in the general population. If there be a tendency for members of the same affected stock to present the same associated defects, which are not characteristics of the anomaly in other stocks, it is clear that the presentation may be unduly influenced by individual family histories; particularly is care needed when, as in aniridia, the condition is rare, relatively few pedigrees are available, and at the same time the defect is dominant in the sense that many members of an affected family tend to manifest it.

Further, I would call attention to the ever present need to bear in mind that two fundamentally different sources of associated defect may be operating in cases of hereditary anomaly, namely (1) that of definite inherent hereditary linkage of which the syndrome of blue sclerotics, brittle bones and oto-sclerosis provides an example; (2) defects may arise in association because one is actually determined by the presence of the other. Thus, for example, some irregularity in the invagination of the lens into the optic cup, during development, may lead to a lenticular anomaly and provide a mechanical interference with the growing forward of the iris, resulting in aniridia associated with some defect of the lens.

It may be questioned why other anomalies of the iris are not included here, such as failure in the development of the mesodermal layers of the iris, heterochromia iridis, persistent pupillary membrane and corectopia; these conditions may present hereditary characters and certainly provide problems of great interest and importance bearing on the pathogenesis of anomalies of the iris, but too few hereditary examples are available to prove of any value to the main purpose of this volume. I would note however that a few pedigrees of mal-development of the anterior layers of the iris are in existence which show no associated cases of aniridia. The published records of aniridia collected here show a few associated cases of mal-development of the anterior layers of the iris, but I do not feel at all sure that the records as a whole can be trusted to reveal any relationship there may be between the two conditions; earlier methods of examination might readily fail to recognise defects confined to the iris stroma. Though the mesodermal and ectodermal layers of the iris develop independently, it is by no means clear that a failure of the former at the appointed time may not in some way inhibit the later development of the ectodermal structure. It seems almost inconceivable that two structures so intimately connected should not have associated developmental determinants.

The question of corectopia too is of some special interest; tables on pp. 431 and 480 will reveal the frequency of its occurrence in association with other defects, and indeed if a collection were made of pedigrees in which corectopia now figures as an associated defect, a considerable amount of material is readily available which might be used to illustrate the hereditary nature of the defect. I do not however propose to analyse my pedigrees from this point of view because—(a) There is no criterion as to what degree of eccentricity in the position of the pupil is really anomalous; the normal pupil is not centrally placed, and though eccentricity such as that illustrated in Plate S, Fig. 5 is certainly anomalous there is no standard as to within what limits with regard to position the normal pupil may lie. (b) Some degree of corectopia, if unaccompanied by other ocular defects, is not of a character to attract attention and it is unlikely that the few pedigrees available provide any measure of the frequency of the defect or of its hereditary characters. (c) In pedigrees showing the occurrence of corectopia in association with other defects we have no assurance that individuals classified as normal with regard to the subject of the pedigree have normally placed pupils. Corectopia becomes of special interest in its association with ectopia lentis and will be again referred to on consideration of that condition. It is not always easy to draw the line between what constitutes a partial aniridia and what is more truly described as an extreme degree of coloboma iridis, but the cases are rare in which any doubt can be felt as to which category they belong; the frequent occurrence of the two conditions in the same pedigree certainly points to some common factor in their pathogenesis. Early accounts of anomalies of the iris are not easy to find, apart from the fabulous reports concerning polycoria in Pliny's *Natural History*; so conspicuous a defect as coloboma iridis must surely have been recognised at an early date, but I find no definite description of a case before the seventeenth century, when Plemp[1], in 1648, saw a man who had an oval pupil in his left eye, but could see as well as other people. In 1673, Bartholinus[2] gave an interesting history of a unilateral case of coloboma iridis, in a boy whose father had a similar bilateral affection; the father's stock carried the defect; it is suggested that the boy owed his right, well-formed eye to his mother, his left eye to his father. Bloch[3], in 1774, and Conradi[4], in 1796, described further hereditary cases; Albinus[5], in 1764, and Tode[6], in 1774, described isolated cases. All these reports provide little more than a mere statement of the occurrence and it is not until the early nineteenth century that several admirable papers were published by Gescheidt[7], discussing, from a wider aspect, the structural anomalies of microphthalmos, irideremia, iridoschisma (coloboma iridis) and corectopia; these papers gave a number of historical references and describe the phenomena from the point of view of developmental and embryological considerations. It is not clear why there should have been a more ready and earlier recognition of coloboma iridis than of the grosser defect exhibited by aniridia, though the latter anomaly is much rarer than coloboma iridis. Writing in 1834 Gescheidt says that hitherto this defect has been so rarely observed that physicians doubt its occurrence in any case, and have suggested that when noted it has been mistaken for a very exaggerated mydriasis. To-day aniridia is rarely seen, whilst coloboma iridis is regarded as one of the most common of all eye anomalies, yet the two conditions are closely allied and we have a better series of pedigrees for the rarer condition than for coloboma iridis.

(a) Aniridia.

Aniridia, of which illustrations are given on Plates P and S, refers to a total absence of iris which, in the opinion of most authorities, never occurs in cases described under this heading; in many cases a careful examination will reveal some evidence of a rudimentary iris in the form of a narrow ring of iris tissue or of one or more tags in isolated positions; even when clinically no vestige of an iris is demonstrable, it is held that on microscopic examination some trace of the structure can invariably be found; thus many writers prefer the use of the synonym irideremia as more accurately describing the condition.

The essential function of the iris is simply concerned with the regulation of the amount of light which enters the eye; there would appear to be no reason then to expect the anomaly of aniridia to be accompanied clinically by very serious disabilities of vision, unless such might be looked for through the effects of dazzling or through the lack of protection to lenticular structures. As a matter of fact it would appear that the patient with this defect commonly presents very grave disabilities throughout life, and we can only seek their explanation in associated defects correlated with the failure in the development of an iris.

[1] *Bibl.* No. 4.   [2] *Bibl.* No. 6.   [3] *Bibl.* No. 10.   [4] *Bibl.* No. 14.
[5] *Bibl.* No. 9.   [6] *Bibl.* No. 11.   [7] *Bibl.* Nos. 18, 20, 23.

It is difficult to obtain any estimate, from the material available, as to the proportion of cases of hereditary aniridia who do retain useful vision; information regarding this factor is only given in 67 of the 237 cases of my collected records, though a further 74 individuals are known to have had associated defects of a character which must assuredly have interfered with vision; of the remaining 96 cases no description is given and I feel unable to hazard any suggestion as to the probable state with regard to vision of these individuals; many of them were not examined by the recorder and the only fact stated concerning them is the presence of aniridia. The path of the collector of pedigrees is commonly beset by one or other of two difficulties: on the one hand a recorder sets out to illustrate the hereditary characters of a disease, but perhaps gives no details of cases and is not always at pains to verify the statements of relations; on the other hand very detailed accounts may be given of several affected and related individuals, but enquiries are not sufficiently widely spread to contribute to the knowledge of the hereditary factors, and no information is given of the normal relations. The difficulty in the present case lies in deciding whether or no we can accept the detailed accounts of individuals as providing a random sample of all cases, or whether individuals free from hampering disabilities, who have not needed to seek ophthalmological aid, tend to occur in excess in the group of cases of which we have no detailed knowledge.

Characteristics of Vision in Cases of Aniridia	No. of Cases	Remarks
Blind, or nearly blind[1]	29	19 cases known to have severe associated defects[2]
Very bad, always bad, bad, very poor	13	10 ,, ,, ,, ,,
Never good, lowered, always rather poor	5	4 ,, ,, ,, ,,
Visual acuity $\frac{6}{24}$—$\frac{6}{36}$	7	4 ,, ,, ,, ,,
,, ,, about $\frac{6}{12}$ with correction	2	1 with cataract
Good at one time, cataract now	3	Ages 42, 34 and 9 years, respectively
Fair	5	Ages 28, 9, 4, 3 and 1½ years, respectively
No marked impairment	1	Lived to middle age
Saw well in a dim light	1	—
Not lowered demonstrably	1	Aged 11 months

[1] Including V. = perception of light, hand movements, or less than $\frac{6}{60}$.

[2] Including cataract, ectopia lentis, corneal opacities, glaucoma, absence of fovea.

The table given here includes all information I can offer concerning the vision in cases of aniridia. It is clear that the common visual defect can generally be explained on grounds not necessarily contributed to by the absence of an iris. Nystagmus, as may be seen from the descriptions of pedigree plates appended, is frequently present, but the real significance of this symptom in cases of aniridia is not altogether clear; it may or may not be an indication of defect in the development of the fovea, which is believed by some observers to be a common accompaniment of aniridia. Photophobia should be a normal characteristic in cases of aniridia and it is a little surprising that complaint from this source is not more general; the commonly associated cataract may mask the symptom. Some observers have been led to the impression that the discs tend to be paler than is normal in cases of aniridia which may indicate some lack of sensitivity to light on the part of patients.

In considering what are the defects commonly found in association with aniridia the following points have some bearing on this question[1]. (*a*) The mesodermal iris, or iris stroma, develops in advance of the posterior pigment layer of ectodermal origin, which at a later stage provides the musculature of the pupillary sphincter. (*b*) The mesodermal structure can only develop subsequently to the separation of the lens from the cornea and its invagination into the optic cup. (*c*) In process of development a spur of mesodermal tissue dips into the optic cup at the margin and forms a temporary vascular structure posterior to the lens which subsequently disappears. On the basis of embryological material available to her, Dr Ida Mann suggests that coloboma iridis may arise from the failure of a portion of this vascular structure to disappear at the appointed time, thus preventing the ectodermal iris from growing forward at the position of the vestige; she further suggests that if aniridia be regarded as a total coloboma iridis, it may result from the retention of the structure throughout. Development of the iris would of necessity be prevented also if the lens failed to separate from the cornea and become invaginated below the margin of the optic cup at the appointed time. Embryologists have provided some evidence that if a structure be prevented from differentiating normally at the proper moment, its further development tends to be inhibited. (*d*) There is a close link in developmental history between the iris stroma and the substantia propria of the cornea. Clearly the associated defects in cases of aniridia, particularly those affecting the lens and cornea, are of special interest from the point of view of the pathogenesis of the anomaly, but only the embryologist is in a position to state what may be deduced from the observed facts.

The table on p. 469 shows what associated defects have been noted in the cases of aniridia of my records, but again I have no means of judging whether the cases described in detail provide a random sample of cases of hereditary aniridia in general, or whether there has been a tendency to describe selected cases who sought aid owing to their multiple defects and severe grade of disability. It will be seen that we have evidence of some, for the most part serious, complicating defect in 118 of our cases. What of the remaining 119 affected individuals? No information is given concerning most of these cases, but there is evidence of examination in 31 of them; of these nystagmus was noted in nine; five further cases were practically blind; three cases were young infants; vision was bad in six cases; only eight cases remain of the 31 who were apparently free from serious disability. We see however that clinically complete aniridia is not incompatible with an otherwise normal eye and useful vision in some individual cases.

I am reluctant to attempt any analysis of the facts in the table here presented; their significance can only be fully appreciated by an examination of the individual histories and of the pedigrees in which they figure; it is not alone the associated defects in the individual, but the family history with the tendency to multiple defects throughout the stock which is so marked a feature in pedigrees of aniridia. It is for the embryologist to consider the source of the extremely common affection of the lens

[1] See Mann, I.: "Coloboma Iridis and its Embryology." *Transactions, Ophthalmological Society of U.K.*, Vol. XLIV, p. 161 *et seq.* London, 1924.

in these cases; some form of cataract, commonly congenital and often of the anterior polar variety, is noted in 70 individuals with or without further defects; ectopia lentis with or without cataract is described in 36 cases; opacities in the cornea would appear

Defects observed in association with Aniridia in the same Individual.

	♂	♀	♂	Total
Cataract	15	15	—	30
„ and ectopia lentis	5	4	—	9
„ ectopia lentis and corneal opacity	—	1	—	1
„ „ and glaucoma	—	2	—	2
„ „ microphthalmos, ptosis, defective teeth	—	1	—	1
„ „ microphthalmos, defective teeth	—	1	—	1
„ and glaucoma	1	1	—	2
„ and corneal opacity	—	2	—	2
„ corneal opacity and pale discs	—	1	—	1
„ „ microphthalmos, coloboma of discs, mental dullness, deafness, defective teeth, talipes varus	1	—	—	1
„ and coloboma iridis	—	1	—	1
„ microphthalmos and blue sclerotics	1	—	—	1
„ „ and mal-developed corneae	1	—	—	1
„ „ and strabismus	1	—	—	1
„ „ ptosis, small discs and retinal vessels	1	—	—	1
„ and blue sclerotics	1	—	—	1
„ blue sclerotics and persistent pupillary membrane	1	—	—	1
„ and strabismus	1	4	—	5
„ strabismus, ptosis and embryontoxon	1	—	—	1
„ ptosis, absent fovea, embryontoxon, cleft palate	—	1	—	1
„ and pale discs	1	1	—	2
„ and absent fovea	1	—	—	1
„ and mental defect	—	1	—	1
„ defective teeth and congenital hernia	1	—	—	1
„ and rickets	—	1	—	1
Ectopia lentis	4	2	8	14
„ and corneal opacity	1	—	—	1
„ and glaucoma	1	—	3	4
„ corneal opacity, mental dullness, rickets	—	1	—	1
„ and microphthalmos, choroidal atrophy, small retinal vessels	—	1	—	1
„ and cretinism	—	1	—	1
Corneal opacity	4	7	—	11
„ and coloboma iridis	—	—	1	1
„ and microcornea, coloboma of disc, strabismus, defective teeth	1	—	—	1
Microphthalmos	1	4	—	5
Microcornea and absent fovea	1	—	—	1
Glaucoma	—	2	—	2
Coloboma of choroid	—	1	—	1
Coloboma of choroid and lens	1	—	—	1
Blue sclerotics and gerontoxon	—	1	—	1
Strabismus	1	—	—	1
Pale discs	1	—	—	1

to be fairly common, but no description of the character of the opacity is given and it is very difficult to say what significance can be attached to this observation. I think the relative rareness of glaucoma is of some interest and importance; it might be expected that a narrow unorganised rudimentary iris would have a tendency to block the filtration angle and lead to glaucoma; such cases as are noted are however commonly secondary in character and it would appear that there is no marked liability to glaucoma in the aniridic patient. An examination of the histories reveals the further fact that the complications in cases of aniridia are generally bilateral and both eyes usually present a similar appearance; moreover the same complications tend to occur in different members of the same stock.

The not uncommon occurrence of aniridia and coloboma iridis in the same stock is of very great interest and importance; I have no fewer than 16 histories in which these two anomalies are associated[1]; the affection of members is usually the more severe one of aniridia with an occasional case only of coloboma iridis, but a striking exception occurs in Fig. 1157, where a history of coloboma iridis in 11 members of five generations exhibits a further two members with aniridia. Figs. 1142, 1144 show cases in which an individual has aniridia in one eye, coloboma iridis in the other; in one case the father and a brother had bilateral aniridia, in the other case the mother had unilateral coloboma iridis. Figs. 1095, 1096, 1104, 1122, 1137 and 1157 provide examples of eight parents with coloboma iridis who between them have 12 children with bilateral aniridia. Single cases of coloboma iridis occur in aniridic sibships, or among the offspring of an aniridic parent, in Figs. 943, 1093, 1104, 1116, 1118, 1120, 1126 and 1138. Fig. 1097 shows an aniridic mother with two sons each showing bilateral coloboma iridis. These cases are very suggestive. I would call attention in this connection to the few examples of aniridia in which coloboma of the choroid has been noted, but would remind the reader that the frequency of cataract and corneal opacities must often interfere with any examination of the fundus.

Aniridia is nearly always bilateral, but the condition is not invariably identical on the two sides; examples of some degree of asymmetry are included in the table below.

Examples of Asymmetry in Aniridia.

Individual	Right Eye	Left Eye
II. 2, Fig. 1125	Complete Aniridia	Small tag up and outwards
II. 2, ,, 1096·	Complete Aniridia	Small tag up and inwards
I. 1, ,, 1092	Narrow band, absent in one place	Complete Aniridia
I. 1, ,, 1145	Narrow rim	Complete Aniridia
III. 2, ,, 1118	Slight tag upwards	Complete Aniridia
III. 2, ,, 1125	Complete Aniridia	Tag outwards
III. 2, ,, 1116	Small outer rim	Wider inner rim, with tags
IV. 5, ,, 1105	Tags up and inwards	Smaller tags up and inwards
II. 1, ,, 1096	Narrow strip on inner side	Tags inwards
III. 6, ,, 1106	A trace below	Some trace throughout
III. 2, ,, 1132	Complete Aniridia	Slight trace
III. 2, ,, 1122	Slight rim below	Complete Aniridia
II. 1, ,, 1142	Coloboma iridis	Aniridia
II. 1, ,, 1144	Coloboma iridis	Aniridia

No single case, to my knowledge, has been recorded in which aniridia in one eye is associated with a normal eye on the other side; my experience, however, is limited to hereditary cases of the anomaly, and I do not know that isolated cases, occurring in

---

[1] See Figs. 943, 1093, 1095, 1096, 1097, 1104, 1116, 1118, 1120, 1122, 1126, 1137, 1138, 1142, 1144, 1157.

otherwise normal stocks, conform in all respects to the clinical characteristics of the group to which my collected cases belong.

Sex-incidence and Inheritance of Aniridia. My material includes 57 family histories; many of these are very imperfect, but, from the point of view of the inheritance of the disease, the pedigrees provide an interesting little series. Perhaps the most remarkable pedigree ever published is the history of aniridia, due to Samuel Risley, published in America in 1915 and reproduced in *The Lancet* in this country; this history extends through four generations and includes 119 individuals of whom no fewer than 113 were said to have aniridia; many large families are represented in which every member was affected; we are told of four members who were normal and of two who were not known to be affected; several members are described who had one eye normal; the age at death is given of a number of individuals; two members of the family only were described in detail. I was unwilling to accept this history without verification, though such cases as that of Galezowski (see Fig. 1103) lent a measure of support to the view that the pedigree did not represent an impossibility. My letter to Dr Risley arrived shortly after his death and was forwarded to his house surgeon, who had obtained the facts of the pedigree. This observer assured me that, though he had only seen two members of the family, he had obtained all particulars with great care and was convinced of their accuracy. Subsequent attempts to get in touch with the family failed and I put the pedigree aside for the time being. Later Dr Lucien Howe, the American ophthalmologist, who was greatly interested in problems of heredity and had himself reproduced this pedigree, told me that on investigation it had proved to be without satisfactory foundation, and that the history should not be accepted without further verification. I put this on record as a warning of the great care needed in accepting pedigrees without due consideration of the methods by which they have been compiled. Had I included Risley's pedigree amongst my little group of examples, it would have completely dominated the picture presented by the inheritance of aniridia.

My material includes 237 examples of aniridia, of whom 97 were males, 97 were females; the sex in 43 cases was not given. The male sex-incidence is thus 50·0 °/₀, or either sex is equally liable to show the defect; it would appear from the table below that each sex is also equally potent as a transmitter of the anomaly.

Parentage in Cases of Aniridia[1].

	♂	♀	♂	Totals	Remarks
Mother affected	33	37	33	103	20 of the 33 ♂ were offspring of two mothers only (Fig. 1103)
Father affected	33	34	10	77	
Both Parents normal	13	12	—	25	In 2 ♂ there were affected members in the father's stock (Fig. 1105)
No knowledge of Parents	18	14	—	32	
	97	97	43	237	

[1] The affected parents in this table include several parents with coloboma iridis.

On examination of the pedigrees it becomes clear that aniridia is usually transmitted to affected individuals by a parent who manifests the defect, but this is not
invariably the case. In a considerable proportion of the cases on record for which
both parents were said to be normal, the information is based on statements by
descendants; probably some of them were in error, or the parent may have had
a less conspicuous affection which might well escape recognition in the family annals;
nevertheless, I think there is no doubt that two parents who appear to have normal
eyes do occasionally have children with aniridia who themselves transmit the defect.
Without giving actual figures, which cannot be trusted in so short a series, I think
definite evidence can be produced in support of the view that the proportion of
affected amongst the offspring is on the average much less when the parentage is
apparently normal than when one or other of them is affected; this certainly is
in favour of the suggestion that the parentage of the two groups has different
potentialities. A further fact of some significance, in the consideration of the nature
of the cases of apparently normal parentage of affected sibships, lies in the rarity
of examples in which a normal member of an affected sibship has been demonstrated
to transmit the defect.

Plates LXX and LXXI certainly present an extremely intriguing group of cases
illustrating the inheritance of aniridia; it provides much of suggestive interest, but it
would be unwise to draw general conclusions from so small a sample of material, which
shows such great diversity in the potency of the hereditary factors in different stocks.

(b) Coloboma Iridis.

Coloboma iridis consists in a localised failure of the iris to develop, resulting in
a cleft at the position of the defect and a resulting anomaly in the shape of the pupil,
which is now no longer circular, but is prolonged into the cleft and may be described
as pear-shaped, key-hole-shaped, U-shaped, Gothic or slit-shaped, depending upon
the nature of the cleft in any particular case. The area of the iris involved varies
considerably; in rare cases it may be of so extensive a character as to be more
fittingly described as a partial aniridia, or again the defect may be represented by
a mere notch in the iris at the pupillary margin. The defect is described as complete
or incomplete according as the cleft extends throughout the width of the iris to the
peripheral limit, or stops short of this; occasionally cases appear which exhibit
a complete coloboma with a narrow bridge of iris tissue crossing the cleft at one
point. Further there may be two or even more colobomata in one iris. Illustrative
examples of various types after von Ammon are shown on Plate A.

This anomaly is described as typical or atypical according to whether the direction
of the coloboma is pointed downwards (including the more commonly observed cases
downwards and slightly inwards), or in other directions. Typical colobomata may
be explained as a result of failure in the closure of the embryological cleft in the
optic cup during development, but examples of this type are not all necessarily thus
produced; atypical colobomata can certainly not be so explained. If then the position
of the cleft is of particular interest from the point of view of the pathogenesis of the

condition, it becomes of interest to note whether typical or atypical colobomata tend to be characteristics of a particular pedigree, and whether the two eyes of an individual are similar in this respect. Further, since aniridia cannot be explained by a failure in the closure of the optic cleft at the appointed time, the association of this anomaly with coloboma iridis in the same individual, or in the same stocks, becomes of some special significance.

The following table gives the position of a coloboma iridis in cases intimately related to individuals with aniridia:

Case with Coloboma Iridis	Direction of Coloboma	Relation with Aniridia
III. 1, Fig. 1126 ♀	Outwards in both	Mother
II. 1, „ 1097 ♂	R. (double) down-in and down-out, L. down-in	Mother
II. 2, „ 1097 ♂	Down-in, in both	Mother
I. 1, „ 1096 ♂	Down-in, in both	Offspring
III. 5, „ 1116 ♂	Inwards, R. and L.	Father
I. 1, „ 1140 ♂	In-up, R. and L.	Offspring
II. 1, „ 1144 ♂	Outwards in R., aniridia in L.	Mother coloboma iridis, downwards
I. 1, „ 1144 ♀	Downwards in R., unilateral	Offspring
II. 2, „ 1122 ♀	Up-out in R., down-out in L.	Offspring
IV. 3, „ 1157 ♂	Down-out, R. and L.	Offspring
III. 5, „ 1157 ♂	Down-out, R. and L.	Offspring
III. 4, „ 1118 ♀	Downwards, R. and L.	Father
I. 1, „ 1095 ♀	Upwards in R., up-out in L.	Offspring
II. 7, „ 1104 ♂	Down-in, R. and L.	Father
I. 1, „ 1137 ♂	Inwards, R. and L	Offspring

It will be agreed that there is an exceptional proportion of atypical colobomata represented in this table; if, however, we may assume that aniridia and coloboma iridis in parent and offspring have a similar determinant, it may be inferred that typical colobomata are by no means invariably due to failure in closure of the optic cleft.

It is unfortunate that information of the direction of the cleft is so frequently not given in my group of hereditary cases. Such figures as I have refer to 91 eyes of 49 individuals and are included in the table below.

Direction of Coloboma	Hereditary Cases. No. of Eyes		Totals	Fichte's Cases*
	Pedigrees not including Cases of Aniridia	Pedigrees including Cases of Aniridia		
Down and In	22	8	30	49
Downwards	16	3	19	52
Down and Out	2	[18]	[20]	2
Up and Out	4	2	6	3
Up and In	2	2	4	5
Outwards	—	3	3	3
Inwards	2	4	6	1
Upwards	2	1	3	—
Totals	50	41	91	115

* *Bibl.* No. 36.

I am unwilling to draw any conclusions from these few figures, but think they are worth recording for the benefit of future workers who may be in a position to add to them. The position with regard to pedigrees including cases of aniridia is dominated by one family history due to Snell (Fig. 1157) in which all affected members had bilateral colobomata directed downwards and outwards; if two cases of aniridia had failed to occur in the last generation of this pedigree, no fewer than 16 of the 18 cases of this entry would have been transferred to the first column. It was noted of aniridia that no single case among my records had a unilateral affection associated with a normal eye on the other side; coloboma iridis, on the contrary, tends to be less symmetrical than aniridia and to occur not infrequently in association with a normal eye in the same individual. So far as can be judged, when commonly no detailed description of both eyes is given, it would appear that colobomata in the two eyes of an individual tend for the most part to lie in the same direction, though they frequently differ in other characteristics; such types of asymmetry as have been noted among my cases can be studied in the table given below. My material includes 119 cases of the defect, less than half the number of cases provided by the pedigrees of aniridia, but many more cases of asymmetry are noted in coloboma iridis, and I find no fewer than 18 cases of the latter anomaly in which the condition was unilateral and probably associated with a normal eye in the same individual. Parsons[1] writes that coloboma iridis is *usually* unilateral; thus it would appear that though hereditary coloboma iridis is much more commonly unilateral than is hereditary aniridia, yet it is bilateral in character much more frequently than are cases of coloboma iridis which are not of hereditary origin; it is true that no description is given in a considerable proportion of my hereditary cases, but I think it unlikely that a unilateral affection would escape notice, and probably 18 in 111 examples amongst hereditary cases of the anomaly is near the true proportion of cases exhibiting unilateral affection with a normal second eye.

The table given on p. 475 includes 22 further examples of asymmetry, of which most are due to differences in extent or shape; indeed in only two cases, apart from those involving double colobomata, is a definite difference of direction noted in the two eyes; II. 2 of Fig. 1122 has a coloboma up-out in the right eye, down-out in the left, and I. 1 of Fig. 1162 has a coloboma down-in in the right eye, up-in in the left. I think we may state that bilateral cases of hereditary origin appear to be nearly always symmetrical with respect to direction. This table accounts then for 40 cases showing some varying degree of asymmetry; of the remaining 71 cases of my series, no details are given for 39 individuals; in 24 cases the direction is noted to be the same in each eye; in 8 cases some indication of symmetry in shape or size is given but no information of the direction of the cleft.

There would appear to be no reason to expect any serious defect in vision in cases of coloboma iridis from this cause alone; indeed good or probably useful vision is indicated in a considerable proportion of my cases; yet a good deal of cataract, often of a congenital variety, is found in association with the defect, which must hamper vision

[1] *Bibl.* No. 175, p. 821.

and sometimes leads to blindness; also, coloboma of the choroid, possibly involving the optic nerve, is a common accompaniment which frequently impairs vision to some extent; such instances of blindness or very bad sight as are noted amongst my cases

Examples of Asymmetry in Coloboma Iridis.

Individual	Right Eye	Left Eye
II. 2, Fig. 1170	Normal	Coloboma, down
II. 3, ,, ,,	Coloboma, down	Rudimentary
II. 4, ,, 1161	Normal	Coloboma iridis
III. 5, ,, ,,	Normal	Coloboma, down, iris lighter than in R. eye
IV. 2, ,, ,,	Normal, iris blue-grey	Coloboma, down-in, iris light brown
IV. 3, ,, ,,	Coloboma, down-in	Normal
II. 2, ,, 1155	Normal	Coloboma iridis
II. 7, ,, ,,	Coloboma iridis	Normal
II. 1, ,, 1151	Normal	Coloboma, down-in
I. 2, ,, 1164	Normal	Small coloboma
I. 1, ,, 1144	Coloboma, down	Normal
II. 1, ,, ,,	Coloboma, out	Aniridia
II. 2, ,, 1158	Normal	Key-hole coloboma, incomplete
II. 5, ,, ,,	Normal	Coloboma, down-in, incomplete
III. 5, ,, ,,	Keyhole coloboma, down, complete with bridge	Pear-shaped coloboma, down, complete
II. 1, ,, 1162	Coloboma, down-in	Normal iris, darker than in R. eye
I. 1, ,, ,,	Coloboma, down-in, slit-shaped	Coloboma, up-in, oval
III. 4, ,, ,,	Coloboma, complete	Coloboma, complete; some atrophy of stroma
I. 1, ,, 1166	Broad, double coloboma, up-in and down-out	Large open U-shaped coloboma
II. 4, ,, ,,	Two eccentric pupils, atrophy of iris	Large triangular coloboma
II. 1, ,, 1142	Coloboma .	Aniridia
II. 2, ,, 1122	Coloboma, up-out, complete	Coloboma, down-out, incomplete
I. 1, ,, 1095	Coloboma, upwards, large	Coloboma, up-out, smaller
I. 1, ,, 1096	Discoloration, down-in	Large coloboma, down-in
I. 1, ,, 1140	Coloboma, up-in, nearly complete	Notch in iris, up-in
III. 2, ,, 1157	Coloboma, down-out	Coloboma, down-out, narrower than in R. eye
IV. 1, ,, ,,	Coloboma, down-out	Coloboma, down-out, wider than in R. eye
II. 1, ,, 1097	Colobomata, down-in and down-out	Coloboma, down-in, incomplete
III. 5, ,, 1116	Complete coloboma	Incomplete
III. 8, ,, 1160	Coloboma, down, incomplete	Double, incomplete, down and down-out
III. 10, ,, 1156	Incomplete coloboma, down-in	Complete, down-in
II. 1, ,, 1149	Coloboma in one iris, notch in the other	
II. 1, ,, 1150	,, up-in in one eye, up-out in the other	
III. 3, ,, 1160	,, definite in one eye, an indication only in the other	
I. 1, ,, 1149	,, down-in in one eye, a pronounced notch down-in in the other	
	Additional cases of unilateral coloboma are noted in II. 3, Fig. 1152, II. 2 and II. 5, Fig. 1159, II. 2, Fig. 1168, and I. 1, Fig. 1169	

can usually be attributed to these causes. It becomes then of interest to note the incidence of associated defects.

There is evidently a considerable liability to associated defect in cases of coloboma iridis, but it would appear to be on the whole of a less severe grade and accompanied by much less functional disturbance than in the case of aniridia or microphthalmos; the entries in the table should be regarded as minimum values in every case and it is difficult to form any estimate as to how far the cases of which no description is given tend to be free from associated defect.

It is perhaps surprising not to find a more general evidence of coloboma of the choroid in these cases; its occurrence is definitely noted in only 21 individuals, but in many cases the fundus was not seen owing to cataract or other causes; a normal

Defects observed in association with Coloboma Iridis in the same Individual.

	♂	♀	♂	Totals
Coloboma of choroid (with or without involvement of disc)	2	6	—	8
,, ,, and cataract	2	—	—	2
,, ,, cataract and microphthalmos	—	1	—	1
,, ,, cataract, microphthalmos and coloboma lentis	1	—	—	1
,, ,, cataract, microphthalmos, strabismus, high-arched palate	1	—	—	1
,, ,, cataract and mental dullness	—	1	—	1
,, ,, and microphthalmos	—	1	—	1
,, ,, microphthalmos and strabismus	—	2	—	2
,, ,, microphthalmos and high-arched palate	—	2	—	2
,, ,, and strabismus	1	—	—	1
,, ,, and high-arched palate	1	—	—	1
Cataract	3	3	—	6
,, and coloboma lentis	1	1	—	2
,, and microphthalmos	1	1	2	4
,, microphthalmos and high-arched palate	1	—	—	1
,, cryptorchidism and mental dullness	1	—	—	1
,, and hazy corneae	1	—	—	1
,, and mental dullness	1	—	—	1
,, and aniridia	—	1	—	1
Microphthalmos and opaque nerve fibres	—	1	—	1
Aniridia	—	—	1	1
Ectopia lentis	—	1	—	1
Persistent pupillary membrane	1	—	—	1
Mental defect	—	1	—	1

fundus is described in 17 cases. When associated with coloboma of the choroid, the iridal cleft lies in a position downwards or downwards and inwards in all the few cases for which information is given. Cataract, often noted early in life, is described in 23 cases; this and the frequency of microphthalmos further indicate that hereditary coloboma iridis is commonly a characteristic of a mal-developed eye and is not, for the most part, an entirely localised defect.

Inheritance and Sex-incidence in Coloboma Iridis. Twenty-seven pedigrees (many of them worth little from the standpoint of heredity) of coloboma iridis are included under Figs. 1147–1173 of Plates LXXI and LXXII; cases also may be sought for under the heading of aniridia. This is a very short series, yet ophthalmologists are agreed that coloboma iridis is one of the most common of all anomalies of the eye. I have endeavoured to find some explanation of this paucity of published pedigrees, and can only conclude that perhaps the anomaly does generally occur in isolated cases, and carries for the most part no hereditary potentiality. Hird, in 1912, collected information on the general characteristics of the anomaly and could trace no sign of heredity in the 16 cases under his personal observation; Usher, agreeing in the common occurrence of the defect, and ever watchful for hereditary characteristics, has been unable to trace any influence of this nature in cases which have been under his care.

The hereditary cases of my series cover 111 individuals, including 52 males, 52 females and 7 of unrecorded sex; the male sex-incidence is thus 50 °/$_o$, as in the case of aniridia.

The defect is most commonly transmitted by an affected parent, but this cannot be stated as a characteristic of the condition in view of the following table showing that some 30 °/$_o$ of the 79 cases, whose parentage was known, had parents who were unaffected. The pedigrees are too few and scanty to consider as a whole, but individual

Parentage in Cases of Coloboma Iridis.

Parentage	♂	♀	♂	Totals
Mother affected	12	7	6	25
Father affected	13	17	—	30
Both Parents normal	13	11	—	24*
Totals	38	35	6	79

* In five of these cases the mother's stock was affected, in one case the father's stock.

cases provide varied interest and are worth some study. A generation is skipped in Figs. 1160, 1172 and 1173, a consanguineous marriage having occurred in one of these cases. In Fig. 1156 two generations are skipped, one consanguineous marriage having occurred in the interval. Figs. 1159 and 1160 provide examples in which a normal member of an affected sibship has transmitted the defect. It is clear that either sex is equally potent in the transmission of the defect.

C. HEREDITARY ECTOPIA LENTIS.

Hereditary ectopia lentis is an anomaly in the position of the lens of the eye, which is no longer centrally placed with regard to the iris but is displaced in almost any direction, though more commonly in some directions than in others. The condition arises as the result of an embryological defect affecting the development of the suspensory ligament of the lens, which may be absent in parts and evidently varies within wide limits in its departure from the normal. In eyes presenting this anomaly the lens may be altogether withdrawn from the pupillary area, or its margin may be seen crossing the pupil; the defect again may be of so slight degree that only upon dilatation of the pupil can the anomaly be demonstrated. In a considerable proportion of cases the lens becomes completely luxated and may be seen lying in the anterior chamber or in the floor of the vitreous; in some cases the mobility of the lens is so marked that it can be seen to swing in position with movements of the head. Obviously the defect must be of a serious nature, not alone through the direct interference to vision occasioned by the misplaced lens, but also from the secondary effects such as cataract or glaucoma, to which the subject must be liable as a result of irritation set up by irregular movements within the eye.

The condition would appear to be among the more common of the hereditary anomalies of the eye if we may judge by the number of published histories. My material consists of 73 pedigrees covering 345 cases of the defect, including 179 males, 142 females and 24 cases of unstated sex. The male sex-incidence thus determined is $55\cdot8 \pm 1\cdot9$, showing some actual excess of males amongst published records of cases, but evidently both sexes are almost equally liable; in certain pedigrees an excess of males may be presented, as in Fig. 1176 due to Vogt, including 13, probably 15, affected males and one or two affected females; other pedigrees show an excess of females, an example of which is shown in Fig. 1178 by Cameron, including 13 females and only one male affected.

It is evident that the defect is almost invariably bilateral, though several cases have been noted in which one lens is said to be in a normal position[1]; moreover the condition is commonly symmetrical in the two eyes. I find the same displacement in

Position of Lens	Symmetrical Displacement			All Cases (No. of Eyes)		
	Males	Females	Totals	Males	Females	Totals
Up and In	14	8	22	38	22	60
Up	8	9	17	23	23	46
Down	8	5	13	23	17	40
Up and Out	8	3	11	22	13	35
Out	6	7	13	17	17	34
In	8	5	13	19	13	32
Down and In	2	5	7	5	17	22
Down and Out	1	4	5	5	13	18
In Anterior Chamber	4	2	6	11	9	20
In Vitreous	4	—	4	13	4	17
Complete Luxation	6	2	8	13	4	17
Tilted	1	—	1	2	1	3
Totals	70	50	120	191	153	344

both eyes in 120 cases; and some degree of asymmetry in 31 males and 29 females of my records; the latter cases include for the most part those in which the asymmetry is of slight degree only or in which one lens has become completely dislocated and is lying in the vitreous or in the anterior chamber; it is evidently very rare for one lens to be displaced in an upward direction (including up-in and up-out) and the other lens to be displaced downwards. The direction of the displacement should, one would think, have considerable interest with regard to the pathogenesis of the anomaly, but it is difficult to see what deduction can be made when the character of the displacement varies within such wide limits and may indeed lie in any direction; all that one can point to is some definite excess of displacements in an upward direction (including up and in, up and out) as compared with those directed downwards (including down and in, down and out). Another point of some particular interest in these cases is the frequent accompaniment of corectopia; the following table includes all the information I have, indicating the frequency of the association in 209 cases. It will be seen that 55 cases show some abnormality of the pupil; this is a considerable proportion, but it is clear

[1] See IV. 2 of Fig. 1220, II. 3 of Fig. 1210, II. 2 of Fig. 1203.

that a marked displacement of the lens may be and most commonly is associated with a normal pupil; only the embryologist is in a position to discuss the probable nature of the association between these two anomalies when it occurs; the occurrence, however, of multiple cases of the association in the same family suggests the possibility of some genetic link between the two factors in these pedigrees rather than a common developmental determinant. In only 26 eyes is the direction of the displacement given

Pupil in Cases of Ectopia Lentis.

Pupil	No. of Cases	Remarks
Normal	43	—
Presumably Normal	111	Cases described, no mention of pupils
Circular, central	6	One pin-point, no reaction; 3 small; 2 react sluggishly
Corectopia	42	Eight cases have one or both pupils pear-shaped or oval; one has a persistent pupillary membrane
Central, not circular	6	One with persistent pupillary membrane
Double	1	—

for the lens and the pupil; in 10 of these the displacement is towards the same direction, in 16 eyes the pupillary eccentricity differs from that of the lens; there would thus appear to be no evidence of a close link determining any parallelism of the direction in the two cases.

With regard to defects or liabilities associated with hereditary ectopia lentis, other than those affecting the pupil, such as occur may perhaps be largely explained as the result of mechanical injury due to the defect itself, and are largely included in the following table under the heading of cataract, with or without accompanying defects; and under secondary glaucoma with or without other defects. The table given on p. 480, including all cases of observed associated defects, leads to the conclusion that the anomaly of ectopia lentis is for the most part strictly limited in its manifestation; it is indeed a little unexpected after an examination of the frequent occurrence of ectopia lentis in cases of aniridia (see p. 469) to find no single case of aniridia noted in my pedigrees of ectopia lentis; it is further noteworthy that, though corectopia and slight departure from the normal shape of pupil are frequent with hereditary ectopia lentis, a definite coloboma iridis is never described.

Certain individual pedigrees show an interesting linkage of ectopia lentis with other conditions. Such is Strebel's[1] pedigree of ectopia lentis with corectopia, high myopia and a liability to heart disease; also two small pedigrees due to Weve[2] and Haas[3] include a few cases all of which are associated with arachnodactyly, but I find no widespread evidence of such linkage; there is moreover little evidence of associated abnormality outside the eye. The table given on p. 480 includes reference to 119 cases of ectopia lentis; my records include a further 111 cases, giving evidence of examination, which show no associated defect, apart from refractive errors, often very high but of doubtful significance, and the very common visual defect which is to be expected.

It would appear that the eyes of cases which present this anomaly are not for the

[1] Fig. 1177.   [2] Fig. 1227.   [3] Fig. 1226.

most part markedly ill-developed or malproportioned eyes, apart from the particular error, and that the accidents which occur, such as cataract or glaucoma, result from

Diseases observed in association with Ectopia Lentis	♂	♀	Totals
Cataract	9	8	17
„ and secondary glaucoma	3	2	5
„ and pupillary anomaly	2	5	7
„ corectopia and secondary glaucoma	1	—	1
„ corectopia, ptosis and strabismus	1	—	1
„ corectopia, mental weakness and high-arched palate	—	1	1
„ anomaly of pupils and mental weakness	1	—	1
„ anomaly of pupils, strabismus and stammering	1	—	1
„ and coloboma lentis	1	—	1
„ secondary glaucoma and mental weakness	—	1	1
„ and corneal maculae	1	—	1
„ and megalocornea	—	1	1
„ and small discs	—	1	1
„ and strabismus	—	1	1
„ hyperthyroidism and rickets	—	1	1
„ nervousness and high-arched palate	—	1	1
Corectopia or anomaly of pupils	14	9	23
„ secondary glaucoma and heart disease	2	—	2
„ and heart disease	4	6	10
„ and phlyctenular keratitis	—	1	1
„ strabismus and cretinism	1	—	1
„ and epispadia	1	—	1
Secondary glaucoma	2	3	5
„ „ and anomaly in pupils	1	—	1
Anomaly in pupils and corneal opacity	1	—	1
„ „ detachment of retina, small lenses and strabismus	—	1	1
Anomaly in discs and retinal vessels	1	1	2
Coloboma lentis	1	1	2
Corneal opacity	1	—	1
Buphthalmos	1	—	1
Megalocornea, rachitis	1	1	2
Strabismus	2	—	2
„ and ?tuberculous glands	—	1	1
Choroiditis	—	1	1
Detached retina and high-arched palate	—	1	1
Arachnodactyly	5	2	7
Glands in neck, ?tuberculous	—	1	1
Tuberculosis and neurosis	—	1	1
Hyperthyroidism	—	1	1
Facial asymmetry	—	1	1
Heart disease	1	2	3
Mental defect	—	3	3
Imbecility with tuberculosis	—	1	1

the nature of the anomaly rather than from a common cause; none the less, the defect is often a most serious handicap, as will be seen from the table below, including such information as I have concerning the vision of affected individuals. It is unfortunate that many cases of my records are described from the point of view of the hereditary relationships and give no details of the functional capacity in individuals; it may well be that there has been a tendency to describe in detail the cases which are under treatment seeking help, and that those not described may present a less severely affected group than the cases included in this table; probably few, if any, cases of blindness would escape record but many cases of good or useful vision might do so. It is evident that there must be great variation in these respects dependent upon the grade of the anomaly; the pupil may be entirely occupied by the lens though it is not accurately centred and troublesome astigmatism may result; or the pupil may be wholly aphakic and a strong convex glass may lead to useful vision; again the margin of the lens may cross the pupil and there may be a choice of vision, with a convex glass through the aphakic section or with a concave glass through the marginal region of the lens, whichever is most suited to the individual patient.

Vision in cases of ectopia lentis	♂	♀	Total
Blind in both eyes	3	3	6
Blind in one eye	7	6	13
"Very bad" or "always bad"	10	17	27
$> \frac{6}{60}$ with correction or finger counting in both eyes	13	10	23
$\frac{6}{60}$ or less in one eye, up to $\frac{6}{18}$ in the other	6	6	12
$\frac{6}{12} - \frac{6}{36}$ in both eyes, with correction	10	8	18
Good, or good 'till middle age	6	4	10
Cataract. No statement of vision	8	11	19

The Inheritance of Ectopia Lentis. A study of the pedigrees on Plates LXXIII—LXXVI will reveal the great variety to be found in the genetic manifestations of this anomaly. Fig. 1193, due to Gunn, illustrates an extreme example of dominance in which no fewer than 17 out of the 22 members of five affected sibships show the anomaly; other examples of dominance, some of them less straightforward in that normal members are seen occasionally to transmit the defect, are Fig. 1205 due to Lewis, Fig. 1216 due to Stanford Morton, Fig. 1177 due to Strebel and Fig. 1176 due to Vogt. The condition may be seen behaving as a recessive, with normal parents and unaffected offspring, in Fecht's case of Fig. 1182 or Franceschetti's case of Fig. 1204. We are most fortunate in having the very interesting histories worked out by Usher and illustrated on Plates LXXIII and LXXIV, showing the appearance of the anomaly in a single case of a large sibship, the offspring of normal parents; in two instances such single cases in a widespread family are seen to transmit the defect to children and grandchildren. Is it chance that the affection rests almost entirely with males through the four generations of Fig. 1176, or almost entirely with females through the four generations of Fig. 1178? What is the outlook for the offspring of the single affected sibship of Usher's pedigree 1190? Is it probable that they will show manifest defect like the children of II. 7 in Fig. 1183, or like those of IV. 7 in Fig. 1174, or can they be trusted to follow the example of Fecht's case or Franceschetti's and behave as recessives are expected to behave?

On examining the pedigrees as a whole, it is clear that the condition is most commonly transmitted to an affected individual by a parent who manifests the defect. The following table shows the type of parentage in 287 individual cases; in 58 cases no information on this point was available. It will be seen that some $75°/_{o}$ of these cases had parents who themselves manifested the defect. A slight excess of the cases of my records owe their defect to their mothers and this, in view of the excess of males in the population, is of some interest; if proving nothing, it supports, so far as it goes, the observation made elsewhere that women, for one reason or another, tend on the whole to be more potent than men as transmitters of hereditary affections, and to bear a heavy responsibility for the amount of hereditary defect in the community.

Parentage	Offspring			
	♂	♀	⚥	Totals
Mother affected	51	52	11	114
Father affected	52	41	7	100
Both Parents normal	41	26	6	73
Totals	144	119	24	287
No knowledge of Parents	35	23	—	58

On examination of the sibships to which individuals of the above table belong I find, as may be seen below, that the affected mother has on the average transmitted the defect to a higher percentage of her children than has the affected father. I cannot lay any stress upon these figures, based as they are upon such small numbers, or attempt any explanation with regard to them, but would refer the reader to p. 284 of this volume, in the section on "Blue Sclerotics and Fragility of Bone"; he will find there some tentative suggestions concerning the relative potency of man and woman in the transmission of hereditary defect, which are applicable to this case of ectopia lentis. Though however there would appear to be some similar genetic relationship determining the proportion of affected offspring resulting from an affected mother and father respectively in the two conditions—blue sclerotics and ectopia lentis—the parallel does not extend to those sibships whose parentage shows no manifest defect; in ectopia lentis, the percentage of this group to be affected is markedly in excess of the corresponding group for blue sclerotics and approximates more closely to that provided by figures for retinitis pigmentosa.

Parentage	No. of Sibships	Offspring			Blue Sclerotics	
		Affected	Normal	Percentage Affected	No. of Sibships	Percentage Affected
Mother affected	(35)	91	58	$61 \cdot 1 \pm 2 \cdot 7$	(91)	$62 \cdot 7 \pm 1 \cdot 8$
Father affected	(32)	77	77	$50 \cdot 0 \pm 2 \cdot 7$	(53)	$53 \cdot 8 \pm 2 \cdot 2$
One Parent affected	(67)	168	135	$55 \cdot 4 \pm 1 \cdot 9$	—	—
Both Parents normal	(27)	63	90	$41 \cdot 2 \pm 2 \cdot 7$	(18)	$24 \cdot 8 \pm 2 \cdot 8$
One Parent affected *	(63)	168	123	$57 \cdot 7 \pm 2 \cdot 0$	—	—

* Excluding four unaffected sibships with one parent affected.

It would be fitting that this volume should be closed with some note of appreciation of the man whose work is thus memorialised. If some sections have appeared to provide little reference to Nettleship's personal contributions, and the whole bears upon one aspect only of his work, I hope it may provide some indication of the far-reaching results of the stimulus to interest in the inheritance of eye diseases which we owe to Nettleship. I would add that for any merits which the volume can claim, warm thanks are due primarily to the Editor who planned and directed the work, to C. H. Usher, who has encouraged by his unfailing and most generous help throughout, and to the Medical Research Council, whose support has materially helped the completion of the project.

NAME INDEX TO THE CHRONOLOGICAL BIBLIOGRAPHY AND TO THE RECORDERS OF PEDIGREES[1]

Adams (188, Fig. 1224), Albinus (9), von Ammon (32, Fig. 1004), Angelucci (Fig. 1006), Arana (237, Fig. 1245), Arlt (37, Figs. 1054, 1057, 1063), Ash (244, Fig. 950), Attlee (213, Fig. 1150), Aurand (259, Fig. 1008), Axenfeld (173, Fig. 1090).

Bahr (204, Fig. 1214), Bartels (245, Fig. 1078), Bartholinus (6), Bartisch (2), Batten (146, Fig. 1145), Baudon (74, Fig. 1242), Beauvieux (197, Fig. 1223), Beger (22, Fig. 1107), Benedict (27, Fig. 1055), Benson (64, Fig. 1091), Bergmeister (164, 228, Fig. 1094), Bernard (265, Figs. 1129, 1135), Blair (160, Fig. 1096), Bloc (Fig. 1152), Bloch (10, Fig. 1159), Bondi (134, Fig. 990), Bowman (33, 48, Figs. 1056, 1235), Brav (288), Breitbarth (116, Fig. 1187), Bresgen (66, Fig. 1181), Brisseau (7), Bronner (154, Figs. 960, 963, 976, 977, 978), Brose (153, Fig. 961), Bruns (141, Fig. 981), Bryant (Fig. 1196), Bussy (242, Fig. 1185).

Calhoun (205, Fig. 1040), Cameron (266, Fig. 1178), Cantonnet (254, Fig. 1028), Carra (142, Fig. 1111), Caudron (91, Fig. 1132), Cederskjöld (24, Fig. 971), Celsus (1), Charles (Fig. 1237), Clark (229, Fig. 1179), Clausen (238, Fig. 1118), Collins (111, 234, Figs. 954, 1141), Conradi (14, Fig. 1171), Cooper (40, Fig. 972), Cornaz (35), Courtney (289, Fig. 1069), Cridland (246, Fig. 1024), Croll (280, Fig. 1117), Cross (106, 122, Figs. 1013, 1086, 1126), Cunha (281 A, Fig. 1143), Cunier (29, Fig. 943), Cunningham (189, Fig. 1105), Cykulenko (282).

de Beck (88, 115, 130, Figs. 1104, 1156), de Benedetti (92, Fig. 1138), de Caralt (276, Fig. 1183), de Haas (283, Fig. 1226), de Lapersonne (158, Fig. 1006), Derby (76, Figs. 996, 1080), Dérer (284, Fig. 1089), d'Ewart (290, Fig. 1124), de Wecker (152), Dixon (39, Fig. 1206), Drinkwater (Fig. 1123), Dumont (93, Fig. 1139), Dürr (100, Fig. 1005), van Duyse (177, Fig. 1136), Dwyer (255, Fig. 1133).

Eha (155, Figs. 1200, 1201, 1208, 1211, 1222), Elliot (247), Erdmann (14 A, Fig. 1154).

Fecht (272, Fig. 1182), Ferbers (197), Fichte (36, Fig. 1151), Fischer (15, Fig. 980), Fleischer (178, 224, Figs. 1001, 1019, 1037), Focachon (26, Fig. 1101), Foster (135), Foxonet (235, Fig. 1188), Franceschetti (273, Figs. 1204, 1220), Frank-Kamenetzki (260, Fig. 1048), Frickhöffer (70, Fig. 1240), Friebis (109, Fig. 1196), Fryer (83, Fig. 1246), Fuchs (Fig. 978).

Galezowski (71, 165, Figs. 1102, 1103), Gallemaerts (256, Fig. 973), Gand (89, Fig. 1121), Gehrung (206, Fig. 1244), Gertz (214, Fig. 986), Gescheidt (18, 20, 23, Figs. 959, 975, 1153), Gifford (267, Fig. 1127), Ginestous (147, Fig. 1243), Gleitsmann (54, Fig. 1169), Golomb (199, Figs. 1014, 1016, 1017, 1018), von Graefe (50), Gredig (268, Fig. 984), Grellois (25), Grimsdale (Fig. 1081), Grönholm (239, Fig. 985), Gros (131), Guillemeau (3), Gunn (195, Fig. 1193), Gutbier (21, Fig. 1107), Gutfreund (183, Fig. 1125).

Haffmans (43), Halbertsma (277, Fig. 1162), Hamilton (169, Fig. 1116), Harlan (55, 85, Figs. 965, 967, 969, 970, 1038), Harman (196, 219, Figs. 948, 1164), Hassler (126, Fig. 1231), Henzschel (17, Fig. 1113), Herrnheiser (101, Fig. 1114), Hessin (207, Fig. 1155), Hill (289, Fig. 1069), von Hippel (184), von Hoffmann (52, Fig. 1148), Holland (257, Fig. 1047), Holm (240, Fig. 1115), Hopf (148, Fig. 1110), Horner (102), Hosford (193, Fig. 1229), Howe (94, Fig. 1045), Hubert (176, Fig. 1218), Huhn (13), Hulme (46, Fig. 1198).

Iwumi (194, Fig. 1241).

Jacobson (90 A, Fig. 1030), James (220, 274, Figs. 1026, 1072, 1085), Johnson (136, Fig. 999), Jones (67, Fig. 1207), Jüngken (19, Fig. 995), Juler (156, 157, Figs. 1092, 1145).

Kagoshima (215), Kauffmann (179, Fig. 1071), Kayser (208, 209, Fig. 983), Kennedy (261, Fig. 1232), Kestenbaum (230), Keyser (57, Fig. 1212), Kirkpatrick (Fig. 1025), Klein (75, Fig. 1029), Knape (166, Fig. 1146), Komoto (269, Figs. 974, 1230), Kretschmer (210, Fig. 1249), Krükow (103), Kummer (53, Fig. 1034).

Lafosse (127, Fig. 957), Lambert (231, Fig. 1236), Lang (86, Fig. 1109), Lange (104), Laqueur (143), La Rue (264, Fig. 1167), Laskiewicz-Friedensfeld (61, Fig. 1108), Lawford (180, 200, Figs. 1033, 1038, 1053, 1059, 1061), Leoz (248, Fig. 1233), Levy (248, Fig. 1233), Lewis, A. C. (216, Fig. 1137), Lewis, G. G. (167, Fig. 1205), Lewis, J. B. (270, Fig. 1120), Licsko (275, Fig. 1093), Lindberg (250, Fig. 1128), Loeb (190, Figs. 1049, 1131, 1230, 1237), Löhlein (201, Figs. 1077, 1084).

McMillan (241, Fig. 982), Magnus (90, Fig. 964), Mann (Fig. 1000), Manz (60), Markow (137), Marlow (161, Fig. 1217), Martin (97, Fig. 947), Mayerhausen (77, Fig. 956), Maynard (132, Fig. 1166), Miles (128, Fig. 1202), Mohr (123, Fig. 1110), Moissonnier (162, Fig. 1098), Mooren (49 A, Fig. 1032), Morano (95, Fig. 979), Morrow (Fig. 1248), Morton (68, Fig. 1216), Mules (80, Figs. 1031, 1221), Muller-Kanberg (117, Fig. 1065), Muralt (51, Figs. 988, 994, 1003, 1009).

Nayar (294, Fig. 1068), Nettleship (98, 174, 191, Figs. 1035, 1041), Neuburger (118), Neuffer (211), Nolte (128 A, Fig. 1066), Nunneley (44, 62, Figs. 962, 1134).

Ourgaud (249, Fig. 1173).

---

[1] Bibliography numbers are placed before pedigree numbers.

BIBLIOGRAPHY[1]

1. CELSUS, A. C.: *Of Medicine, in eight Books.* Translated by James Greive. London, 1756.' [Gives an interesting early account which appears to distinguish between cataract and glaucoma, pp. 344—345.]

BARTISCH, G.: 'Οφθαλμωδουλεια, *das ist Augendienst.* Dresden, 1583.

GUILLEMEAU, J.: *Traité des Maladies de l'Œil.* Paris, 1585.

2. PLEMP, V. F.: *Ophthalmographia sive Tractatio de Oculo.* Lovanii, 1648.

5. RIOLAN, J.: *A sure Guide; or the best and nearest Way to Physick and Chyrurgery.* Englished by N. Culpeper, London, 1671 ["The Disease of the Chrystalline Humor in respect of its Scituation has no name, but if it be somewhat higher and flatter than ordinary, it provides a symptom whereby all things appear double." This is an interesting early account of ectopia lentis].

6. BARTHOLINUS, T.: *Acta Medica & Philosophica Hafniensia.* Hafniae, 1673. [A case of Coloboma iridis is described on p. 62 under the title of *Oculorum Affectus et Vulnera.*]

7. BRISSEAU, P.: *Traité de la Cataracte et du Glaucoma.* Paris, 1709. [A thesis of considerable interest from the historical standpoint, stating that glaucoma is not a disease of the lens and differs fundamentally from cataract.]

8. SAINT-YVES, C. DE: *Nouveau Traité des Maladies des Yeux.* Paris, 1722.

9. ALBINUS, B. S.: *Academicarum Annotationum Liber Sextus.* Leidae, 1764. [Lib. VI, Cap. iii, p. 49, gives a section entitled "De miro quodam oculorum vitio" in which is described a case of Coloboma iridis associated with an oval Cornea.]

10. BLOCH, D. M. E.: *Medicinische Bemerkungen.* Berlin, 1774. [An early case of hereditary Coloboma iridis is described under the heading of "Längliche Pupillen." See Fig. 1159.]

11. TODE, J. C.: De vitiosa utriusque oculi pupilla. *Collectanea, Societatis medicae Havniensis.* Vol. II, p. 146. Havniae, 1774. [An early account of Coloboma iridis, downwards and outwards, in a boy aged 8 whose parents and brothers showed no similar defect.]

12. PELLIER DE QUENGSY, G.: *Recueil de Mémoires et d'Observations.* Montpellier, 1783. See Fig. 1152.

13. HUHN, O.: *Observationum medicarum ac chirurgicarum Fasciculus.* Gottingae, 1788. [Observatio V, pp. 24–37, *De prolapsu lentis crystallinae in cameram anteriorem oculi et variis oculorum affectionibus,* describes what is probably an early account of a case of the spontaneous dislocation of the lens into the anterior chamber in a microphthalmic eye.]

14. CONRADI, G. C.: *Handbuch der pathologischen Anatomie.* Hannover, 1796. [An example of hereditary Coloboma iridis is described, p. 517. See Fig. 1171.]

---

[1] Memoirs not seen have an asterisk attached to their index number. In certain instances hereditary cases are cited by an author to whom they have been communicated by ophthalmological colleagues.

14A. ERDMANN, F.: Coloboma iridis. *Zeitschrift f. Natur- und Heilkunde.* Bd. IV, Heft 3, S. 501—504. Dresden, 1826. See Fig. 1154.

15. FISCHER, C. E.: Ueber die jetzt vorkommende deforme Bildung der Augen zweier Landkinder. *Journal der practischen Heilkunde.* Bd. LXV, Supplement Heft d. Jahrgangs 1827, S. 27. Berlin, 1827. See Fig. 980.

16. ROSAS, A.: *Handbuch der theoretischen und practischen Augenheilkunde.* Wien, 1830. [A case of hereditary Coloboma iridis is described. Bd. I, S. 283. See Fig. 1168.]

17. HENZSCHEL.: Vorlaufige Notiz über den Irismangel bei drei Geschwistern. *Zeitschrift f. d. Ophthalmologie.* Bd. I, S. 52—54. Dresden, 1831. See Fig. 1113.

18. GESCHEIDT, A.: Ueber Microphthalmos oder' die angeborne Kleinheit der Augen. *Zeitschrift f. d. Ophthalmologie.* Bd. II, S. 257—278. Dresden, 1832. See Figs. 959, 975.

19. *JUNGKEN, J. C.: *Die Lehre von den Augenkrankheiten.* Berlin, 1832. See Fig. 995. [Reference to case taken from Zahn, Bibl. No. 168.]

20. GESCHEIDT, A.: Die Irideremie, das Iridoschisma und die Corectopie, die drei wesentlichsten Bildungsfehler der Iris. *Journal d. Chirurgie u. Augen-Heilkunde.* Bd. XXII, S. 267—300, 398—435. Berlin, 1834.

21. *GUTBIER, S.: *De Irideremia seu defectu iridis congenito.* Dissertation. Gothae, 1834. See Fig. 1107.

22. BEGER, J. H.: Beitrage zur Lehre von der Irideremia von Carron du Villards und Gutbier. *Zeitschrift f. d. Ophthalmologie.* Bd. V, Heft 1, S. 78—81. Heidelberg und Leipzig, 1835. See Fig. 1107.

23. GESCHEIDT, A.: Anatomische Untersuchung zweier mit Iridoschisma (Coloboma Iridis) behafteter Augen bei einem sechsmonatlichen Kinde. *Zeitschrift f. d. Opththalmologie.* Bd. IV, Hefte 3 und 4, S. 436—440. Heidelberg und Leipzig, 1835. See Fig. 1153.

24. CEDERSKJÖLD: Ein Fall von Microphthalmus. *Zeitschrift f. d. Ophthalmologie.* Bd. V, Heft 3, S. 369. Heidelberg und Leipzig, 1836. See Fig. 971.

25. GRELLOIS, E.: *Dissertation sur l'Hydrophthalmie.* Thèse. Paris, 1836.

26. FOCACHON, A.: *De l'Absence congéniale et complète de l'Iris.* Thèse. Strasbourg, 1840. See Fig. 1101.

27. BENEDICT, T. W. G.: *Abhandlungen aus dem Gebiete der Augenheilkunde.* Breslau, 1842. [An example of hereditary glaucoma is given, pp. 123—132. See Fig. 1055.]

28. SCHWARZ: Pupilla praeternaturalis marginalis congenita. *Schmidts Jahrbücher.* Bd. XXXVII, S. 327—328. Leipzig, 1843. See Fig. 1225.

29. CUNIER, F.: Microphthalmie et Surdi-mutité héréditaires. *Annales d'Oculistique.* T. XIII, pp. 30—34. Bruxelles, 1845. See Fig. 943.

30. PÉTREQUIN, J. E.: Note sur la Microphthalmie. *Annales d'Oculistique.* T. XIII, pp. 27—80. Bruxelles, 1845. See Fig. 958.

31. STOEBER, V.: Absence de l'Iris chez le Père et l'Enfant. *Annales d'Oculistique.* T. XV, pp. 250—251. Bruxelles, 1846. See Fig. 1112.

32. VON AMMON, F. A.: *Klinische Darstellungen der Krankheiten und Bildungsfehler des menschlichen Auges.* Berlin, 1847. See Fig. 1004.

33. BOWMAN, W.: *Lectures on the Parts concerned in the Operations on the Eye, and on the Structure of the Retina.* London, 1849. See Fig. 1235.

34. PRICHARD, A.: Cases of Congenital Defects of the Iris. *Provincial Medical and Surgical Journal.* Vol. XII, pp. 512—514. London, 1849. See Figs. 1130, 1144.

35. CORNAZ, E.: *Quelques Observations d'Abnormités congéniales des Yeux et de leurs Annexes.* Bruxelles, 1850.

36. FICHTE, E.: Zur Lehre von den angeborenen Missbildungen der Iris. *Zeitschrift f. rationelle Medicin.* Bd. II, S. 140—197. Heidelberg, 1852. See Fig. 1151.

37. ARLT, F.: *Die Krankheiten des Auges für praktische Ärzte.* Prag, 1853. [Hereditary glaucoma is referred to in Bd. II, S. 190—209. See Figs. 1054, 1057, 1063.]

38. STELLWAG VON CARION, C.: *Die Ophthalmologie vom naturwissenschaftlichen Standpunkte.* Erlangen, 1856. [Reference to hereditary glaucoma will be found Bd. I, S. 436. See Fig. 1058.]

39. DIXON, J.: Abnormal position of the Crystalline Lens occurring in four Members of the same Family. *Royal London Ophthalmic Hospital Reports.* Vol. I, pp. 54—57. London, 1857. See Fig. 1206.

40. COOPER, W.: Microphthalmos. *Royal London Ophthalmic Hospital Reports.* Vol. I, pp. 110—116. London, 1858. See Fig. 972.

41. SIPPELL, F. W. T.: *Die spontane Luxation der Linse und ihre angeborene Ektopie.* Dissertation. Marburg, 1859.

42. STREATFIELD, J. F.: Coloboma iridis: hereditary and rare Cases. *Royal London Ophthalmic Hospital Reports.* Vol. I, pp. 153—155. London, 1859. See Figs. 1160, 1172.

43. HAFFMANS, J. H. A.: Beiträge zur Kenntniss des Glaucoms. *Archiv f. Ophthalmologie.* Bd. VIII, S. 124—178. Berlin, 1861.

44. NUNNELEY, T.: Congenital Malformation of the Eyes in three Children of one Family. *Lancet.* Vol. II for 1861, pp. 569—570. London, 1861. See Fig. 962.

44A. PAGENSTECHER, H. A.: *Klinische Beobachtungen aus der Augenheilanstalt zu Wiesbaden.* Wiesbaden, 1861. See Figs. 1060, 1062.

45. PAMARD, A.: *Du Glaucome.* Paris, 1861.

46. HULME, E. C.: Malposition and Cataractous State of the Lenses occurring in four Members of the same Family; Clinical Remarks. *Lancet.* Vol. II for 1862, p. 618. London, 1862. See Fig. 1198.

47. WILDE, W. R.: *An Essay on the Malformations and Congenital Diseases of the Organs of Sight.* London, 1862.

48. BOWMAN, W.: Ophthalmic Miscellanies. *Royal London Ophthalmic Hospital Reports.* Vol. V, pp. 1—15. London, 1866. See Fig. 1056.

49. SCHROTER, P.: Ein Fall von vererbter Irideremie. *Klinische Monatsblätter f. Augenheilkunde.* Bd. IV, S. 100—103. Erlangen, 1866. See Fig. 1100.

49A. MOOREN, A.: *Ophthalmiatrische Beobachtungen.* Berlin, 1867. See Fig. 1032.

50. GRAEFE, A. VON: Beiträge zur Pathologie und Therapie des Glaukoms. *Archiv f. Ophthalmologie.* Bd. XV, Abth. iii, S. 108—252. Berlin, 1869. [The inheritance of glaucoma is discussed p. 228.]

51. MURALT, W. VON: *Ueber Hydrophthalmus Congenitus.* Dissertation. Zurich, 1869. See Figs. 988, 994, 1003, 1009. [We are much indebted to the University Librarian at Zürich who sent a copy of this paper and enabled us to abstract the cases given.]

52. HOFFMANN, H. VON: *Ueber ein Colobom der inneren Augenhäute ohne Colobom der Iris.* Dissertation. Frankfurt, 1871. See Fig. 1148.

53. KUMMER: Beobachtung einer Glaucomfamilie. *Correspondenzblatt f. Schweizer Aerzte.* J. I, S. 280. Bern, 1871. See Fig. 1034.

54. GLEITSMANN, E.: *Ueber ein Colobom der Chorioidea.* Dissertation. Greifswald, 1873. See Fig. 1169.

55. HARLAN, G. C.: Report of an Examination of the Eyes of 167 Inmates of the Pennsylvania Institution for the Instruction of the Blind. *American Journal of Medical Sciences.* Vol. LXV, pp. 410—419. Philadelphia, 1873. See Figs. 965, 967, 969, 970.

56. WILLIAMS, E.: Rare Cases with practical Remarks. *Transactions, American Ophthalmological Society,* Vol. II, pp. 291—293. New York, 1873. See Figs. 1194, 1209.

57. KEYSER, P. D.: Congenital hereditary Dislocation of both Lenses. *Medical and Surgical Reporter.* Vol. XXXI, p. 213. Philadelphia, 1874. See Fig. 1212.

58. PAGE, H.: Transmission through three Generations of Microphthalmos, Irideremia and Nystagmus. *Lancet.* Vol. II for 1874, pp. 193—194. London, 1874. See Fig. 1106.

59. PFLUGER, E.: Beidseitiges chronisches Glaukom bei zwei Brüdern von 19 und 20 Jahren. *Klinische Monatsblätter f. Augenheilkunde.* Bd. XIII, S. 111—114. Stuttgart, 1875. See Fig. 1052.

60. MANZ, W.: Die Missbildungen des menschlichen Auges. *Graefe-Saemisch's Handbuch der ges. Augenheilkunde.* Bd. II, S. 58—144. Leipzig, 1876.

61. LASKIEWICZ-FRIEDENSFELD, A. I.: Angeborener Irismangel, verbunden mit Trübung der brechenden Medien. *Klinische Monatsblätter f. Augenheilkunde.* Bd. XV, S. 319—332. Rostock, 1877. See Fig. 1108.

62. NUNNELEY, J. A.: Cases of Irideremia totalis. *Lancet.* Vol. I for 1877, p. 754. London, 1877. See Fig. 1134.

63. SCHNABEL, J.: Beiträge zur Lehre vom Glaucom. *Archiv f. Augen- und Ohrenheilkunde.* Bd. VI, S. 118—158. Wiesbaden, 1877. See Fig. 1073.

64. BENSON, A. H.: Report of Dr Rainsford's Case of congenital Irideremia of both Eyes. *British Medical Journal.* Vol. II for 1878, p. 359. London, 1878. See Fig. 1091.

65. WORDSWORTH, J. C.: Congenital Displacement of both Lenses in six Members of a Family. *Medical Press and Circular.* Vol. XXV, New Series, p. 110. London, 1878. See Fig. 1206.

66. BRESGEN, H.: Zur Heredität der Linsenanomalien. *Centralblatt f. praktische Augenheilkunde.* Bd. III, S. 104. Leipzig, 1879. See Fig. 1181.

67. JONES, H. MACNAUGHTON: Symmetrical Corectopia with Dislocation of the Lens. *Dublin Journal of Medical Science.* Vol. LXVII, pp. 102—103. Dublin, 1879. See Fig. 1207.

68. MORTON, A. STANFORD: Congenital Displacement of both Lenses occurring in several members of one Family. *Royal London Ophthalmic Hospital Reports.* Vol. IX, pp. 435—439. London, 1879. See Fig. 1216.

69. PUFAHL, M.: Ueber Corectopie. *Centralblatt f. praktische Augenheilkunde.* Bd. III, S. 293—300. Leipzig, 1879. See Fig. 1195.

70. FRICKHÖFFER, C.: *Ueber Corectopie.* Dissertation. Bonn, 1880. See Fig. 1240.

71. GALEZOWSKI, X.: Iridérémie ou Absence Congénitale de l'Iris. *Recueil d'Ophtalmologie.* T. II, pp. 122—124. Paris, 1880. See Fig. 1103.

72. *RAVA, G.: Estrazione doppia di Cataratta felicemente esequita. *Annali di Ottalmologia.* Vol. IX, p. 281. Pavia, 1880. See Fig. 955. [Abstract of case in *Centralblatt f. praktische Augenheilkunde.* Bd. IV, S. 456. Leipzig, 1880.]

73. SCHENKL: Zur Erblichkeit des Glaucoms. *Prager medicinische Wochenschrift.* Bd. V, S. 413. Prag, 1880. See Fig. 1051.

74. BAUDON: Luxation Congénitale double du Cristallin en haut et en dedans. *Centralblatt f. praktische Augenheilkunde.* Bd. V, S. 261—262. Leipzig, 1881. See Fig. 1242.

75. KLEIN, S.: *Lehrbuch der Augenheilkunde.* Wien und Leipzig, 1881. See Fig. 1029.

76. DERBY, H. C.: Three Cases of Hydrophthalmus treated with Iridectomy. *Archives of Ophthalmology.* Vol. XI, pp. 37—40. New York, 1882. See Figs. 996, 1080.

77. MAYERHAUSEN, G.: Directe Vererbung von beiderseitigem Microphthalmus. *Centralblatt f. praktische Augenheilkunde.* Bd. VI, S. 97—106. Leipzig, 1882. See Fig. 956.

78. SCHAUMBERG, C. F.: *Casuistischer Beitrag zu den Missbildungen des Auges.* Dissertation. Marburg, 1882. See Fig. 953.

79. STREATFIELD, J. F.: Observations on some Congenital Diseases of the Eye. Buphthalmos. *Lancet.* Vol. I for 1882, p. 264. London, 1882. See Fig. 1020.

80. MULES, P. H.: Two Instances of Heredity. *Ophthalmic Review.* Vol. II, pp. 48—49. London, 1883. See Figs. 1031, 1221.

81. *RAMPOLDI, R.: Tre Sorelle con Buftalmo Congenito. *Annali di Ottalmologia.* Vol. XII, p. 272. Pavia. 1883. See Fig. 1002. [Reference in *Nagels Jahresbericht f. d. Jahr* 1883.]

82. WAGNER, W.: Einiges über Glaucom in Anschluss an einen Bericht über meine Erkrankung an Glaucom. *Archiv f. Ophthalmologie.* Bd. XXIX, S. 280—302. Berlin, 1883.

83. FRYER, B. E.: Two Cases of Double Congenital Symmetrical Ectopia lentis in Sisters. *American Journal of Ophthalmology.* Vol. I, pp. 54—55. St Louis, 1884. See Fig. 1246.

84. RAMPOLDI, R.: Due notevoli osservazioni di glaucoma. *Annali di Ottalmologia.* Anno XIII, pp. 347—351. Pavia, 1884. See Fig. 1046.

85. HARLAN, H.: A Case of hereditary Glaucoma. *Journal of the American Medical Association.* Vol. V, pp. 285—286. Chicago, 1885. See Fig. 1038.

86. LANG, W.: Congenital Aniridia. *Transactions, Ophthalmological Society of U.K.* Vol. V, p. 207. London, 1885. See Fig. 1109.

87. PFLÜGER, E.: Microcephalie und Microphthalmie. *Archiv f. Augenheilkunde.* Bd. XIV, S. 1—11. Wiesbaden, 1885. See Fig. 946.

88. DE BECK, D.: A rare family History of Congenital Coloboma of the Iris. *Archives of Ophthalmology.* Vol. XV, pp. 8—23. New York, 1886. See Fig. 1156.

89. *GAND: Aniridie. Luxation congénitale des Cristallins: *Bulletin de la Clinique nationale ophtalmologique de l'Hospice des Quinze-Vingts.* T. III, p. 246. Paris, 1885. See Fig. 1121. [Abstract of case taken from *Revue générale d'Ophtalmologie.* T. v, p. 51. Paris, 1886.]

90. MAGNUS, H.: *Die Jugend-Blindheit.* Wiesbaden, 1886. See Fig. 964.

90A. JACOBSON, J.: Beitrag zur Lehre vom Glaucom. *Archiv f. Ophthalmologie.* Bd. XXXII, Abth. iii, S. 96—168. Berlin, 1886. See Fig. 1030.

91. CAUDRON, V.: Une Famille d'Anirides. *Revue générale d'Ophtalmologie.* T. VI, pp. 16—18. Paris, 1887. See Fig. 1132.

92. *DE BENEDETTI, A.: Irideremia totale congenita; Ectopia lentis congenita con Lussazione spontanea del Cristallino e Glaucoma consecutivo. *Annali di Ottalmologia.* T. XV, pp. 184, 399. Pavia, 1886—7. See Fig. 1138. [Abstract of case taken from *Nagels Jahresbericht der Ophthalmologie.* Bd. XVII, S. 222. Tübingen, 1887.]

93. *DUMONT: Aniridie. Luxation Congénitale des Cristallins en haut et en bas: Œil droit Irido-choroïdite glaucomateuse. *Bulletin de la Clinique nationale ophtalmologique de l'Hospice des Quinze-Vingts.* T. V, p. 98. Paris, 1887. See Fig. 1139. [Abstract of case taken from *Revue générale d'Ophtalmologie.* T. VI, p. 18. Paris, 1887.]

94. Howe, L.: A family History of Blindness from Glaucoma. *Archives of Ophthalmology.* Vol. xvi, pp. 72—76. New York, 1887. See Fig. 1045.

95. *Morano: Caso di Anoftalmo congenito. *Annali di Ottalmologia.* T. xv, p. 70. Pavia, 1886—1887. See Fig. 979. [Abstract of case taken from *Nagels Jahresbericht der Ophthalmologie.* Bd. xvii, S. 227. Tübingen, 1887.]

96. Thompson, J. L.: Observations on Displacement of the Crystalline Lens from Congenital and other Causes. *Journal of the American Medical Association.* Vol. ix, pp. 674—677. Chicago, 1887. See Fig. 1215.

97. Martin, F.: *Uber microphthalmus.* Dissertation. Erlangen, 1888. See Fig. 947.

98. Nettleship, E.: On the Prognosis in Chronic Glaucoma. *Royal London Ophthalmic Hospital Reports.* Vol. xii, pp. 72—100. London, 1888. See Fig. 1041.

99. Theobald, S.: A Case of double congenital Irideremia in a Child whose Mother exhibited a congenital Coloboma of each Iris. *Journal of the American Medical Association.* Vol. xi, p. 172. Chicago, 1888. See Fig. 1095.

100. Dürr and Schlegtendal: Funf Fälle von Hydrophthalmus congenitus. *Archiv f. Ophthalmologie.* Bd. xxxv, Abth. ii, S. 88—170. Berlin, 1889. See Fig. 1005.

101. Herrnheiser, I.: Aniridia Congenita. *Wiener klinische Wochenschrift.* Bd. ii, S. 118—119. Wien, 1889. See Fig. 1114.

102. Horner, F.: *Die Krankheiten des Auges im Kindesalter,* in Gerhardt's *Handbuch der Kinderkrankheiten.* Bd. v, Abth. ii, S. 339. Tübingen, 1889.

103. *Krukow: Notiz über d. Glaukom auf Grund von 1430 Fällen desselben. *Westnik Oftalmologii.* Vol. vi, p. 327. Kiev, 1889. Abstract in *Jahresbericht d. Ophthalmologie.* Bd. xx, S. 354—355. Tübingen, 1890.

104. *Lange: Ueber Glaukom. *Westnik Oftalmologii.* Vol. vi. Moscow, 1889. Abstract in *Jahresbericht d. Ophthalmologie.* Bd. xx, S. 355—361. Tübingen, 1890.

105. Weyert, F.: Zur Hereditat der Opticus-Colobome. *Klinische Monatsblätter f. Augenheilkunde.* Bd. xxviii, S. 325—331. Stuttgart, 1890. See Fig. 1163.

106. Cross, F. R.: Hydrophthalmos. *Transactions, Ophthalmological Society of U.K.* Vol. xi, pp. 224—240. London, 1891. See Figs. 1013, 1086.

107. Priestley Smith: *On the Pathology and Treatment of Glaucoma.* London, 1891.

108. Schweigger, C.: Glaucom und Sehnervenleiden. *Archiv f. Augenheilkunde.* Bd. xxiii, S. 203—271. Wiesbaden, 1891. See Fig. 1074.

109. Friebis, G.: Double Congenital Dislocation of the Lens. *Journal of the American Medical Association.* Vol. xix, pp. 277—278. Chicago, 1892. [In a discussion following this paper hereditary cases are referred to by Dr Bryant and Dr Morrow. See Figs. 1196, 1248.]

110. Zirm, E.: Beiderseitige Ectopia lentis bei zwei Geschwistern, combinirt mit Anomalien des Knochen-Systems. *Wiener klinische Wochenschrift.* Bd. v, S. 310—311. Wien, 1892. See Fig. 1239.

111. Collins, E. Treacher: Congenital Defects of the Iris, and Glaucoma. *Transactions, Ophthalmological Society of U.K.* Vol. xiii, pp. 128—139. London, 1893. See Fig. 1141.

112. Ray, J. M.: Hereditary and congenital Eye Diseases. *Ophthalmic Record.* Vol. ii, pp. 467—471. Nashville, 1893. See Figs. 1049, 1064.

113. Somya, J. R.: Ueber erbliches Glaukom. *Klinische Monatsblätter f. Augenheilkunde.* Bd. xxxi, S. 390—394. Stuttgart, 1893. See Fig. 1043.

114. Story, J. B.: Cases of Glaucoma in young People. *Ophthalmic Review.* Vol. xii, pp. 69—79. London, 1893. See Fig. 1079.

115. de Beck, D.: Addenda to an Article, *Rare family History of Coloboma of the Iris.* *Archives of Ophthalmology.* Vol. xxiii, pp. 264—269. New York, 1894. See Fig. 1156.

116. Breitbarth, E.: *Beitrag zur Kenntniss der Ectopia pupillae.* Dissertation. Giessen, 1894. See Fig. 1187.

117. Muller-Kannberg: Zur Casuistik der Opticus-Colobome. *Klinische Monatsblätter f. Augenheilkunde.* Bd. xxxii, S. 173—177. Stuttgart, 1894. See Fig. 1065.

118. Neuburger, S.: Beitrag zur Altersstatistik des Glaucoms. *Centralblatt f. praktische Augenheilkunde.* Bd. xviii, S. 13—15. Leipzig, 1894.

119. Pfannmuller, F.: *Beitrag zu den Colobomen des Auges.* Dissertation. Giessen, 1894. See Fig. 1170.

120. Pflüger, L.: *Uber Megalocornea und infantiles Glaucom.* Dissertation. Zürich, 1894. See Figs. 989, 992.

121. Priestley Smith: On an Instance of hereditary Glaucoma and its Cause. *Ophthalmic Review.* Vol. xiii, pp. 215—226. London, 1894. See Fig. 1044.

122. CROSS, F. R.: Congenital Anomalies of the Iris. *Clinical Sketches.* Vol. I, pp. 104—106. London, 1895. See Fig. 1126.

123. MOHR, W.: *Über hereditäre Irideremie.* Dissertation. Jena, 1895. See Fig. 1110.

124. SOUS, G.: Ectopie du Cristallin. *Annales d'Oculistique.* T. CXIV, pp. 390—391. Paris, 1895. See Fig. 1234.

125. TIFFANY, F. B.: Ectopia lentis. *Journal of the American Medical Association.* Vol. XXV, pp. 796—798. Chicago, 1895. See Fig. 1189.

126. HASSLER: Ectopie congénitale bilatérale et symétrique du Cristallin. *Lyon Médical.* T. LXXXI, pp. 177—182. Lyon, 1896. See Fig. 1231.

127. LAFOSSE, V.: Bilateral Anophthalmus and Epicanthus in a Child whose Mother presented a Congenital Absence of the right Eyeball. *Archives of Ophthalmology.* Vol. XXV, pp. 49—50. New York, 1896. See Fig. 957.

128. MILES, H. S.: A number of Lens Cases, illustrating Heredity. *Annals of Ophthalmology and Otology.* Vol. V, pp. 542—546. Chicago, 1896. See Fig. 1202.

128A. NOLTE, F.: *Beitrag zu der Lehre von der Erblichkeit von Augenerkrankungen.* Dissertation. Marburg, 1896. See Fig. 1066.

129. STEPHENSON, S.: Irideremia in two Brothers. *Transactions, Ophthalmological Society of U.K.* Vol. XVI, pp. 184—185. London, 1896. See Fig. 1099.

130. DE BECK, D.: A Family History of Irideremia and Coloboma iridis: Cataract Operation on two Members. *Transactions, American Ophthalmological Society.* Vol. VII, pp. 117—128. Hartford, 1897. See Fig. 1104.

131. GROS, E. L.: *Étude sur l'Hydrophthalmie ou Glaucome infantile.* Paris, 1897.

132. MAYNARD, F. P.: Two Cases of Coloboma iridis in Mother and Son, with monocular Polycoria also in the Son. *Indian Medical Gazette.* Vol. XXXII, pp. 456—458. Calcutta, 1897. See Fig. 1166.

133. PELTESOHN: Beiderseitige congenitale hereditäre (familiäre) Ectopia lentis. *Centralblatt f. praktische Augenheilkunde.* Bd. XXI, S. 113—114. Leipzig, 1897. See Fig. 1213.

134. BONDI, M.: Zwei seltene Fälle von angeborenem Megalophthalmus. *Wiener medizinische Presse.* Bd. XXXIX, S. 1041—1046. Wien, 1898. See Fig. 990.

135. FOSTER, M. L.: Congenital Irideremia. *Archives of Ophthalmology.* Vol. XXVII, pp. 593—615. New York, 1898.

136. JOHNSON, W. B.: Buphthalmia; an interesting series of Cases occurring in the same Family. *Transactions, American Ophthalmological Society.* Vol. VIII, pp. 308—312. Hartford, 1898. See Fig. 999.

137. *MARKOW, J.: Beitrag zur Glaukomstatistik. *Westnik Oftalmologii.* Vol. XVIII, p. 729. Moscow, 1897. Abstract in *Jahresbericht d. Ophthalmologie.* Bd. XXVIII, S. 481—482. Tübingen, 1898.

138. PARKER, E. F.: Five Cases of congenital, bilateral symmetrical Displacement of the Lens of the Eye in three successive Generations of one Family. *Journal of the American Medical Association.* Vol. XXXI, pp. 708—710. Chicago, 1898. See Figs. 1199, 1211. [In a discussion following this paper a hereditary case is referred to by Dr Starkey. See Fig. 1219.]

139. REBER: Microphthalmie compliquée d'Hypermétropie excessive et d'Anomalies de la Macula, observée chez trois Sœurs. *Annales d'Oculistique.* T. CXIX, pp. 445—446. Paris, 1898. See Fig. 966.

140. WILDER, W. H.: Cases of Hereditary Ectopia lentis. *Journal of the American Medical Association.* Vol. XXXI, pp. 710—711. Chicago, 1898. See Fig. 1197.

141. BRUNS, H. D.: A microphthalmic Family. *American Journal of Ophthalmology.* Vol. XVI, pp. 68—70. St. Louis, 1899. See Fig. 981.

142. CARRA, V.: Un nuovo Caso di Aniridia còngenita. *Policlinico.* Anno V, pp. 239—240. Roma, 1899. See Fig. 1111.

143. LAQUEUR, L.: Bemerkungen über die Natur des entzündlichen Glaukoms. *Archiv f. Ophthalmologie.* Bd. XLVII, Abth. iii, S. 631—643. Leipzig, 1899.

144. ROGMAN, A.: A propos de la Pathogénie du Glaucome chronique simple. Une Famille de Glaucomateux. *La Clinique ophtalmologique.* T. V, pp. 73—75. Paris, 1899. See Fig. 1039.

145. SCHÜSSELE, W.: *Über die Beziehungen des primären Glaukoms zu Geschlecht, Lebensalter und Refraktion.* Dissertation. Tübingen, 1899.

146. BATTEN, RAYNER D.: Congenital Aniridia and Displacement of Lenses with Glaucoma. *Transactions, Ophthalmological Society of U.K.* Vol. XX, p. 192. London, 1900. See Fig. 1145.

147. GINESTOUS, E.: Luxation congénitale bilatérale du Cristallin. *Recueil d'Ophtalmologie.* T. XXII, pp. 282—283. Paris, 1900. See Fig 1243.

148. Hopf, O.: *Zur pathologischen Anatomie des angeborenen Irismangels.* Dissertation. Jena, 1900. See Fig. 1110.

148 A. Pinckard, C. P.: Ectopia lentis; a Report. *Journal of the American Medical Association.* Vol. xxxiv, p. 146. Chicago, 1900. See Fig. 1186.

149. Scherenberg, K.: *Beitrag zur Lehre vom reinen Mikrophthalmus.* Dissertation. Tübingen, 1900. See Fig. 951.

150. Selz, E.: *Eine Colobom-Familie.* Dissertation. Jena, 1900. See Fig. 1161.

151. Tiffany, F. B.: Congenital Aphakia and Irideremia. *Journal of the American Medical Association.* Vol. xxxiv, pp. 1043—1044. Chicago, 1900. See Fig. 968.

152. de Wecker, L.: Le Glaucome en Orient. *Annales d'Oculistique.* T. cxxiv, pp. 45—51. Paris, 1900.

153. Brose, L. D.: Congenital right-sided Anophthalmus with left-sided Microphthalmus. *Archives of Ophthalmology.* Vol. xxx, pp. 12—13. New York, 1901. See Fig. 961.

154. Bronner, A.: Two Families with congenital Microphthalmus and Cataract. *Ophthalmic Review.* Vol. xxi, pp. 207—210. London, 1902. See Figs. 960, 963, 976, 977, 978.

155. Eha, L.: *Beitrag zur Kasuistik der Ectopia lentis congenita.* Dissertation. Tübingen, 1902. See Figs. 1200, 1201, 1208, 1211, 1222.

156. Juler, H.: Aniridia. *Transactions, Ophthalmological Society of U.K.* Vol. xxii, pp. 195—198. London, 1902. See Fig. 1145.

157. Juler, H.: Aniridia. *Ophthalmic Review.* Vol. xxi, pp. 22—23. London, 1902. See Fig. 1092.

158. de Lapersonne, F.: Hydrophtalmie et troubles cardiovasculaires. *Archives d'Ophtalmologie.* T. xxii, pp. 565—573. Paris, 1902. See Fig. 1006.

159. Venneman, E.: Remarques au Sujet de Cas de Buphtalmos. *Annales d'Oculistique.* T. cxxviii, pp. 137—142. Paris, 1902. See Fig. 1021.

160. Blair, C. and Potter, B.: Two Cases of Aniridia and one of Coloboma of the Iris in the same Family. *Transactions, Ophthalmological Society of U.K.* Vol. xxiii, pp. 261—262. London, 1903. See Fig. 1096.

161. Marlow, F. W.: Buphthalmos in a Subject of Congenital Dislocation of the Crystalline Lens. *Archives of Ophthalmology.* Vol. xxxii, pp. 470—472. New York, 1903. See Fig. 1217.

162. Moissonnier, M. and Fouchet, G.: Aniridie familiale. *Archives d'Ophtalmologie.* T. xxiii, pp. 648—655. Paris, 1903. See Fig. 1098.

163. Ridley, N. C.: Congenital Anophthalmos. *Ophthalmic Review.* Vol. xxii, p. 55. London, 1903. See Fig. 1147.

164. Bergmeister, R.: Zwei Fälle von angeborener Irideremie. *Archiv f. Ophthalmologie.* Bd. lix, Heft i, S. 31—45. Leipzig, 1904. See Fig. 1094.

165. Galezowski, X.: Aniridie congénitale. *Recueil d'Ophtalmologie.* Vol. xxiv, pp. 148—155. Paris, 1904. See Fig. 1102.

166. *Knape, E. N.: Aniridia bilateralis bei Vater und Sohn. *Wochenschrift f. Therapie u. Hygiene des Auges.* Bd. for 1904, p. 273. Dresden, 1904. Abstract in *Ophthalmoscope.* Vol. ii, p. 325. London, 1904. See Fig. 1146.

167. Lewis, G. G.: Hereditary Ectopia lentis with Reports of Cases. *Archives of Ophthalmology.* Vol. xxxiii, pp. 275—284. New York, 1904. See Fig. 1205.

168. Zahn, E.: *Ueber die hereditären Verhältnisse bei Buphthalmus.* Tübingen, 1904. See Figs. 993, 997, 998, 1010, 1011, 1015, 1165.

169. Hamilton, T. K.: A Family with Irideremia. *Ophthalmoscope.* Vol. iii, pp. 481—488. London, 1905. See Fig. 1116.

170. Reis, W.: Untersuchungen zur pathologischen Anatomie und zur Pathogenese des angeborenen Hydrophthalmus. *Archiv f. Ophthalmologie.* Bd. lx, S. 1—18. Leipzig, 1905. See Fig. 1007.

171. Sattler, R.: Juvenile Glaucoma. *Transactions, American Ophthalmological Society.* Vol. x, pp. 519—521. Hartford, 1905. See Figs. 1076, 1082.

172. Vogt, A.: Dislocatio lentis spontanea als erbliche Krankheit. *Zeitschrift f. Augenheilkunde.* Bd. xiv, S. 153—165. Berlin, 1905. See Fig. 1176.

173. Axenfeld, T: Drei Geschwister mit familiärem Glaukoma simplex juvenile. *Münchener medizinische Wochenschrift.* Bd. liii, S. 1938. München, 1906. See Fig. 1090.

174. Nettleship, E.: Some Hereditary Diseases of the Eye. *Ophthalmoscope.* Vol. iv, pp. 493, 549. London, 1906. See Figs. 1035, 1041.

175. Parsons, J. H.: *The Pathology of the Eye.* London, 1904—1906.

176. TERRIEN F. and HUBERT: Ectopie bilatérale du Cristallin congénitale dans trois et peut-être quatre Générations. *Recueil d'Ophtalmologie.* T. XXVIII, pp. 721—726. Paris, 1906. See Fig. 1218.

177. VAN DUYSE: Aniridie incomplète (Iris rudimentaire). *Archives d'Ophtalmologie.* T. XXVII, pp. 1—9. Paris, 1907. See Fig. 1136.

178. FLEISCHER, B.: [Report of Description of a Case of hereditary Glaucoma.] *Verhandlungen d. Gesellschaft Deutscher Naturforscher u. Ärzte.* Bd. LXXIX, S. 250. Dresden, 1907. See Fig. 1037.

179. KAUFFMANN, F.: Zur Statistik der Vererbung von Augenkrankheiten. *Wochenschrift f. Therapie u. Hygiene des Auges.* Bd. XI, S. 68. Dresden, 1907. See Fig. 1071. [We are much indebted to Dr H. Goldschmidt of Berlin for obtaining a copy of this paper for us.]

180. LAWFORD, J. B.: Examples of hereditary primary Glaucoma. *Royal London Ophthalmic Hospital Reports.* Vol. XVII, pp. 57—68. London, 1907. See Figs. 1033, 1036, 1053, 1059, 1061.

181. ROCHON-DUVIGNEAUD, A.: Describes a case of Ectopia lentis in mother and child in the discussion following a paper by Terrien F. and Hubert. *Archives d'Ophtalmologie.* T. XXVII, p. 31. Paris, 1907. See Fig. 1247.

182. WALLENBERG, T.: Hydrophthalmus. *Deutsche medizinische Wochenschrift.* Bd. XXXIII, S. 1275. Berlin, 1907. See Fig. 1088.

183. GUTFREUND: Zwei Fälle von Irideremia congenita. *Wiener klinische Wochenschrift.* Bd. XXI, S. 1283. Wien, 1908. See Fig. 1125.

184. VON HIPPEL, E.: Die Missbildungen und angeborenen Fehler des Auges. *Graefe-Saemisch Handbuch d. ges. Augenheilkunde.* 2. Aufl. Bd. II, S. 1—136. Leipzig, 1908.

185. POLTE, L.: Several Cases of congenital Anomaly of the Iris. *Archives of Ophthalmology.* Vol. XXXVII, pp. 699—700. New York, 1908. See Fig. 1097.

186. SCHMIDT-RIMPLER, H.: Glaukom und Ophthalmomalacie. *Graefe-Saemisch Handbuch d. ges. Augenheilkunde.* 2. Aufl. Bd. VI, Abth. I, Kap. VII. Leipzig, 1908.

187. SNELL, S.: Coloboma of Iris in each Eye occurring in five Generations. *Transactions, Ophthalmological Society of U.K.* Vol. XXVIII, pp. 148—150. London, 1908. See Fig. 1157.

188. ADAMS, P. H.: A Family with congenital Displacement of Lenses. *Transactions, Ophthalmological Society of U.K.* Vol. XXIX, pp. 274—275. London, 1909. See Fig. 1224.

189. CUNNINGHAM, J. F.: A Case of Aniridia with a Family History of the Condition in four Generations. *Transactions, Ophthalmological Society of U.K.* Vol. XXIX, pp. 131—133. London, 1909. See Fig. 1105.

190. LOEB, C.: Hereditary Blindness and its Prevention. *Annals of Ophthalmology.* Vol. XVIII, pp. 1—47. St Louis, 1909. See Figs. 1049, 1131, 1230, 1237.

191. NETTLESHIP, E.: Some Hereditary Diseases of the Eye. *Transactions, Ophthalmological Society of U.K.* Vol. XXIX, pp. lvii—cxcviii. London, 1909.

192. WALLENBERG, T.: Erbliches juveniles Glaukom. *Zeitschrift f. Augenheilkunde.* Bd. XXIV, S. 468. Berlin, 1910. [Glaucoma was observed in four generations of one family; all cases resulted in blindness; the onset occurred at the same period of life in all the affected members. No details of the pedigree are given.]

193. HOSFORD, STROUD: Congenital Dislocation of both Lenses with Corectopia in six Members of a Family of seven. *Transactions, Ophthalmological Society of U.K.* Vol. XXXI, pp. 50, 51. London, 1911. See Fig. 1229.

194. IWUMI: A Case of Luxation of the Lens into the Anterior Chamber in Congenital Ectopia lentis. *Nippon Gankakai Zashi.* May 1911. See No. 215. [Abstract of Case in *Klinische Monatsblätter f. Augenheilkunde.* Bd. I, S. 269. Stuttgart, 1912. See Fig. 1241.]

195. GUNN, A. RUGG: Complete Congenital Dislocation of the Lens: A Family History. *Ophthalmoscope.* Vol. X, pp. 193—195. London, 1912. See Fig. 1193.

196. HARMAN, N. BISHOP: Congenital Cataract. *Treasury of Human Inheritance.* Vol. I, pp. 156—157. London, 1912. See Fig. 948.

197. BEAUVIEUX, M. J. C. J.: Étude sur les Déplacements congénitaux du Cristallin. *Archives d'Ophtalmologie.* T. XXXIII, pp. 16—35. Paris, 1913. See Fig. 1223.

198. FERBERS, H.: *Beitrag zur Kasuistik des Hydrophthalmus congenitus und Megalophthalmus congenitus.* Dissertation. Leipzig, 1913.

199. GOLOMB, J.: *Zur Aetiologie, Pathogenese und Therapie des Hydrophthalmus congenitus.* Dissertation. Berlin, 1913. See Figs. 1014, 1016, 1017, 1018.

200. LAWFORD, J. B.: Note on hereditary primary Glaucoma. *Royal London Ophthalmic Hospital Reports.* Vol. XIX, pp. 42—44. London, 1913. See Figs. 1033, 1036.

201. LÖHLEIN, W.: Das Glaukom der Jugendlichen. *Archiv f. Ophthalmologie*. Bd. LXXXV, S. 393—488. Berlin, 1913. See Figs. 1077, 1084.

202. STREBEL, J.: Korrelation der Vererbung von Augenleiden (Ektopia lentium cong., Ektopia pupillae, Myopie) und Herzfehlern in der Nachkommenschaft Schleuss-Winkler. *Archiv f. Rassen- u. Gesellschafts-Biologie*. Bd. X, S. 470—478. Leipzig, 1913. See Fig. 1177.

203. STUELP, O.: Über familiären Mikrophthalmus congenitus bei 8 von 14 Geschwistern. *Archiv f. Ophthalmologie*. Bd. LXXXVI, S. 136—140. Berlin, 1913. See Fig. 944.

204. BAHR.: Ektopie der Linse mit Linsenkolobom in drei Generationen. *Klinische Monatsblätter f. Augenheilkunde*. Bd. LII, S. 129. Stuttgart, 1914. See Fig. 1214.

205. CALHOUN, F. P.: Hereditary Glaucoma (Simplex). *Journal of the American Medical Association*. Vol. LXIII, pp. 209—215. Chicago, 1914. See Fig. 1040.

206. GEHRUNG, J. A.: Congenital Dislocation of the Lenses in Brother and Sister. *Archives of Ophthalmology*. Vol. XLIII, pp. 271—272. New York, 1914. See Fig. 1244.

207. HESSIN: Fünf Geschwister mit Kolobomen der Iris und Chorioidea. *Klinische Monatsblätter f. Augenheilkunde*. Bd. LII, S. 728—729. Stuttgart, 1914. See Fig. 1155.

208. KAYSER, B.: Über den Stammbaum einer Familie mit Vererbung von Megalocornea nach dem Hornerschen Vererbungstypus. *Archiv f. Rassen- u. Gesellschafts-Biologie*. Bd. XI, S. 170—173. Leipzig, 1914. See Fig. 983.

209. KAYSER, B.: Megalokornea oder Hydrophthalmus? *Klinische Monatsblätter f. Augenheilkunde*. Bd. LII, S. 226—239. Stuttgart, 1914. See Fig. 983.

210. KRETSCHMER: Angeborene Linsenverschiebung bei Vater und Sohn. *Centralblatt f. praktische Augenheilkunde*. Bd. XXXVIII, S. 8. Leipzig, 1914. See Fig. 1249.

211. NEUFFER, R.: Ueber die Beziehungen des primären Glaukoms zu Geschlecht, Lebensalter und Refraktion. Dissertation. Tübingen, 1914.

212. WISSMANN: Reports a case of hereditary ectopia lentis at a meeting of the Vereinigung Südwestdeutscher Augenärzte, Dec. 7, 1913. See *Klinische Monatsblätter f. Augenheilkunde*. Bd. LII, S. 129. Stuttgart, 1914. See Fig. 1238.

213. ATTLEE, J.: Coloboma of Iris in Mother and Child. *Proceedings, Royal Society of Medicine, Sect. of Ophthalmology*. Vol. VIII, Part III, pp. 125—126. London, 1915. See Fig. 1150.

214. GERTZ, O.: Demonstration zweier Fälle von Megalocornea congenita (Horner). *Klinische Monatsblätter f. Augenheilkunde*. Bd. LIV, S. 331—332. Stuttgart, 1915. See Fig. 986.

215. *KAGOSHIMA: [The Statistical Phase of Glaucoma] *Nippon Gankakai-Zashi*, 1915. Abstract in *Ophthalmology*. Vol. XII, p. 791. Milwaukee, 1916.

216. *LEWIS, A. C.: A Case of complete bilateral Irideremia in a Child whose Father has bilateral Coloboma of the Iris. *Ophthalmic Record*. Vol. XXIV, p. 134. Chicago, 1915. [Abstract of case in *Klinische Monatsblätter f. Augenheilkunde*. Bd. LIV, S. 697. Stuttgart, 1915.] See Fig. 1137.

217. SPICER, W. T. HOLMES: Spontaneous Dislocation of the Lens into the Anterior Chamber in three Members of the same Family. Ectopia of the Pupils. Extraction of the Dislocated Lenses. *Transactions, Ophthalmological Society of U.K.* Vol. XXXV, pp. 353—356. London, 1915. See Fig. 1210.

218. THOMSEN, C.: Ueber die Vererbung des Mikrophthalmus mit und ohne Katarakt. *Klinische Monatsblätter f. Augenheilkunde*. Bd. LIV, S. 236—249. Stuttgart, 1915. See Fig. 945.

219. HARMAN, N. BISHOP: Congenital Absence of the Sphincter of the Iris of each Eye. *West London Medical Journal*. Vol. XXI, pp. 44—45. London, 1916. See Fig. 1164.

220. JAMES, R. R.: Trephining for Glaucoma. *Ophthalmic Review*. Vol. XXXV, pp. 131—144. London, 1916. See Figs. 1072, 1085.

221. SEEFELDER, R.: Ueber die Beziehungen der sog. Megalokornea und des sog. Megalophthalmus zum Hydrophthalmus congenitus. *Klinische Monatsblätter f. Augenheilkunde*. Bd. LVI, S. 227—231. Stuttgart, 1916.

222. *RING, G. O.: Concerning Coloboma of the Iris in association with Congenital Cataract. *Ophthalmic Record*. Vol. XXVI, pp. 113—116. Chicago, 1917. See Fig. 1149. [Abstract of the case taken from *Archives of Ophthalmology*. Vol. XLVI, p. 392. New York, 1919. Also from the discussion on Shannon's paper. See Bibl. No. 223.]

223. SHANNON, C. E. G.: Two Cases of Congenital Coloboma of Iris and Choroid. *Transactions, American Ophthalmological Society*. Vol. XV, pp. 43—56. Philadelphia, 1917. See Figs. 1122, 1149, 1158.

224. FLEISCHER, B.: Ueber die Trepanation beim Hydrophthalmus congenitus. *Klinische Monatsblätter f. Augenheilkunde*. Bd. LXI, S. 152—174. Stuttgart, 1918. See Figs. 1001, 1019.

225. PETER, L. C.: Buphthalmia. *Transactions, College of Physicians of Philadelphia*. Vol. XL, pp. 240—241. Philadelphia, 1918. See Fig. 1012.

226. PLOCHER, R.: Beitrag zum juvenilen familiären Glaukom. *Klinische Monatsblätter f. Augenheilkunde.* Bd. LX, S. 592—620. Stuttgart, 1918. See Figs. 1023, 1037.

227. SPIECE, W. K.: A Case of Ectopia lentis with Family History. *American Journal of Ophthalmology.* Ser. 3, Vol. I, pp. 681—683. Chicago, 1918. See Fig. 1203.

228. BERGMEISTER, R.: Über Polykorie und verwandte seltenere Irisanomalien. *Zeitschrift f. Augenheilkunde.* Bd. XLI, S. 82—106. Berlin, 1919.

229. CLARK, C. F.: Coloboma and so-called Congenital Dislocation of the Lens. *Archives of Ophthalmology.* Vol. XLVIII, pp. 475—484. New York, 1919. See Fig. 1179.

230. KESTENBAUM, A.: Ueber Megalocornea. *Klinische Monatsblätter f. Augenheilkunde.* Bd. LXII, S. 734 — 752. Stuttgart, 1919.

231. LAMBERT, W. E.: Two Cases of Congenital Dislocation of the Lenses. *Archives of Ophthalmology.* Vol. XLVIII, p. 84. New York, 1919. See Fig. 1236.

232. VOGT, A.: Vererbter Hydrophthalmus beim Kaninchen. *Klinische Monatsblätter f. Augenheilkunde.* Bd. LXIII, S. 233. Stuttgart, 1919. See Fig. 1022.

233. WAARDENBURG, P. J.: Aangeboren Ooggebreken als Oorzaak van Halfblindheid en Blindheid. *Genetica.* Deel I, pp. 209—284. 'S-Gravenhage, 1919. See Fig. 1142.

234. COLLINS, E. TREACHER: Megalocornea and Microcornea. *Transactions, Ophthalmological Society of U.K.* Vol. XL, pp. 132—142. London, 1920. See Fig. 954.

235. FOXONET, J.: Glaucome double, consécutif à l'Ectopie congénitale du Cristallin, avec Luxation dans la Chambre antérieure du Cristallin gauche. Extraction des deux Cristallins dans leur Capsule. Guérison. *Annales d'Oculistique.* T. CLVII, pp. 616—624. Paris, 1920. See Fig. 1188.

236. USHER, C. H.: Enlarged Corneae in Goldfish. *Transactions, Ophthalmological Society of U.K.* Vol. XL, pp. 125—132. London, 1920.

237. *ARANA: [Congenital Ectopia lentis in two Members of the same Family]. *España Oftalmologica.* Vol. VI, pp. 130—131. Malaga, 1921. [Abstract of case taken from *Zentralblatt f. d. ges. Ophthalmologie.* Bd. VIII, S. 39. Berlin, 1923. See Fig. 1245.]

238. CLAUSEN, W.: Aniridia congenita und Heredität. *Klinische Monatsblätter f. Augenheilkunde.* Bd. LXVII, S. 116—117. Stuttgart, 1921. See Fig. 1118.

239. GRÖNHOLM, V.: Ueber die Vererbung der Megalokornea nebst einem Beitrag zur Frage des genetischen Zusammenhanges zwischen Megalokornea und Hydrophthalmus. *Klinische Monatsblätter f. Augenheilkunde.* Bd. LXVII, S. 1—15. Stuttgart, 1921. See Fig. 1115.

240. HOLM, E.: Ein anatomisch-untersuchter Fall von Aniridie. *Klinische Monatsblätter f. Augenheilkunde.* Bd. LXVI, S. 730—735. Stuttgart, 1921. See Fig. 1115.

241. McMILLAN, L.: Anophthalmia and Maldevelopment of the Eyes: four Cases in the same Family. *British Journal of Ophthalmology.* Vol. V, pp. 121—122. London, 1921. See Fig. 982.

242. ROLLET and BUSSY: Deux Cas d'Ectopie familiale des Cristallins. *Lyon Médical.* T. CXXX, pp. 1066—1067. Lyon, 1921. See Fig. 1185.

243. USHER, C. H.: A Pedigree of Microphthalmia with Myopia and Corectopia. *British Journal of Ophthalmology.* Vol. V, pp. 289—299. London, 1921. See Fig. 942.

244. ASH, W. M.: Hereditary Microphthalmia. *British Medical Journal.* Vol. I for 1922, pp. 558—559. London, 1922. See Fig. 950.

245. BARTELS: Glaucoma chron. heredit. climactericum. *Zeitschrift f. Augenheilkunde.* Bd. XLVIII, S. 298. Berlin, 1922. See Fig. 1078.

246. CRIDLAND, B.: Chronic Glaucoma at 20 years of age. *Transactions, Ophthalmological Society of U.K.* Vol. XLII, pp. 310—311. London, 1922. See Fig. 1024.

247. ELLIOT, R. H.: *A Treatise on Glaucoma.* London, 1922.

248. *LEOZ, G.: Angeborene und familiäre Subluxation beider Linsen nach untenaussen mit ciliarer Diplokorie. *Archivos de Oftalmologia Hispano-Americanos.* Vol. XXII, pp. 177—189. Madrid, 1922. [Abstract of case taken from *Zentralblatt f. d. ges. Ophthalmologie.* Bd. VIII, S. 39—40. Berlin, 1923. See Fig. 1233.]

249. OURGAUD: Un Cas d'Anophtalmie bilatérale. *Archives d'Ophtalmologie.* T. XXXIX, pp. 574—575. Paris, 1922. See Fig. 1173.

250. LINDBERG, J. G.: Beitrag zur Kenntnis der kongenitalen sog. Aniridie. Fälle totaler und partieller Aniridie und ein "Aniridie" Fall mit beibehaltener Iris in einer und derselben Familie. *Klinische Monatsblätter f. Augenheilkunde.* Bd. LXX, S. 133—138. Stuttgart, 1923. See Fig. 1128.

251. SNELL, A. C.: Hereditary Glaucoma simplex (Juvenile Glaucoma). *New York State Journal of Medicine.* Vol. XXIII, pp. 151—154. New York, 1923. See Figs. 1075, 1083.

252. VELHAGEN, C.: Atypische Coloboma iridis congenitum beim Vater, Aniridia congenita bei den Kindern. *Münchener medizinische Wochenschrift*. Bd. LXX, S. 469—470. München, 1923. See Fig. 1140.

253. VOGT, A.: Weitere Ergebnisse der Spaltlampenmikroskopie des vorderen Bulbusabschnittes. *Archiv f. Ophthalmologie*. Bd. CXI, S. 91—127. Berlin, 1923. See Fig. 1042.

254. CANTONNET, A.: Glaucome familial. *Annales d'Oculistique*. T. CLXI, p. 213. Paris, 1924. See Fig. 1028.

255. DWYER, H. L.: Aniridia in five Generations. *Journal of the American Medical Association*. Vol. LXXXIII, p. 1587. Chicago, 1924. See Fig. 1133.

256. GALLEMAERTS, E.: Anophtalmie congénitale et familiale. *Annales d'Oculistique*. T. CLXI, pp. 490—496. Paris, 1924. See Fig. 973.

257. HOLLAND, H. T.: Hereditary Glaucoma affecting three Generations. *Indian Medical Gazette*. Vol. LIX, p. 408. Calcutta, 1924. See Fig. 1047.

258. USHER, C. H.: A Pedigree of Congenital Dislocation of Lenses. *Biometrika*. Vol. XVI, pp. 273—282. Cambridge, 1924. See Fig. 1175.

259. AURAND: Deux Cas de Glaucome infantile chez deux Frères. *Archives d'Ophtalmologie*. T. XLII, pp. 630—631. Paris, 1925. See Fig. 1008.

260. FRANK-KAMENETZKI, S. G.: Eine eigenartige hereditäre Glaukomform mit Mangel des Irisstromas und geschlechtsgebundener Vererbung. *Klinische Monatsblätter f. Augenheilkunde*. Bd. LXXIV, S. 133—150. Stuttgart, 1925. See Fig. 1048.

261. *KENNEDY, E. W.: Complete ectopia lentis. *New York State Journal of Medicine*. Jan. 1925. New York, 1925. See Fig. 1232.

262. PETER, R.: Über die Corneagrösse und ihre Vererbung. *Archiv f. Ophthalmologie*. Bd. CXV, S. 29—48. Berlin, 1925.

263. RÖTTH, A. VON: Über die Vererbung der Linsenektopie. *Archiv f. Augenheilkunde*. Bd. XCV, S. 78—83. München, 1925. See Fig. 1180.

264. SPENCER, F. R. and LA RUE, C. L.: Familial Defects of Lens and Iris. *American Journal of Ophthalmology*. Vol. VIII, pp. 731—732. Chicago, 1925. See Fig. 1167.

265. BERNARD, R. J.: *Contribution à l'Étude de l'Aniridie Congénitale*. Thèse. Paris, 1926. See Figs. 1129, 1135.

266. CAMERON, E. P.: An interesting Example of Hereditary Dislocation of the Lens occurring in four successive Generations. *British Journal of Ophthalmology*. Vol. X, pp. 384—386. London, 1926. See Fig. 1178.

267. GIFFORD, S.: Congenital Aniridia. *American Journal of Ophthalmology*. Vol. IX, p. 548. Chicago, 1926. See Fig. 1127.

268. GREDIG, C.: Eine neue Vererbungsart der Megalocornea. *Archiv der Julius Klaus-Stiftung*. Bd. II, S. 79—89. Zurich, 1926. See Fig. 984.

269. KOMOTO, J.: Detachment of Retina with Coloboma of Iris and Choroid. *American Journal of Ophthalmology*. Vol. IX, pp. 414—415. Chicago, 1926. See Fig. 974.

270. LEWIS, J. B.: Aniridia in four Generations. *Medical Journal of Australia*. Vol. I for 1926, p. 489. Sydney, 1926. See Fig. 1120.

271. ZENTMAYER, W.: Congenital bilateral symmetric Dislocation of the Lens. *American Journal of Ophthalmology*. Vol. IX, pp. 376—377. Chicago, 1926. See Fig. 1228.

272. FECHT, W.: Über familiare Linsenluxation. *Zeitschrift f. Augenheilkunde*. Bd. LXII, S. 162—168. Berlin, 1927. See Fig. 1204.

273. FRANCESCHETTI, A.: Ectopia lentis et pupillae congenita als rezessives Erbleiden und ihre Manifestierung durch Konsanguinitat. *Klinische Monatsblätter f. Augenheilkunde*. Bd. LXXVIII, S. 351—362. Stuttgart, 1927. See Figs. 1204, 1220.

274. JAMES, R. R.: A Pedigree of a Family showing Hereditary Glaucoma. *British Journal of Ophthalmology*. Vol. XI, pp. 438—443. London, 1927. See Fig. 1026.

275. LICSKO, A.: Vererbte Irisatrophie. *Klinische Monatsblätter f. Augenheilkunde*. Bd. LXXVIII, S. 708. Stuttgart, 1927. See Fig. 1193.

276. *DE CARALT, D.: Hereditäre Ektopie der Linsen. *Archivos de Oftalmologia Hispano-Americanos*. Bd. XXVIII, S. 65 et seq. Madrid, 1928. See Fig. 1183.

277. HALBERTSMA, K. T. A.: Ueber einige erbliche familiare Augenerkrankungen. *Klinische Monatsblätter f. Augenheilkunde*. Bd. LXXX, S. 794—812. Stuttgart, 1928. See Fig. 1162.

278. PETRES, J. VON: Beiträge zur Megalokornea. *Klinische Monatsblätter f. Augenheilkunde*. Bd. LXXXI, S. 404. Stuttgart, 1928. See Fig. 987.

PLATE LXIV.   DESCRIPTIONS OF PEDIGREE PLATES   495

279. WEIZENBLATT: Megalocornea. *Zeitschrift f. Augenheilkunde.* Bd. LXV, S. 356. Berlin, 1928. See Fig. 991.

280. CROLL, L. J.: Aniridia occurring in three Generations. *Archives of Ophthalmology.* Vol. II for 1929, pp. 699—700. Chicago, 1929. See Fig. 1117.

281. WERNER, S.: Zur Kenntnis des erblichen juvenilen Glaukoms. *Acta Ophthalmologica.* Bd. VII, S. 162—168. Copenhagen, 1929. See Fig. 1067.

281 A.*CUNHA, E. B.: Aniridia congenita. *Brazil-medico.* No. 13, 1930. Rio de Janeiro, 1930. See Fig. 1143.

282. *CYKULENKO, K.: [On the Relation of Glaucoma to Sex and Age]. *Russk. Oftalmologii. Ž.* Vol. XII, pp. 17—23, 1930.

283. DE HAAS, H. L.: Demonstration von Bruder und Schwester mit Arachnodaktylie. *Klinische Monatsblätter f. Augenheilkunde.* Bd. LXXXV, S. 438—439. Stuttgart, 1930. See Fig. 1226.

284. *DÉRER, J.: [Family Juvenile Glaucoma]. *Oft. Sbornik.* Vol. V, 1930. Abstract taken from *Klinische Monatsblätter f. Augenheilkunde.* Bd. LXXXV, S. 852. Stuttgart, 1930. See Fig. 1089.

285. ROSENGREN, B.: Studien über die Tiefe der vorderen Augenkammer mit besonderer Hinsicht auf ihr Verhalten beim primären Glaukom. *Acta Ophthalmologica.* Vol. VIII, pp. 99—136. Copenhagen, 1930.

286. WEVE, H. J. M.: Ueber Arachnodaktylie. *Klinische Monatsblätter f. Augenheilkunde.* Bd. LXXXV, S. 438. Stuttgart, 1930. See Fig. 1227.

287. WOLFE, E.: A microphthalmic Family. *Proceedings, Royal Society of Medicine, Sect. of Ophthalmology,* Vol. XXIII, Part I, pp. 623—625. London, 1930. See Fig. 949.

288. BRAV, A.: The Incidence of Glaucoma among the Jews. *American Journal of Ophthalmology.* Vol. XIV, pp. 48—50. St. Louis, 1931.

289. COURTNEY, R. H. and HILL, E.: Hereditary Juvenile Glaucoma Simplex. *Journal of the American Medical Association.* Vol. XCVII, pp. 1602—1609. Chicago, 1931. See Figs 1069, 1070.

290. D'EWART, J.: The Problem of Aniridia. *British Medical Journal.* Vol. I for 1931, p. 284. London, 1931. See Fig. 1124.

291. SANDER, P.: A Case of Microphthalmos. *British Journal of Ophthalmology.* Vol. XV, pp. 22—23. London, 1931. See Fig. 952.

292. ULIANITSKY, Y. I.: [A Case of Familial Congenital Aniridia]. *Russk. Oftalmologii. Ž.* Vol. XI, p. 671. 1930. Abstract taken from *Archives of Ophthalmology.* Vol. V, p. 297. Chicago, 1931. See Fig. 1119.

293. VAIL, D. T.: Adult hereditary anterior Megalophthalmus sine Glaucoma. A definite Disease Entity. *Archives of Ophthalmology.* Vol. VI, pp. 39—62. Chicago, 1931.

294. WRIGHT, R. E. and NAYAR, K. K.: Trephining in the Treatment of Congenital Glaucoma. *British Journal of Ophthalmology.* Vol. XV, pp. 166—172. London, 1931. See Fig. 1068.

DESCRIPTIONS OF PEDIGREE PLATES[1]

MICROPHTHALMOS

PLATE LXIV. Fig. 942. *Usher's Case.* Microphthalmos associated with corectopia and myopia in four males and seven females of three generations. I. 1, G. W., was reported by II. 3, II. 10 and III. 9 to have had small eyes; in June 1890 he was noted at the Aberdeen Royal Infirmary to have "myopia, choroidal atrophy, tremulous iris, striae and posterior polar cataract, large staphyloma posticum"; he was illegitimate.

II. 3, G. W., aged 49 (1895), always near sighted, complained that the vision of his right eye had been failing for one week; he had right internal concomitant strabismus; corneae were small with transverse diameters of 9·5 mm.; refraction was myopic, more than 11 D. in the right eye; with correction, 25 D. in the horizontal meridian in the left eye; with correction R. V. = $\frac{3}{36}$, L. V. = $\frac{6}{8}$; pupils were eccentric towards the nasal side; iridodonesis was present; a posterior staphyloma with choroidal atrophy surrounded the disc in each eye; no vitreous opacities. In 1904 R. V. = hand movements; T. = + 1; anterior chamber was shallow; pupil was oval and reacted to light; the left eye had normal tension; neither eye moved fully outwards. Further examinations are described and in 1920 there was no perception of light in either eye, no nystagmus, much corneal opacity; R. T. was normal, L. T. = + 2.

II. 10, aged 41 (1897), complained of attacks of inflammation in his right eye during a year; the sight of this eye had failed suddenly in boyhood; corneae were small with a transverse diameter of 10 mm.; R. V. = no perception of light, cornea nebulous; the left eye had myopia of 20 D., L. V. with correction = $\frac{6}{60}$; pupils were ectopic, far upwards and inwards; irides were tremulous; the right fundus was not seen, the left showed a myopic crescent; R. T. = + 1, L. T. was normal; the left lens was hazy.

[1] p.l. is frequently used as an abbreviation of "perception of light".

III. 9, Mrs A. W., the only daughter of II. 3, aged 21 (1896), had always been near sighted; corneae were small and clear; refraction was myopic, 11 D. in the vertical, 13 D. in the horizontal meridian for the right eye, 14 D. and 9 D. being the corresponding measurements for the left; with correction R. V. = $\frac{6}{36}$, L. V. = $\frac{6}{24}$; large myopic crescents were noted. In 1920 R. V. = L. V. = $\frac{2}{60}$ with − 11 D. in each; corneal transverse diameters measured 9 or 9·5 mm., pupils were ectopic, up-in, and were not quite circular; no nystagmus; no iridodonesis; the irides were pale grey with a darker peripheral zone; lenses were clear excepting a few small dots below; discs were normal, but were surrounded by large areas of choroidal atrophy; some vitreous opacity was noted; tension was normal; anterior chambers not very shallow; eye movements full; when the upper lid was raised and the patient looked down, the eyeball appeared to be of a fair size. III. 30, Mrs M., aged 41 (1921), daughter of II. 10, had had a gastro-enterostomy performed for dilated stomach; the corneal transverse diameter in each eye measured 9 mm. and the eyeballs were smaller than normal; constant rotatory nystagmus was noted; R. V. with − 12 D. Sph. = $\frac{2}{60}$, L. V. = no perception of light; pupils were equal; irides were bluish with much yellow stroma; left iris was tremulous, not the right; pupils were markedly eccentric, up-in; the left lens was opaque and partially dislocated into the vitreous; the right lens was clear, no opacities in the right vitreous, a large area of complete choroidal atrophy surrounded the right disc; tension was normal in each eye; vision had deteriorated since an examination in 1907. III. 31 died unmarried, aged 31; at the age of 13 (1893) she had been admitted into an asylum for the blind, where she remained for three years; she was totally blind for some years before her death and is reported to have had small eyes and nystagmus; she is known to have had high myopia and a secondary cataract in the left lens. III. 32, Mrs McP., aged 21 (1903), had corneal transverse diameters of 10 mm.; the right eye was hypermetropic, about 5 D., the left eye myopic, about 7 D.; with correction R. V. = $\frac{6}{12}$, L. V. = $\frac{3}{60}$; pupils, nearly circular, contracted readily and were ectopic up-in; no iridodonesis; rotatory nystagmus was noted; lenses had peripheral dot opacities; the right iris had an incomplete corona at the nasal side where it was slate colour; fundi and tension were normal; a pupillary membrane was seen crossing the lower part of the right pupil, also fine pigmented dots on the lens capsule; this patient had convergent concomitant strabismus of the left eye; anterior chambers were deep down-out, shallow up-in. III. 33, J. W., aged 12 (1897), had a corneal transverse diameter of 8 mm. in each eye; refraction in both eyes was myopic, 7–10 D.; R. V. = $\frac{6}{60}$, L. V. = $\frac{6}{60}$ with correction; pupils were markedly ectopic, up-in, they contracted to light and accommodation and were not circular; lateral nystagmus was noted; myopic crescents were seen in the fundi; in the left eye an opacity was seen in the vitreous; partial ptosis was present; the palatal arch was rather high.

IV. 6, A. W., aged 2 (1907), had corneal transverse diameters of 9·5 mm.; not very high myopia was increased to 10 D. in each eye at the age of 7; pupils were markedly ectopic, up-in; rotatory nystagmus was present. At the age of 15 (1920) lenses were clear; a posterior staphyloma of choroidal atrophy was noted in each eye; eyeballs looked small but appeared to be of larger size when exposed by raising the lid; anterior chambers were of uniform depth, not shallow; no iridodonesis was present; there was a slow rotatory nystagmus. IV. 7 was seen aged 6 (1912) and again in 1920; she was an albino; a slight degree of myopia had increased by the age of 14 to about 8 D. in each eye; R. V. = L. V. = $\frac{6}{36}$ with correction; corneal transverse diameters measured 10 mm.; pupils, not quite circular, were markedly ectopic, up-in; lenses were clear; no iridodonesis was present; irides were bluish grey with a darker peripheral zone; fundi were typically albinotic and hair very fair; fine rotatory nystagmus was present; anterior chambers were of moderate depth.

IV. 23, aged 3 years, had small corneae, the transverse diameter of each measuring 9 mm.; also the whole eyeball was too small; no nystagmus was present and no iridodonesis; lenses were clear; anterior chambers were of equal and usual depth; discs were normal and fundi pale; refraction was hypermetropic in the right, myopic in the left eye; pupils were ovoid in shape and markedly ectopic, upwards and inwards.

II. 2, aged 65 (1914), had high myopia, diffuse lens opacity, and normal tension in the right eye; the left eye had vision reduced to perception of light, iridodonesis, a lens dislocated into the lower part of the vitreous chamber, a large posterior staphyloma of complete choroidal atrophy, much retinal pigmentation at the periphery of the fundus and tension of + 1; the optic disc was of good colour and not cupped. III. 8, the son of II. 2, aged 24 (1910), had in his right eye myopia of 22 D. and V. = $\frac{3}{60}$ with correction, in the left eye myopia of 18 D. and V. = $\frac{6}{12}$ with correction; each fundus showed extensive myopic changes. IV. 2 was a deaf-mute, III. 34 was mentally affected and died in a lunatic asylum. IV. 13 had epicanthus. II. 9 died in childhood. IV. 1 died aged 3 years. There was no coloboma of lens, iris, choroid, optic nerve, or eyelid in any of the affected members of this family. No consanguinity. Bibl. No. 243.

Fig. 943. *Cunier's Case.* Four cases of microphthalmos in a pedigree associated with other defects. III. 3, the normal daughter of a microphthalmic mother, married III. 2 who was normal, but whose grandfather I. 1 was a deaf mute; there were from this marriage three normal sons and two daughters with bilateral microphthalmos. Of these daughters IV. 4, aged 23, was also a deaf mute and had a complete absence of iris. IV. 5, aged 26, had nystagmus; she was married and had a son V. 1, aged 3 years, with bilateral microphthalmos; V. 1 was also a deaf mute and had a coloboma of the right iris; he further had congenital talipes equinus and small ill-developed upper limbs relatively to the rest of the body. No consanguinity recorded. Bibl. No. 29.

Plate LXIV.   DESCRIPTIONS OF PEDIGREE PLATES ·   497

Fig. 944. *Stuelp's Case.* Microphthalmos in eight members of a sibship of fourteen. The mother, I. 2, was healthy, had good sight and lived to the age of 80 years; by her first husband she had two children who saw well, a son, aged 69 (1913) and very vigorous, and a daughter, II. 2, who died from heart failure at the age of 60. By her second husband, who was alcoholic and who appears to have been suspected to have had a syphilitic infection, I. 2 had fourteen children, eight of whom were born blind; she had no miscarriages. Of these children II. 3 saw well but died from convulsions aged 1½ years; II. 4, aged 61 (1913), had never been seriously ill; he had complete ptosis and his eyes were about half the normal size with markedly small corneae; he was married and had three healthy children and two healthy grandchildren who saw well. II. 6, aged 59, and II. 7, aged 57, were both blind and were unmarried. II. 8 was blind and died, aged 5 years, from "Unterleibsdrüsen." II. 9 was blind and died, aged 2 years, from "Brustfieber." II. 10 saw well but died, aged 1 year, following vaccination. II. 11 saw well but died, aged 3, from "Brustwasser." II. 12 saw well but died, aged 9 months, from diarrhoea. II. 13, aged 51, saw well and had nine children and four grandchildren, none of whom were microphthalmic, but several of them died young. II. 15 was blind and died soon after birth. II. 17 was blind; he had from two marriages five children who saw well. II. 19 aged 43, was healthy, he and his six children saw well. II. 21 was blind and died, aged 5 months, from diarrhoea. All cases of microphthalmos known to have occurred in this family were members of a single sibship. No consanguinity. Bibl. No. 203.

Fig. 945. *Thomsen's Case.* I. 2 was born blind. II. 2 had markedly small eyes; he was married to a mentally defective woman; of their children, III. 2 had bilateral cataract, III. 3 saw very badly, III. 4 had bilateral cataract with eyes of normal size. III. 2 had children who were very short sighted. III. 4 married his second cousin, who was mentally very unstable, and had five children, of whom IV. 2, aged 10, had normal eyes; IV. 3, aged 8, had very small eyes and bilateral cataract; IV. 4, aged 4, also had very small eyes and bilateral cataract; IV. 5, aged 2, had bilateral cataract but normal sized eyes; IV. 6, aged 7 months, had bilateral microphthalmos and cataract. III. 6, the mother of this sibship, and her forbears were free from all eye anomalies, but her mother, II 4, was mentally defective and her half sister, III 8, was an imbecile. Consanguinity. Bibl. No. 218.

Fig. 946. *Pflüger's Case.* III. 1, Emma B., aged 11, had a markedly asymmetric skull and some degree of microcephaly which was chiefly conspicuous in the frontal region; she also had a not very pronounced though definite microphthalmos; the corneae were somewhat elliptic, vertical diameter 9 mm., horizontal diameter 10 mm.; she had a very marked horizontal nystagmus and absolute failure of central fixation; corneae were transparent, irides normal, R. lens normal, L. lens showed a cortical opacity; both fundi exhibited a coloboma of the choroid and of the optic nerve. III. 2 had normal eyes. III. 3 died two hours after birth; this child was hydrocephalic. II. 2, the mother of III. 1, had a deformity of the skull and eyes similar to that of III. 1 but of a less marked character; both corneae were smaller than normal—vertical diameter 10 mm., horizontal diameter 11 mm.—she had no colobomata. II. 3, aged 35, had a normal skull but showed a slight degree of microphthalmos in each eye with corneal diameters of 10 mm.; her fundi were normal. I. 1, the father of II. 2, was said to have abnormal eyes, but he was not seen and no indication of the nature of the abnormality is given. No consanguinity recorded. Bibl. No. 87.

Fig. 947. *Martin's Case.* Microphthalmos in thirteen members of three generations. I. 1 and 2, of whom no information could be obtained, had two sons with very small eyes and other children whose eyes were of normal size. II. 2 had a daughter, III. 2, and a granddaughter, IV. 1, who each had small eyes. II. 4 had three daughters with microphthalmos of whom III. 5, aged 47 (1888), had corneae with diameters of 7 mm.; her lids and cilia were normal; media were clear; irides were brown with normal pupils; the right fundus was normal, the left papilla was white and excavated; R. V. = $\frac{12}{30}$, refraction emmetropic; the left eye was blind. This patient lost the vision of her left eye suddenly, when in child-bed, seven years previously. Of the children of III. 5, one son had eyes of a normal size. IV, 4, aged 16, had cornea measuring 7 mm.; he had slight epicanthus; irides were brown, media transparent, pupils reacted normally; refraction was emmetropic, vision was good and fields were full. IV. 5, aged 14, was backward in bodily development though mentally normal; she had had occasional attacks resembling epilepsy; her corneae measured 7 mm. in breadth, 6·5 mm. in height; she also had epicanthus, more marked on the left side; irides were blue, the right pupil showing a trace of pupillary membrane; media were transparent, fundi normal, refraction emmetropic, vision good and fields full. IV. 6, aged 11, was healthy but had microphthalmos and slight epicanthus; his irides were blue, media clear, fundi normal; refraction was high hypermetropia but vision was good and fields were full. IV. 7, aged 7, had corneae measuring 6·5 mm. in width, 5·5 mm. in height; he also had epicanthus to a more marked degree than his siblings; he had high hypermetropia but vision was good, and in other respects his eyes were normal; irides were brown.

III. 7, a microphthalmic sister of III. 5, had children with eyes of a normal size. III. 9, another affected sister of III. 5 had five children of whom two had small eyes. III. 4 had completely normal eyes. No other developmental defects were known to have occurred in the family. No consanguinity recorded. Bibl. No. 97.

Fig. 948. *Bishop Harman's Case*. Microphthalmos in four members of two generations, associated with anterior polar cataract; the eyeball was very small in these cases with a corneal diameter measuring 7 to 7·5 mm.; the irides were poorly developed and the pupil eccentric in the cases seen; on the front of the lens was a plaque of dense white tissue; the condition was bilateral and was associated with a marked internal squint; constant nystagmus was noted; the affected members were mentally below the average, one of them, also an unaffected sister, died in an asylum; vision of the affected cases was very poor. I. 2 and 4 were remembered by their descendants but the state of their eyes was unknown; I. 2 had two normal children; I. 4 appears to be the source of the defect in the family. I. 8, aged 73, was a healthy old lady, she and her seven living siblings had good eyes. II. 3 was dead but had had good eyes; II. 4, also dead, was said to have had "tiny eyes and a terrible squint"; these two siblings were unmarried. Of the sibship II. 5—9 only II. 9 was married, other members had normal eyes; II. 8 died in a lunatic asylum. II. 9 died, aged 40, of paralysis, in an asylum; he had "very small eyes, bad squint, sight extremely bad, like his two daughters, III. 3 and 9." II. 10 was healthy with normal eyes. III. 2, aged 24, was normal and had one normal child. III. 3, aged 20, was affected; vision = p. l. only, and she was in a blind asylum. III. 4—6 were normal. III. 7 and 8 died, aged one year ten months, and eight weeks respectively; they had normal eyes. III. 9, aged 12, was affected and was in a blind school; she had a high arched palate and badly placed teeth with normal dental enamel; she had a small head and defective intelligence. No consanguinity recorded. Bibl. No. 196, p. 156.

Fig. 949. *Wolff's Case*. Microphthalmos in five siblings; all were high hypermetropes with little or no astigmatism, and all had fairly good vision at one time; some pseudoneuritis was noted and some ptosis associated with narrow palpebral fissures of about 2·1 cm. in length; the orbits were small with a vertical height of only 2·5 cm. and the eyes were said to be deeply set; it seems likely therefore that the eyes were truly microphthalmic even though the corneal diameter measured about 10 mm. in transverse diameter, which is small but not necessarily anomalous. An orbital height of 2·5 cm. is definitely anomalous; Dr Morant calculates, from a series of 17th century London skulls, that the probability of finding one female with an orbit of such a height or less is six in a million. The parents of the affected sibship were first cousins whose mothers were sisters; no evidence of other cases of anomaly in the family could be found.

III. 1, Elizabeth, had R. V. with + 15 D. sph. = $\frac{6}{18}$ = L. V.; the remains of a hyaloid artery were noted in the left eye near the disc. III. 10, George, had R. V. = L. V. = $\frac{6}{9}$ with $\dfrac{\text{D. sph.} + 14\cdot5}{\text{D. cyl.} + 1\cdot5}$. III. 13, Edward, had R. V. with + 15 D. sph. = $\frac{6}{9}$, L. V. with + 15·5 D. sph. = $\frac{6}{9}$. III. 3, Rose, was in Canada and was said to wear glasses. III. 5, Ivy, had the left canaliculus slit for epiphora at the age of five years; seven years ago she suddenly lost the vision of her R. eye; when seen later she had no p. l. in this eye and a cupped disc; later a secondary cataract developed; L. V. with $\dfrac{\text{D. sph.} + 13}{\text{D. cyl.} + 1\cdot5} = \frac{6}{12}$; two years ago this patient had an attack of subacute glaucoma in the L. eye, which was trephined; a cataract developed and was extracted; operation was complicated by the deeply sunken position of the globe in the orbit; after twice needling L. V. with + 22 D. = $\frac{3}{36}$. Three of this family, III. 5, 8, and 10, had only two upper incisors; III. 5 had four abnormally small lower incisors; III. 10 had supernumerary teeth and was reported to have had two rows. III. 3, III. 10 and several normal members of the family were married and had normal children. III. 6 had epileptic fits as a child and was unmarried. None of the cases in this sibship showed corectopia. III. 9, the twin brother of III. 8, died. A grandfather of the affected sibship had cataract; he had previously been in the Navy and had reading glasses of + 3 D. sph. Consanguinity. Bibl. No. 287.

Fig. 950. *Ash's Case*. Microphthalmos in eleven males of three generations; all the affected members were born blind and all were free from other congenital or acquired defect except one affected member of the sibship, IV. 4—8, who was epileptic. No description of the microphthalmic eyes is given. There was no history or evidence of syphilis in the family. No consanguinity. Bibl. No. 244.

Plate LXV. Fig. 951. *Scherenberg's Case*. Microphthalmos in three siblings; their three brothers, the second, third and fifth born in the family, had normal eyes; the parents were examined and found to have normal eyes; no eye disease was known to have occurred in the mother's family; a first cousin of the father, II. 6, a daughter of the latter, III. 7, and a niece, III. 9, were born with very "bad eyes"; no details could be obtained regarding the nature of the defect in II. 6, III. 7 and III. 9.

III. 1, Sophie Sch., aged 36, had seen very badly since childhood; she had never been seriously ill or had any inflammatory affection of the eyes; she was not quite normal mentally; her skull showed no abnormality, the orbits were of normal size and the annexes of the eye were normal; she had two small eyes in orbits so roomy that it was almost possible to touch the posterior pole with the forefinger; the horizontal and vertical diameters of the cornea measured 8 mm. in the right, 10 mm. in the left eye; the corneae were clear and transparent, the irides of normal structure but showed a pigmented border at the pupillary margin; the pupils were small but reacted briskly; the anterior chambers were very shallow; media were clear; the papillae were pale and a little swollen, also there were some yellowish white flecks

Plate LXV.   DESCRIPTIONS OF PEDIGREE PLATES   499

to be seen on the fundi; the maculae were intact, colour vision was normal, there was no contraction of the visual fields, tension was normal; refraction was highly hypermetropic; R.V. with + 10 D. = $\frac{5}{60}$, L.V. with + 16 D. = $\frac{5}{60}$.

III. 4, Karl Sch., aged 24, was normal mentally and had never been seriously ill, but he had seen badly since his youth; he had a normal skull with small eyes sunken in a relatively large orbit; this case differs from the last in that the corneae were large relatively to the size of the eyeballs, the horizontal and vertical diameters measured 11 mm. and 10·5 mm. respectively for each cornea; the anterior chambers were very shallow; this patient, like his sister, had high hypermetropia and hyperaemic papillae; fields of vision and colour perception were now normal, though he had complained of green vision at one period; R.V. with + 14 D. = $\frac{5}{60}$, L.V. with + 14 D. = $\frac{5}{60}$. III. 6, Anna Sch., aged 20, had a normal skull and very small eyeballs sunk in orbits of normal size; her corneae measured 10 mm. in the horizontal, 9 mm. in the vertical diameters; she had high hypermetropia and hyperaemic papillae, as in her sister, III. 1; the anterior chambers were shallow; pupils were small but reacted well; media were clear; R.V. with + 14 D. = $\frac{5}{60}$. L.V. with + 12 D. = $\frac{5}{60}$. No consanguinity. Bibl. No. 149.

Fig. 952. *Sander's Case.* III. 2, aged 23 days, was a well-developed baby with normal eyelids; her eyeballs were very small, about 9 mm. in diameter; each eye had a small transparent cornea measuring not more than 4 mm. in horizontal, 2 mm. in vertical diameters; some bluish grey colour could be seen through the cornea, but no pupil nor design of iris, nor anterior chamber could be defined; the movements of both eyeballs and eyelids were normal; sensibility was normal. At the age of 9 years this girl was of normal intelligence; the eyes had not enlarged but the corneae were less transparent; the child was blind. III. 2 was the second child of her mother; the first child was born with "no eyes," under eyelids which could be opened; this child had died from some acute infection. The parents, II. 1 and 2, were healthy young people; the mother, an Italian, attributed the defect in III. 1 to the fact that she had watched an operation upon her mother for glaucoma in her second month of pregnancy; the operation was not successful and the eye had been lost. No consanguinity recorded. Bibl. No. 291.

Fig. 953. *Schaumberg's Case.* III. 1, Moritz D., aged 29, had never suffered from inflammatory eye affections, but had not seen well since childhood; soon after birth his family had noted the marked smallness of his eyes; R.V. = $\frac{1}{4}$, L.V. = $\frac{1}{6}$; refraction was hypermetropic but vision was not improved by correction; the left disc was a vertical oval, the right disc was a horizontal oval; no further anomalies are noted. The patient said that his maternal grandfather, also one of his brothers, III. 2, had very small eyes; four of his siblings had normal eyes and saw well. No consanguinity recorded. Bibl. No. 78.

Fig. 954. *Treacher Collins's Case.* Microphthalmos in three generations. III. 1, Grace B., seen aged 27, had a cornea in each eye with horizontal and vertical diameters measuring 8 mm.; no opacities were seen in the corneae; fundi were normal; there were scattered dots of opacity in the posterior part of each lens leading to some lowering of vision; R.V. = $\frac{6}{12}$; L.V. = $\frac{6}{24}$. II. 2, the father of Grace B., also had small eyes with corneae measuring 9 mm. in diameter. II. 2 said that he had two sons with normal eyes, but that his father had had very small eyes. No consanguinity recorded. Bibl. No. 234.

Fig. 955. *Rava's Case.* Microphthalmos in five members of three generations. II. 2, aged 50, had eyes which were less than two-thirds of the normal in size, her corneal vertical diameter measured 7 mm.; her mother and one of her three sisters were similarly affected, all had good sight earlier in life but developed cataract, in each case at the same age; two sisters of II. 2 had normal eyes. Two sons of II. 2 were also microphthalmic; they had defective vision; one of them had a bilateral broad coloboma iridis upwards and saw with his right eye; the other had nystagmus with very bad vision and was deaf. No consanguinity recorded. Bibl. No. 72.

Fig. 956. *Mayerhausen's Case.* Microphthalmos in three members of three generations. II. 2, J. G., aged 53, had always had very bad sight, but it had become worse so that it was now difficult to find her way about the streets; she had bilateral microphthalmos and ptosis; her bulbs were about two-thirds of the normal size and the corneae measured about 7½ mm. in diameter; the anterior chambers were very deep; the left pupil was circular but was displaced inwards, the right pupil was oval; it was not possible to examine the fundus on account of a marked nystagmus and the very small pupils; tension was normal: II. 2 had nine children, of whom six with normal eyes died at the ages of 18 weeks, 1 year, 2 years, 2½, 6, and 8 years respectively; of the three living children III. 1, aged 17, and III. 2, aged 12, had normal eyes; III. 3, aged 10, had the same anomaly as his mother. Thus August G., aged 10, had marked nystagmus, his bulbs were somewhat larger than his mother's but definitely microphthalmic, his corneae were smaller than his mother's; he further had posterior capsular cataract in each eye. II. 1 had normal eyes.

I. 2, aged 83, the mother of II. 2, saw well until the age of 40, two years later she had a bilateral operation for cataract; she had slight ptosis and her bulbs were about three quarters of the normal size; her right cornea measured 10 mm. in horizontal, 9 mm. in vertical diameter; the right pupil was markedly eccentric inwards; discs were very small; nystagmus was not present. No consanguinity recorded. Bibl. No. 77.

Fig. 957. *Lafosse's Case.* III. 1, seen aged 2½ years, was well developed and in good health apart from his eyes, but he had not yet walked; he had epicanthus, more marked on the right side than the left; eyelids were normal; palpebral fissures were rather small; upon opening the lids no trace of eyeball could be found; the orbits were well formed but rather small; lachrymal apparatus was normal; the child was walking and fairly intelligent at a later date. A younger sister was normally developed. The mother, II. 2, had nystagmus in the right eye; on the right side her eyelids were well formed but smaller than on the left, the orbit also was smaller; the right eyeball was rudimentary, the size of a small pea, with some slight power of movement; lachrymal apparatus was normal. II. 2 attributed her anomaly to an accident which happened to her mother during pregnancy; she was in good health but with less than average intelligence. No consanguinity. Bibl. No. 127.

Fig. 958. *Stoeber's Case.* (Taken from Pétrequin.) Microphthalmos in a mother and in her two sons. II. 2, aged 32, was born with the left eye much smaller than the right; this eye also showed a coloboma iridis downwards and a corectopia downwards; the cornea was very small and there was no contractility in the iris; she stated that no member of her family had previously shown the defect, though her father had lost an eye from an accident. II. 2 by a normal husband had two sons, of whom III. 1, aged 7, had bilateral microphthalmos, III. 2, aged 4, was microphthalmic in the right eye only. No consanguinity. Bibl. No. 30.

Fig. 959. *Gescheidt's Case.* A male, aged 42, with microphthalmos, had bluish white sclerotics and gerontoxon; also his pupils were displaced inwards; of his two brothers one had normal eyes, the other, II. 3, was very short-sighted. II. 3 had two children who were blind in one eye. The paternal uncle of II. 2 had two blind children. No consanguinity recorded. Bibl. No. 18.

Fig. 960. *Bronner's Case.* Microphthalmos in two males and four females of three generations. II. 2 had bilateral congenital microphthalmos, cataract and nystagmus, the right eye was lost after cataract extraction; she had four children, two males and two females, of whom two were dead, all had had bilateral microphthalmos and cataract, two had also nystagmus and convergent strabismus; irides were normal in all; cataracts in all had been removed but vision remained very defective. I. 1 was reported to have had eyes similar to those of II. 2, "very small and which were always on the move, and vision very bad." No consanguinity recorded. Bibl. No. 154.

Fig. 961. *Brose's Case.* III. 1, aged 5 days, the first baby of her parents, had no trace of a right eyeball; a small rudimentary left eye, as large as a pea, was found; there was a small transparent cornea through which an iris could be detected by its bluish colour; no pupil could be seen; the eyebrows, eyelashes and tear ducts were normal; in other respects the child was normally developed. The mother, II. 1, attributed the defect to the shock she received on looking at the face of a relative's dead child during her second month of pregnancy. The father and his four siblings had good sight and presented no anomaly, but their father, I. 1, was born without a right eye; I. 1 saw well with his left eye. No consanguinity recorded. Bibl. No. 153.

Fig. 962. *Nunneley's Case.* Microphthalmos in two sisters, aniridia in their brother. II. 2, aged 15, had both globes smaller than normal, they were somewhat flattened and rather soft to the touch; sclerotic coats were vascular, corneae conical, irides thin and tremulous, pupils considerably displaced towards the nasal side and very imperfect in action; both eyes were myopic. II. 1, elder sister to II. 2, had a similar congenital condition of her eyes but of a less severe degree. II. 3, aged 13, had a total absence of iris in both eyes; fundi normal; he found a strong light unpleasant; lenses were clear when he was first seen, but cataract in the right lens was seen later fully formed.

Parents had good sight. Some years ago Nunneley had operated on a maternal first cousin to II. 1—3 for congenital cataract. No consanguinity recorded. Bibl. No. 44.

Fig. 963. *Bronner's Case.* Microphthalmos in a male and in four of his eight children. I. 2, aged 48 (1902), had had microphthalmos associated with cataract and with lateral nystagmus from birth; no other member of the man's family was affected; the cataracts were both extracted, but with correcting glasses barely $\frac{6}{60}$ vision was obtained; he had eight children of whom II. 1, still-born, II. 2, aged 21 (1902), II. 4 and II. 7 had normal eyes; II. 3, aged 18, had microphthalmos, cataract, nystagmus and converging strabismus of the left eye; II. 5, 6 and 8 had microphthalmos, cataract and nystagmus. The eyes and the corneae were very small and the anterior chamber shallow, no coloboma of the iris or choroid was present. I. 3 had normal eyes. There was no history of alcoholism or of syphilis in the family. No consanguinity recorded. Bibl. No. 154.

Fig. 964. *Magnus's Case.* Microphthalmos in eight of the sixteen children of a man by two wives who were sisters. The parents were normal and unrelated; all the affected children were born blind. No consanguinity. Bibl. No. 90, p. 36.

PLATE LXV.   DESCRIPTIONS OF PEDIGREE PLATES   501

Fig. 965. *Harlan's Case.* Microphthalmos in the eldest member of a sibship of five, the offspring of first cousins. II. 1 had eyes about the size of a cranberry; the corneae were opaque and bluish white, very like the sclerotics; they measured 2·5 lines in diameter; V. = perception of light; one brother was born blind; no other case of blindness was known to have occurred in the family. Consanguinity. Bibl. No. 55.

Fig. 966. *Reber's Case.* Microphthalmos in three sisters of a sibship of five; the parents and two siblings, aged 6 and 2 years respectively, had normal eyes. The three affected sisters were aged 10, 8 and 2 years respectively ; only the eldest sister is described; she had had an alternating convergent strabismus since the age of 3 years; her two globes were small and sunken; the anterior chambers were shallow; the optic nerves were normal, the macular and perimacular regions were occupied by a greyish disc, with ill-defined limits, of a diameter equal to about that of the papilla; the macular reflex was absent; this patient had hypermetropia of 14 D. in each eye. It is not clear from the history of this case whether the two younger sisters also had high hypermetropia and defect in the macular area. No consanguinity recorded. Bibl. No. 139.

Fig. 967. *Harlan's Case.* II. 1 had small eyeballs with corneal diameters measuring 4 lines; his right lens was opaque, the left lens had a small white speck on the surface of the capsule; L.V. $= \frac{2 0}{1 0 0}$, with $+ \frac{1}{3}$ D.; pupils were small and nystagmus was present. II. 2 had similar eyes with a coloboma iridis downwards in the right; R.V. $= \frac{1 0}{7 0}$; the left eye had an occluded pupil. One of the five sisters of II. 1 and 2 had microphthalmos; two brothers had normal eyes. The father, I. 2, had normal eyes; the mother had some anomaly in one eye. No consanguinity recorded. Bibl. No. 55.

Fig. 968. *Tiffany's Case.* Microphthalmos and aphakia in a mother and three of her seven children; all the eyes of the affected members were microphthalmic and had no lens, except a small rim in the peripheral region which was opaque; in the two affected boys the left eye was smaller than the right. I. 1 had nystagmus and iridodonesis; her pupils were displaced towards the nasal and inferior quadrant, and only responded slightly to a mydriatic. II. 1 was emmetropic and had R.V. = L.V. = $\frac{2 0}{2 0}$. II. 2 and II. 3 in addition to their other defects had bilateral convergent strabismus and a high degree of myopia; the vision of the elder boy was $\frac{5}{2 0 0}$ in each eye, and of the younger boy was $\frac{5}{3 0 0}$ in each eye; these boys were bright and well developed. II. 4, aged 24, had an opaque cornea in the right eye which was shrunken and totally blind; in the left eye T. = + 3 and the eye was nearly blind; the right eye was enucleated; there was no iris in either eye. The affected boys had brown eyes like their normal father, the affected mother had blue eyes as had her children with good vision. No consanguinity. Bibl. No. 151.

Fig. 969. *Harlan's Case.* Microphthalmos in a female whose father was born blind and was said to have eyes "just like her own"; her mother had good vision; three of her four brothers and one of her three sisters were born blind; the three youngest members of her sibship had perfect sight. II. 4 had quantitative vision only, her right corneal diameter measured about 3 lines, the left about 2½ lines (the normal value is about 5 lines); pupils were irregular and immovable; corneae were dotted over with numerous white specks in the deeper layers. No information is given as to the nature of the blindness in the four siblings thus affected. No consanguinity recorded. Bibl. No. 55.

Fig, 970. *Harlan's Case.* Microphthalmos associated with other defects in two members of a sibship of seven; no other case of blindness was known to have occurred in the family. II. 1 had small eyes with cataractous lenses; the corneae were partially opaque, the right was flat, the left was staphylomatous; the irides were mere narrow rims. One brother was said to have similar eyes. No consanguinity recorded. Bibl. No. 55.

Fig. 971. *Cederskjöld's Case.* Microphthalmos in a woman and in three of her children. I. 1 had very small eyes; she died from puerperal fever at the birth of her fourth child; her three eldest children all had unusually small eyes and each of them, also their mother, developed cataract. No consanguinity recorded. Bibl. No. 24.

Fig. 972. *Cooper's Case.* Microphthalmos in three siblings; the parents were well developed and free from all ocular defects; no anomaly had been known to occur in the eyes of any of the ancestors; the mother attributed the defect in her children to a maternal impression—when pregnant with her first child she had seen a man in the street with very small and peculiar eyes—"this man's face was in my thoughts night and day until my confinement." II. 1, aged 12, height 3 feet 11½ inches, had never more than a few imperfect teeth which mostly dropped out soon after their appearance, when seen he had three ill-developed stumps; the child was subject to headaches and was seldom without a discharge from the ears; the globes of his eyes were extremely small, each palpebral fissure measuring only ¾ inch in length, and were in constant irregular motion; the corneae measured little more than $\frac{2}{2 0}$ inch in diameter; the irides were an irregular strip of hazel colour, entirely deficient in parts and without the slightest action; lenses were clear but an opaque spot was noted on the anterior capsule in each eye; vision was very bad. II. 2, aged 9, had no teeth, for those which had occasionally appeared dropped out; her eyes were very like those of II. 1; there were a few irregular shreds of hazel-coloured iris in each eye; some haziness of the external half of the right cornea was noted; lenses were clear but there was an opaque patch on the anterior capsule of each. II. 3, aged 7, had smaller eyes than II. 1 or II. 2; the iris was absent along the upper border of each eye; central opacities were noted in the anterior capsule of each lens; vision was apparently better than that of her affected siblings. II. 4, aged 15 months, was normal in all respects with eyes of full size and well-developed teeth. No consanguinity recorded. Bibl. No. 40.

Fig. 973. *Gallemaerts's Case*. I. 2, aged 30, was healthy with normal eyes. I. 1, aged 33, was well and had had no miscarriages, but she had a microphthalmic eye on the left side; the eyelid could be opened to show a deeply set very reduced globe in the back of the conjunctival sac. I. 1 and 2 had three children of whom II. 1, aged 9 years, was examined and had normal eyes. II. 2, aged 2 years, had on the right side a palpebral fissure measuring 12 mm. in length; at the back of the conjunctival sac a very small microphthalmic eye could be identified; no iris could be seen through the very undeveloped cornea; on the left side the orbit was deeply sunken, the palpebral fissure measured 10 mm. in length, the conjunctival sac was scarcely noticeable; no trace of ocular globe could be discovered. II. 3 died aged 3 months; no trace of globe could be found in either eye during life; post mortem examination showed in the right orbit a small nodule consisting of a mass of pigmented cells in a fibrous capsule; no trace of cornea, lens or optic nerve was recognisable; the left orbit showed no trace of a rudimentary eye. Examination of the brain revealed gross defects including an absence of the chiasma and optic nerves; the external geniculate bodies were not differentiated; quadrigeminal bodies were rudimentary. No consanguinity recorded. Bibl. No. 256.

Fig. 974. *Komoto's Case*. I. 1, Mrs O., had microphthalmos of the right eye with coloboma of the iris and choroid; she had three children of whom the eldest, a boy aged 5, had a microphthalmic right eye with coloboma of the iris and choroid, also a hare-lip; the second son was normal; the third child, a girl aged 2 months, had both eyes microphthalmic to a high degree and it was doubtful whether she had any sight. No consanguinity recorded. Bibl. No. 269.

Fig. 975. *Gescheidt's Case*. Microphthalmos in two brothers. I. 1 was healthy and normal; I. 2 had senile cataract. II. 2, aged 22, had very small eyes and was suffering from capsular cataract; he had an oval pupil and a gerontoxon. II. 1 had eyes which were still smaller than his brothers; he also had a capsular cataract. Both brothers had some abnormality in the development of the skull. No consanguinity recorded. Bibl. No. 18.

Fig. 976. *Priestley Smith's Case*. Microphthalmos and glaucoma in a woman and in her father. II. 1 had lost one eye from primary glaucoma; her corneae were 10·5 mm. in diameter. No consanguinity recorded. Bibl. No. 154 (cited).

Fig. 977. *Argyll Robertson's Case*. Microphthalmos in a boy, aged 6 to 8 years, the diameter of the eyes being about two-thirds of the normal; the child had cataract and showed nystagmus. I. 2 had microphthalmos but no nystagmus, and there is no note of his having cataract. No consanguinity recorded. Bibl. No. 154 (cited).

Fig. 978. *Fuchs's Case*. Unilateral microphthalmos in a father and son; no further information is given. No consanguinity recorded. Bibl. No. 154 (cited).

Fig. 979. *Morano's Case*. A child, aged 3 months, of healthy parents, had bilateral congenital anophthalmos; four older siblings had been born with the same condition; all the five children died in the first year of life. No consanguinity recorded. Bibl. No. 95.

Fig. 980. *Fischer's Case*. A brother and sister had the left eyeball entirely missing; the right eyeball in each was the size of a pea and useless. No consanguinity recorded. Bibl. No. 15.

Fig. 981. *Bruns's Case*. Microphthalmos in three siblings. The father, I. 1, aged about 35, was healthy and had good vision; the mother, I. 2, was short and stout, a rather dull, mild temperament, with good general health but suffered acutely from headaches; she spoke in a vague way of "fainting spells" with loss of consciousness which might be epileptic or hysterical; she was aged about 30; V. = $\frac{20}{40}$; she had a mixed astigmatism but no abnormality in the media or fundi. These parents had seven children of whom II. 1, 2 and 6 were in good health and saw well; II. 4 was still-born and there was no knowledge regarding his eyes; II. 3, aged 5, and II. 7, aged 5 months, were microphthalmic; in both cases the eyelids were closed and deeply sunken in the orbits; the four orbits contained four little shrunken globes not bigger than very small green peas; on each globe there was a miniature cornea through which a dark bluish iris could be partially seen; through pin-head pupils it was thought that chalky white opaque lenses could be seen; in none of the orbits could a trace of any other sac or swelling be discovered. A third child of the sibship, II. 5, was said to be similarly affected. No consanguinity recorded. Bibl. No. 141.

Plate LXVI, Fig. 982. *Usher's Case*. In 1921 a paper entitled "Anophthalmia and mal-development of the Eyes" was published by Lewis McMillan in the *British Journal of Ophthalmology*; an account is therein given of the four affected children, VI. 28—31, in the family of A. C. in the Benderloch, a district of

Plate LXVI.   DESCRIPTIONS OF PEDIGREE PLATES   503

Argyllshire. It seemed desirable to obtain a record of the subsequent history of this family and to investigate the nature of the stock from which it had arisen. The complete family consists of ten children, of whom VI. 28, Charlotte C. (Plate Q, Fig. 1), aged 16, pale faced and rather depressed, menstruates; mental condition satisfactory; height 5′ 2″; high palate; fingers normal; with either ear hears a watch at 15″. R. eyeball is very small and set far back in the orbit; it has a considerable range of movement; it is pale grey except at the part representing the cornea, which has a small dark centre and a greenish appearance just to the temporal side of the dark spot; there is an ill-defined anterior staphyloma which includes the pupillary area; tension normal; R.V. = perception of light; no cyst in lower lid; puncta lacrinalia and caruncle are present; eyelashes normal; palpebral fissure considerably smaller than on the left side; the orbit is smaller than on the left side; a rough measurement, taken at the orbital margin, gave in the vertical direction 25 mm. for the right side and 28 mm. for the left, in the horizontal direction 28 mm. for both. L.V. = $\frac{6}{12}$, refraction estimated low hypermetropia; horizontal diameter of cornea 10 mm.; coloboma of iris down-in; fundus normal; eye movements full. Examined at her home, 15th May, 1931.

VI. 29, John C. (Plate Q, Fig. 2), aged 14, is mentally backward and imbecile and dirty; answers usually in monosyllables that are jerked out; height 4′ 4″, weight 69 lb.; has general convulsions, these began on 12th May, 1930, and there have been 26 altogether; palate and fingers normal; hears quite well. In the right orbit no trace of an eyeball can be felt; the puncta lacrinalia are present and the lashes are normal in appearance; the palpebral fissure is smaller than on the left, its horizontal measurement is 11 mm., on left side 20 mm.; the vertical measurement when lids are held apart is 10·5 mm., on left side 18 mm.; the right orbit is obviously smaller than the left one; vertical direction measures 10 mm. in right and 14 mm. in left, horizontal direction gives 14 mm. in right and 24 mm. in left. Left eyeball is small and set far back in the orbit; it is pale grey with a darkish area anteriorly, probably uveal tissue seen through opaque corneal tissue; no cyst in either lower lid, puncta lacrinalia, caruncle, and lashes normal; L.V. = no p. l. Examined on 16th May, 1931, in Argyll and Bute District Mental Hospital, Lochgilphead, with Dr Donald Ross, medical superintendent, who kindly gave permission for the examination.

VI. 30, Charles C. (Plate Q, Fig. 3), aged 13, pale faced, height 4′ 9″, sits in a curious attitude with head down and neck markedly bent; his replies, which are usually "yes" or "no," are sudden, abrupt, and loud and were well described by the district nurse when she likened them to a bark; he is dirty, palate normal, uvula bifid in some degree; fingers normal. The right eyeball, set well back in the orbit, is the size of a large pea; it is grey in colour, smooth, cornea indistinguishable from rest of eyeball; palpebral conjunctiva appears reddish in contrast with the grey eyeball; movements of eyeball much restricted; no evidence of perception of light; puncta lacrinalia and caruncle present; lashes normal; palpebral fissure 22 mm. in length and 15 mm. vertical measurement with lids drawn apart; orbital vertical measurement is 22 mm., horizontal measurement 33 mm. Left orbit contains no eyeball as far as can be determined by palpation; no cyst in lower lid; puncta and caruncle are present; lashes normal; palpebral fissure is much smaller than that on right side, it measures 14 mm. in length and 7 mm. at widest part when lids are held apart; orbit measured 18 mm. vertically and 27 mm. horizontally. The orbital measurements must only be taken to show very roughly the relative sizes of the orbits. Hearing equal on each side, namely recognition at 1′ of the feeble tick of a watch. This case was examined at his home on 15th May, 1931, and shows some mental defect.

VI. 31, Margaret C. (Plate Q, Fig. 4), aged 12, height 4′ 7½″; mental condition satisfactory though she is not clever; menstruates; hears watch at 1′ with each ear; taste: recognised peppermint and some other flavours in sweetmeats; smell is apparently quite satisfactory. Right eyeball is small and pale grey; no pupil or iris recognisable, though anteriorly there is a darker area; tension normal; no perception of light; no cyst in lower lid; puncta lacrinalia and caruncle present; orbital measurements: vertical 20 mm., horizontal 24 mm. Left eye, V. = $\frac{6}{12}$ not fully, wearing a convex glass[1], reads 1 J. slowly at 9″; eye movements full; constant fine lateral nystagmus; pupil circular, contracts to light; iris greenish yellow, has no coloboma; horizontal diameter of cornea cannot be measured accurately owing to nystagmus, it appears to be 10 or 11 mm.; puncta lacrinalia and caruncle present; lashes normal; ophthalmoscopic examination, no coloboma of choroid present; owing to a small pupil and nystagmus further particulars were not obtained; palate and fingers normal; orbital measurements: vertical 24 mm., horizontal 26 mm. This case was examined on 18th May, 1931, at The Royal Blind Asylum and School, Edinburgh, by kind permission of Dr George Mackay. Mr W. M. Stone, superintendent, kindly supplied some of the information regarding this child.

As regards the next 3 children, VI. 32, Allan C., VI. 33, Cissie C., and VI. 34, Edward C., who died of diphtheria in April 1929. Allan and Cissie were of school age; a visit to their school mistress elicited the information that they were both able to read letters as well as other children; both were intelligent; Cissie had blue eyes and Allan brown eyes; Cissie blinked, otherwise nothing unusual was noticed about their eyes. The district nurse, who knew the children and also their mother, gave similar reports. Edward's

[1] On 20th March, 1929, Dr George Mackay found L.V. = $\frac{6}{6}$, with +2 D. sph. = $\frac{6}{5}$, and on 8th December, 1930, L.V. with +2 D. sph. = $\frac{1}{5}$.

iris was dark brown and his vision full. It may therefore be accepted that the eyes and vision of VI. 32, 33 and 34 were normal. These children were mentally and physically sound[1].

VI. 35, Alexandrina C. (Plate Q, Fig. 5), aged 3, is mentally quite normal; height 3′ 3″; R. V. good, picks up small objects without hesitation using either eye; iris brown, no coloboma; no nystagmus; fundus oculi normal; lashes, puncta lacrimalia, and caruncle normal; L. V. good; iris brown, no coloboma; refraction estimated low degree of hypermetropia in each eye; fundus oculi normal; puncta lacrimalia, caruncle and lashes normal; hearing quite good; palate and fingers normal. Examined at her home on 15th May, 1931.

VI. 36, Johanna C. (Plate Q, Fig. 6), aged 2, height 2′ 8½″; mental state said to be good; palate and fingers normal; palpebral fissures are very small, owing to child's restlessness no attempt made to measure these or the orbits; in palpation nothing could be felt in the orbit, clinically the eyes are absent, yet the puncta lacrimalia and eyelashes are present; hearing is satisfactory. Examined at her home on 15th May, 1931.

VI. 37, male (Plate Q, Fig. 7), aged 2 months (31st August, 1931), reported by Dr MacNicol to be quite normal. When seen on the above date pupils were equal, eye movements full; iris blue, no coloboma; lids normal; face, hands and feet normal.

In this family of ten, five are males and five females, ocular defects are present in two of the former and in three of the latter. The four oldest members, two females and two males, have ocular defects, and the males are also mentally affected. The next three children in order of birth, two males and one female, now dead, had no ocular defect and were mentally and physically sound. The eighth child, a female, has normal eyes and is mentally and physically sound. The ninth child has double anophthalmos. The youngest child is normal. Seven of the children are alive to-day including all those with ocular defects. Three of the normal children died from diphtheria within a few days of each other two years ago. None of the cases shows cysts in connection with the small eyeballs. None of the cases is deaf. In neither parent nor in any of the children are there signs of syphilis. There is no polydactylism, hare-lip, cleft palate, nor any other congenital malformation present in any of the children, excepting the ocular conditions. Although the palpebral fissure is small where there is anophthalmos, the puncta lacrimalia, the caruncle and the eyelashes are always present. In the cases where an eyeball is absent on one side, but present on the other side, and in cases with a small eyeball on one side and a full-sized or nearly full-sized eyeball on the other side, the palpebral fissure and the orbit are smaller on the side of the absent or of the smaller eye than on the other side. In none of the children, nor in either parent, is there a coloboma of the choroid. In one eye of the first born child there is a coloboma of the iris. In the two totally blind males a striking attitude with tilted head is frequently assumed when they are sitting; this is well shown in Fig. 2 of Plate Q; their oldest sister occasionally sits in a similar posture. The teeth of four of the affected children were examined and appeared to be sound. VI. 36 had all of her milk incisors and canines and six molars. VI. 28 had all of her incisors, canines, bicuspids and eight molars. VI. 30 had some teeth extracted; in both jaws incisors and canines were intact; in the lower jaw were three bicuspids and two molars, in the upper jaw were four bicuspids and two molars. VI. 31 had some teeth extracted; she has the usual numbers of incisors and canines; in the upper jaw are four bicuspids and two molars, in the lower jaw are two molars. V. 44, Jessie C. (Plate Q, Figs. 7, 8), mother of VI. 28—37, illegitimate child of IV. 41, Jessie C., and IV. 106, Donald C., is aged 37 (1931) but looks older; height 5′ 2″; mental condition normal; R. V. = L. V. reads 1 J. at 9″; refraction, low degree of hypermetropia in both; irides brown; fundi normal; movements of eyeballs full; no colobomata. Wasserman reaction and Kahn test both negative. Was given an excellent character by her aunt, under IV. 42, and her grandmother, III. 80.

V. 27, Alexander C. (Plate Q, Fig. 9), aged 43 (1931), father of VI. 28—37, looks healthy; height 5′ 4″; railway workman; palate and fingers normal; mentally sound. R. V. = L. V. reads 1 J. at 9″; refraction, low degree of hypermetropia; fundi normal; movements of eyeballs full; irides blue; no colobomata. It was said that V. 27 had bouts of drinking. The maternal grandmother, Jessie C., IV. 41, after the birth of V. 44, married her second cousin, IV. 77, and had a family of three, V. 45—47, none of whom is married; the oldest of them is a nurse and all are reported to be normal. IV. 41 died. The maternal grandfather, IV. 106, a sailor, died at the age of 40, from malignant disease of the liver; he was married, and had four healthy children, of whom none is married, and the youngest is still at school age. The paternal grandmother, Jessie C., IV. 24, was said to be addicted to drink; she is peculiar, lives apart from her husband and entirely by herself. The paternal grandfather, John C., IV. 21, was said to look so mad and wild that his appearance frightened children; he is aged 74 and only speaks Gaelic; lives apart from his wife, entirely by himself; works occasionally; is not quite normal mentally but not altogether certifiable. An elder brother of IV. 21, who died aged 90, was also named John but was referred to as Ian.

The maternal great-grandmother, Jessie McP. (Mrs Alex. C.), III. 80, aged 82, is exceptionally robust and has a retentive memory, but has a considerable degree of deafness. The maternal great-grandmother III. 87, Christina M., is the youngest of five siblings; her two brothers and two sisters left the district when young and could not be traced.

[1] Reported on 29th April, 1929, by the School Medical Officer of the Argyll County Education Authority to Dr George Mackay.

Plate LXVI.   DESCRIPTIONS OF PEDIGREE PLATES   505

Of the maternal great-grandfathers, III. 20, Alex. C., died aged 56; III. 83, Sam C., a shepherd, was sound bodily and mentally; he and his brother John were the only members of this sibship. Of the paternal great-grandparents, III. 14, Christina MacP., had a sister III. 15 who was "funny"; III. 8 was Flora McL. (Mrs C.); III. 13, Alex. C., was a "character" and probably not altogether normal; his brother and two sisters are all dead; III. 7, Archie C., is described as a bright and clever man by his son, but III. 80 said he was quick tempered, had head jerkings and on one occasion had attempted to drown his mother; III. 7 was believed to be related to III. 13.

Of other ancestors of VI. 28—37 in the direct line who were known are II. 33, Janet R. and her husband Duncan McP.; II. 17, Catherine C. and her husband II. 12, Archie C., who died at a great age; II. 9, Annie C. and her husband II. 8, Alex. McP. who lived to an old age; II. 7, Catherine McI., and her husband II. 6, John C.; II. 4, John McL ; II. 1, Donald C., came as herd laddie from Lochaber and is not related to Archie C., II. 12, to Sam C., III. 83, or to Donald C., I. 8; these members of the stock, also II. 36, gamekeeper, I. 14, I. 13, Jessie S., I. 12, John McP., weaver, I. 11, Mary McM.; I. 8, Donald C., I. 4, Alex. C., and I. 1, Duncan C., were known not to have had mal-developed eyes or deformity of any part of the body.

It will be seen from the pedigree that sixteen cases of certifiable mental defect have occurred in the stock and nineteen cases of less severe grade of departure from the normal; thus some grade of mental defect is widespread in the families of both parents of the affected sibship VI. 28—37. Notes on the mental state of all these cases are given in the *Annals of Eugenics*, Vol. v, pp. 56—8 and will not be repeated here.

Sixty-six members of the pedigree have been personally examined by the recorder; also a large proportion of the living members and some of those deceased are well known to Dr Fergussson, who has supplied much of the information that has been obtained concerning the relatives of the Benderloch family.

There is little to relate of the other members of the pedigree. No mal-formation of the eyes or other parts has been seen, or reported, in any of the relatives of the affected children of the sibship VI. 28—37. In generation II, the three males under II. 5 were drowned when carrying seaweed in a boat. II. 16, Margaret C., married II. 15, Alasdair C.; II. 29 went to Australia. The three males under III. 10 went to Montreal. III. 23 went to Australia. III. 25, Marion C., "shortsighted," is unmarried. III. 31, Flora C., is the only member of her sibship who married. III. 41, Archie C., married an epileptic wife and had three epileptic grandchildren. One female under III. 73 died in infancy. IV. 22 was ill for a year before his death at the age of 14. IV. 38 died in infancy. IV. 45 is in New York. One male under IV. 49 became "queer" after a head injury. One male under IV. 49 died aged 16. IV. 53, Archie H., married his first cousin IV. 61 who is described as "fushionless"; they have three children of whom one is mentally defective, of a possibly certifiable grade. None of IV. 64 is known to have married. The elder of IV. 88 was killed in the war. One female under IV. 93 died young. IV. 102 is in Canada; he is married but has no children. No mental defect or deformity has occurred in sibship IV. 95—102. One male under V. 10 died of measles aged 9. V. 32 died in infancy. Two males under V. 26 died in infancy. V. 35—40 is a sibship containing two mentally affected cases, the offspring of an insane mother, IV. 36. V. 49—51 are not in Scotland. The sibship V. 57—64 are all healthy except V. 63 who died at 18 months. V. 68 has an illegitimate son, VI. 39. V. 73—77, the children of Ann C., are all well but the three eldest are regarded as dull. V. 100, Mrs A., "highly strung," had a still-born child. One male under V. 99 died of pulmonary tubercle. Members of V. 104 are all healthy and see well; none is married; they are in Australia. Three males and one female of VI. 18 died young. One female of VI. 18 and one under VI. 22 died in infancy. VI. 41 was killed in the war. VI. 43 was drowned. VI. 50 died a few hours after birth. VI. 51, a dead child removed with forceps, no evidence of syphilis in the placenta. As indicative of the comparatively large number of people in the district with the same name is the occurrence of twenty-three matings in which the forty-five people concerned had the same name before mating and in only one instance was consanguinity known. In one instance the maiden names of a man's first and third wives were the same as his own surname. The following are among the non-consanguineous matings in which both partners had the same family name before marriage. Ian C., I. 7, and Annie C.—John C. II. 10, and Miss C.—Archie C., II. 12, and Caroline C.—Charles C., II. 13, and Catherine C.—Alasdair C., II. 15, and Margaret C.—Janet C., II. 24, and John C.—Hugh C., III. 1, and Sarah C, II. 30. —Donald C., III. 18, and Ailie C., III. 19, also Christina C., III. 50.—Dugald C., III. 28, and Maggie C.— John C., IV. 21, and Jessie C.—Annie C., IV. 28, and Donald C.—Jessie C., IV. 36, and Donald C.— Duncan C., IV. 58, and Flora C.—Ann C., IV. 59 and IV. 60.—Donald C., IV. 106, and Jessie C., IV. 41.— Alexander C., V. 27, and Jessie C , V. 44—Sam C., V. 102, and Jessie C., IV. 89.

Dr Roderick R. MacNicol, Taynuilt, and Dr Duncan Fergusson, Salen, Loch Sunart, have given valuable and indispensable help in collecting the facts of this pedigree. Consanguinity. Here first published.

MEGALOCORNEA

Fig 983. *Kayser's Case.* Megalocornea in sixteen members of five generations; only males are affected; with one exception the transmission has been through unaffected females of the stock. The pedigree has been very fully worked out and evidently no trouble has been spared to ensure the maximum of accuracy and completeness in the investigation; the condition of affected individuals was readily noted by the family themselves and by the laity in the district of Calw in Wurttemberg in which they mostly lived; the cases were interviewed whenever possible and information concerning members of generations I and II was obtained from their still living children or grandchildren of generation III.

I. 1, Joh. Ulrich G., 1772—1845, appears with great probability to have been the source of the anomaly in the family, and he is thus exceptional in that he transmitted the condition directly to his son II. 12, 1810—1891; so far as can be judged from statements of relatives only, no direct descendants of II. 12 show the anomaly; his two married daughters, first and second wives to the same man, went to America and all the grandchildren, IV. 14—20, were in America and reported to be normal. The descendants of the only brother of I. 2 were followed as far as possible for three generations, his one married daughter appears to have had no affected sons or grandsons. Of the twelve children of I. 1 and 2, II. 3 died aged 9, II. 6 died aged 4, II. 7, 11, and 18 died under one year of age, II. 8 died aged 2, II. 9 married, went to America and could not be traced; thus the only son of I. 1 who survived one year was the affected II. 12.

V. 73, Albert K., aged $2\frac{1}{2}$ years, was born with large eyes; his mother said that she had no doubt at the birth of her children whether they had "Calwer Augen" or not; the eyes of V. 73 were free from inflammation and vision was good; there was no photophobia; corneae were markedly prominent so that the eyes suggested exophthalmos, they were clear, showing no opacities or rupture of Descemet's membrane; corneal diameters measured 13·5 mm.; depth of anterior chamber was 5 mm.; pupils were small and reacted normally; there was no tremor of the iris; media were clear; discs were not excavated; vessels were normal; tension was not raised. The mother, IV. 68, had normal eyes. V. 71, Max K., aged 6, was born with large eyes which were healthy and free from inflammation; at the age of 3 years he had a catarrhal conjunctivitis; vision was good with no photophobia; corneae were markedly prominent, showing no opacities and no rupture of Descemet's membrane; corneal diameters measured 13·5 mm.; depth of anterior chamber was 5 mm.; iris showed no tremor; pupils were narrow and reacted well; discs were not excavated; tension normal.

V. 7 and 8 were twins of whom V. 7 died at birth; both twins were noticed at birth to have large eyes; V. 8, E. M., aged 6, was robust, healthy and intelligent; his eyes showed no inflammation and no photophobia; corneae were clear; right corneal diameter measured 14·5 mm., the left was 14 mm.; depth of anterior chamber was 4·5 mm.; iris showed no tremor; pupils were narrow and reacted normally; discs showed no excavation; Tension = 17 mm. Hg (Schiotz); R. V. = $\frac{6}{7}$, L. V. = $\frac{6}{8}$. The mother, IV. 7, had normal eyes. V. 86, K. M., aged 7, was born with large eyes; there was no inflammation in the eyes; corneae were prominent and completely clear; depth of anterior chambers was 4·5 mm.; corneal diameters measured 13·5 mm.; pupils were not dilated and showed normal reactions; media were clear; discs were not excavated; tension was not raised; V. 86 and his mother had slight myopia, his grandfather (? maternal) had myopia of 10 D.; otherwise the mother, IV. 81, had healthy and normal eyes. V. 83 also was born with large eyes; he appeared to be healthy and robust to the age of 3 years when he died from pneumonia.

V. 11, A. B., aged 22, saw well and considered that he had normal eyes; R. V. = L. V. = $\frac{6}{9} - \frac{6}{7}$ with + 1·5 D.; right corneal diameter measured 12 mm., left diameter was only 11 mm.; corneae were clear; depth of right anterior chamber was 3 mm., that of left anterior chamber was only 2 mm.; no abnormalities were found; tension in right eye was 14 mm. Hg (Schiotz). Kayser evidently fixes 12 mm. as his lower limit for the corneal measurement in megalocornea; on this standard the pedigree is not altogether comparable with that of Gredig who takes 13·0 mm. as his lower limit. V. 37, E. Z., aged 22, was not examined; his mother considered that he had normal eyes though they were perhaps larger than those of his siblings; the siblings, and mother, IV. 41, had normal eyes. IV. 47, Louis O., aged 38, was born with large eyes; he saw well and had no difficulty at school until the age of 17, when he had a corneal ulcer in the left eye, this had healed with a large scar so that vision was markedly contracted; the right cornea was prominent and measured 13 mm. in diameter; the anterior chamber was almost 5 mm. deep; the cornea was clear, pupil normal, iris without tremor; pressure was certainly not raised. The mother, III. 33, had normal eyes. IV. 43, Jakob O., aged 43, was not examined; he wrote that he had eyes like those of his brother, IV. 47; he had never had trouble with his eyes; his six children had normal eyes and saw well.

III. 38, Johannes Pf., aged 68, was born with large eyes; he had never had trouble with his eyes until recently when he noticed a diminution in vision; both eyes were free from inflammation; corneae were prominent with diameters of 14·5 mm.; anterior chambers were 4·5 mm. deep; corneae were clear, irides had a slight tremor; pupils were normal and reacted well; bilateral incipient cataract, more marked in the left lens, was noted; the right disc was not excavated; tension in the left eye was 18 mm. Hg (Schiotz); the mother of III. 38 was said to have had normal eyes. III. 41, Jakob Pf., aged 63, had seen well until the age of 40 when a diminution of vision was noted; at 52 he had acute glaucoma and senile incipient

PLATE LXVI.   DESCRIPTIONS OF PEDIGREE PLATES   507

cataract in the left eye; corneal diameter on the right measured 14·5 mm., on the left 14·2 mm.; at 59, III. 41 had glaucoma in the right eye complicated by cataract; operation for cataract was performed but the resulting vision was scarcely perception of light.

III. 7, Friedrich K., aged 85, was said by his daughter to have large eyes; he saw well in his youth but at the age of 44 received some injury to his eye through a wooden stick; the lens was luxated and was removed; twelve years later he had pain in the other eye and it was found that the lens was cataractous and was luxated into the anterior chamber; the patient ultimately became completely blind; the megalocornea was noted in hospital. III. 9, Heinrich K., appears also to have been blind in old age but no details were obtainable. Of II. 12, his niece III. 33, who often stayed in his house, reported that he had the large family eyes and never up to old age complained of his eyes or vision. Information regarding I. 1 was based on family tradition. No consanguinity recorded. Bibl. Nos. 208, 209.

Fig. 984. *Gredig's Case.* Megalocornea in eleven males and two or three females in four generations; only cases in which the corneal diameter measured 13·00 mm. or more are described as megalocornea; a number of members of the family whose corneal measurements were 12—13 mm. are regarded as within the normal limits. The recorder has a common standard for the two sexes, but if III. 2, with a corneal diameter of 13·00 mm. be regarded as anomalous for a male, it seems to me doubtful whether the corresponding measurement in his daughter of 12·75 mm. can be placed in the normal category; I have therefore entered IV. 1 in my chart as ? anomalous. Evidently great care has been taken in the preparation of this pedigree and in the measurements, which were taken wherever possible with a Wessely's keratometer; information concerning members who were dead, or inaccessible, was based on repeated enquiries from relatives and from photographs. The condition, as judged from this pedigree, is exhibited by both sexes but occurs predominantly in the male, if we may accept the recorder's common standard for the two sexes; both sexes transmit the defect; four or perhaps five males have affected offspring and it is unlikely that their wives were carriers, for the condition is rare and no consanguineous marriages had occurred; the family were living in the Canton of Zurich but III. 14 was married to a woman from another Canton and the wife of III. 19 was Italian.

The following measurements on individual cases are given:

Case	Age	Corneal Diameters in mm.	
		Right	Left
III. 15, Paul No.	47	14·50	14·50
III. 18, Otto No.	40	14·25	14·00
III. 14, Alfred No.	55	13·25	13·25
III. 17, August No.	44	13·25	13·25
III. 19, Leopold No.	56	13·25	13·25
IV. 10, Fritz No.	18	13·25	13·25
III. 25, Johanna M. No.	36	13·00	13·00
III. 2, Hermann Be.	—	13·00	13·00

All individuals of generations I and II, also III. 21 and 22, were dead at the time of the investigation. No consanguinity. Bibl. No. 268.

Fig. 985. *Grönholm's Case.* Megalocornea in eleven males and two females of three generations. The "kuppelförmigen Augen" of the affected members of this family were evidently a conspicuous feature, and the condition when present could be recognised by parents at the birth of their children; the recorder has had the family under observation for many years and shows how in these cases the cornea has enlarged slightly with the growth of the individual. Thus at the age of 4 years the cornea of V. 31 measured 13·5 mm., at the age of 9 the diameter was 14 mm.; in V. 34 at the age of 2 years the cornea measured 12 mm., at 6 years the measure had increased to 12·5 mm.; in V. 26 at 11 months the corneal diameter was 12·5 mm., at five years it had become 13 mm.; in V. 25 the corneal diameter measured 13 mm. at 1½ years and was unchanged at the age of 3½ years. In all the affected eyes the corneo-scleral margin was clear and circular; there were no signs of previous inflammation of the eyes; the sclera was white and opaque; the cornea, as seen with the split lamp and corneal microscope, was free from opacities; the corneae showed no signs of stretching or thinning; the anterior chambers were always unusually deep; the breadth of the iris in these cases was larger than normal; the pupils were usually circular and showed normal reactions; the ocular tension, visual fields and colour sense were normal in all the eyes examined. The enlargement belonged to the corneae and not to the globe of the eye; there was no exophthalmos; no case of hydrophthalmos or glaucoma had occurred in the family. Two of the cases, V. 32 and 33, had zonular cataract when seen at the ages of 4 and 3 years respectively; their only sister, V. 30, also had zonular cataract, she had not enlarged corneae. Nine cases were examined and only one of these had $\frac{6}{6}$ vision, as will be seen from the table below.

Case	Age	Horizontal Diameter of Cornea in mm.		Visual Acuity		Remarks
		Right	Left	Right	Left	
IV. 16	40	12·5	12·5	$\frac{6}{8}$	$\frac{6}{6}$	Tremulous irides
IV. 19	39	13·0	13·0	$\frac{6}{10}$	$\frac{6}{10}$	
V. 25	3	13·0	13·0	—	—	Saw well. Died aged 5
V. 26	5	13·0	13·0	$\frac{5}{7.5}$	$\frac{5}{7.5}$	
V. 29	10	13·0	13·0	$\frac{5}{10}$	$\frac{5}{10}$	—
V. 31	4	14·0	14·0	$\frac{5}{7.5}$	$\frac{5}{7.5}$	Tremulous irides
V. 32	7	14·0	14·0	$\frac{5}{7.5}$	$\frac{5}{7.5}$	Zonular cataract; tremulous irides
V. 33	6	12·0	12·0	$\frac{5}{7.5}$	$\frac{5}{7.5}$	,, ,, ,, ,,
V. 34	6	12·5	12·5	$\frac{5}{7.5}$	$\frac{5}{7.5}$	,, ,, — ,,

The family comes of an old Finlandish stock though I. 1 was a Swede. Nothing was known of the eyes of I. 1 and 2, but it was known that their children and the descendants of their three daughters had normal eyes and produced no case of megalocornea. I. 4 was believed to have been normal; a sketch of him was seen and enquiries were made amongst his relations; he had a number of normal descendants by his first wife. I. 5 was an only child; no information was available concerning her eyes or those of her father; the children of I. 4 and 5 were all known to be without megalocornea; II. 5 died young, II. 6 had only normal descendants, II. 8 and 9 were unmarried. The source of the megalocornea in the descendants of II. 2 and 4 is thus indefinite but the recorder thought it probably came through I. 5.

The children of II. 2 and 4 were mostly dead but many enquiries were made concerning them and photographs were examined; three of the nine brothers in this large family were believed to have megalocornea, they each had normal offspring; their two married sisters however, III. 11 and 15, had affected sons. IV. 8 was not examined, his sister said he had "Kuppelaugen." Two affected members of the family, III. 18 and IV. 19, married their first cousins within the affected stock; the wife of III. 18 had normal parents, the wife of IV. 19 had an affected father; III. 18 and 26 had seven unaffected children, one daughter of whom, IV. 23, had all her five sons affected, one of them perhaps doubtfully so. IV. 19 and 34 had two affected daughters and one normal son.

This is an interesting pedigree most carefully prepared and illustrated in the original account by very striking photographs of four of the affected individuals. Consanguinity. Bibl. No. 239.

Fig. 986. *Gertz's Case.* Megalocornea in two brothers whose two maternal uncles showed the same anomaly; the mother of the patients and her two sisters had normal eyes, as had the children of these two sisters and of the anomalous brothers; there was a tradition of similar cases of megalocornea at an earlier date in the family history, but definite information regarding them could not be found. II. 1, aged 16, was noticed at birth to have eyes which were "unheimlich gross"; the corneae are now (1915) circular with a diameter of 1·8 cm.; they were clear with a normal corneo-scleral margin; anterior chambers were very deep (5·5 mm.); lens and vitreous were clear; irides showed some tremor but were otherwise normal; R. V. with some correction for astigmatism was $\frac{6}{12}$; L. V. with correction = $\frac{6}{9}$; tension = 18 mm. Hg (Schiötz). II. 2, aged 9 years, presented the same anomaly; his corneal diameters measured 1·6 cm.; depth of anterior chambers 5·5 mm.; R. V. = L. V. = $\frac{6}{18}$ with correction; tension = 16 mm. Hg (Schiötz). No further abnormality was found in II. 1 and 2; their two sisters, II. 3 and 4, had normal eyes. No consanguinity recorded. Bibl. No. 214.

Fig. 987. *Petres's Case.* Megalocornea in a father and in two of his sons; the corneal diameters measured from 13 to 16 mm. No statement is made regarding other members of the family. No consanguinity recorded. Bibl. No. 278.

Fig. 988. *Muralt's Case.* Megalocornea in Gottlieb M., Albert M. and Edward M., aged 26, 24 and 20 years respectively; in each of the brothers the anterior chambers were very deep, irides tremulous, pupils rather wider than normal; the intraocular pressure was not raised in any case and there was no excavation of the papilla; for II. 1, R. V. = $\frac{1}{2} - \frac{2}{3}$, L. V. = $\frac{1}{2}$. The parents and one sister of the affected brothers had normal eyes. No consanguinity recorded. Bibl. No. 51.

Fig. 989. *Pflüger's Case.* Megalocornea in five siblings. II. 1, E. M., aged 44, had had very large eyes since birth; both eyes were the same size; until ten years ago he had been able to see quite well, then a progressive diminution of vision was first noticed; five years ago the left eye was operated on for cataract but vision was not improved and the left eye was now phthisical; corneal diameter in the right eye measured 18 mm.; tension was not raised; the anterior chamber was very deep; iris and lens were tremulous

PLATE LXVI.   DESCRIPTIONS OF PEDIGREE PLATES   509

the lens was partially opaque; R. V. = fingers at $1\frac{1}{2}$ m.; there was an opaque ring at the limbus of the cornea but the centre was clear. The parents of II. 1 had normal eyes, but all his four siblings were reported to have eyes which were larger than normal and had always been so. No consanguinity recorded. Bibl. No. 120.

Fig. 990. *Bondi's Case.* II. 1, A. S., aged 17, was noted to have large eyes at birth; the whole eyeball appeared to be enlarged, but the anomaly was most marked in the corneae, with horizontal diameters of 17 mm., vertical diameters of about 16 mm.; the anterior chambers were at least 5 mm. deep; pupils were central and reacted promptly; both pupils showed a remnant of a persistent pupillary membrane; corneae, lenses and vitreous were clear; myopic astigmatism was noted in the right eye, simple myopia of about 2 D. in the left; R. V. with – 2·0 D. Sph. = $\frac{5}{10}$, L. V. = $\frac{5}{6}$; fields were full; colour and light sense normal. None of the siblings of II. 1 nor his parents showed similar anomalies; all had good vision; one sister, with normal sized eyes, had a son, III. 1, who was noted at birth to have large eyes.

III. 1, A. W., aged 12, had a right eye markedly larger than his almost normal left eye; he complained of no visual difficulties; both bulbs were definitely enlarged; the right cornea was normal apart from its size, which measured $15\frac{1}{2}$ mm. in the horizontal, 15 mm. in the vertical diameter; the anterior chamber was very deep—about 5 mm.—iris was normal, pupil circular and prompt in reaction; there was no trace of a persistent pupillary membrane; lens and vitreous were clear, fundus normal; R. V. = $\frac{6}{8}$; the left cornea had a horizontal diameter of 13 mm., vertical diameter of $12\frac{1}{2}$ mm.; the anterior chamber was deeper than normal; vision was reduced to $\frac{6}{12}$ owing to a small central corneal scar; fields were full, colour and light sense normal. Two siblings of III. 1 had normal eyes. No consanguinity recorded. Bibl. No. 134.

Fig. 991. *Weizenblatt's Case.* Megalocornea in I. 2 and in his brother, also in two of his children, of whom one was a daughter; only one case was examined. II. 2, aged 33, had wide lid clefts and not particularly large globes, but her corneae were enlarged in all their measurements; R. horizontal diameter = 16 mm., L. measurement = 15·8 mm.; the corresponding vertical diameters measured 15·5 mm. and 16 mm. respectively; anterior chambers were extraordinarily deep; an embryontoxon was noted in each eye. No consanguinity recorded. Bibl. No. 279.

Fig. 992. *Pflüger's Case.* II. 1, aged 14, had always been healthy and had never had inflammation in his eyes; he had bilateral megalocornea; the anterior chambers were deep, the irides slightly tremulous; there was an opaque marginal ring on each cornea resembling arcus senilis; tension was normal; pupils reacted well; fundi were normal; R. V. with – 1·0 D. = $\frac{6}{12}$, L. V. with – 0·75 D. = $\frac{6}{9}$. The parents of II. 1 had normal eyes; they had had thirteen children of whom four died young; two of the living siblings of II. 1 also had large eyes. No consanguinity recorded. Bibl. No. 120.

BUPHTHALMOS

Fig. 993. *Zahn's Case.* Buphthalmos in four siblings and in two of their cousins. II. 1, Johannes P. seen aged 9 years, had buphthalmos affecting the left eye only; the condition had been first noticed at a very early age. II. 2, Katharine P., was dead but was reported to have had large eyes. II. 3, 5, 6, and II. 9 had good eyes; II. 4 was still-born but was said to have had normal eyes. II. 7, August P., seen aged 10 months, had bilateral buphthalmos which had been present since birth. II. 8, Agnes P., seen aged 2 years, had a similar bilateral affection which had been noticed very shortly after birth. The parents of this sibship were first cousins. The only other members of the family known to suffer from any eye disease are two cousins to the affected siblings of whom II. 10, Anna Sch., was seen, aged 9 months, to have bilateral buphthalmos; the condition had been noticed at birth. II. 11, Karl Sch., was examined and reported to have the same condition. II. 12, Marie Sch., was dead but was reported to have had good eyes. II. 13, Richard Sch., had good eyes. The parents of the sibship II. 10—13 were not related. Consanguinity. Bibl. No. 168.

Fig. 994. *Muralt's Case.* Buphthalmos in three members of a sibship of nine; the parents were healthy and saw well. II. 2, Johannes H., aged 20, was mentally and physically rather backward, but there was no definite abnormality apart from his eyes; his right eye was now reduced to the state of phthisis bulbi; at birth both eyes had been abnormal in size; the left eye now had horizontal and vertical corneal diameters of 14 and $14\frac{1}{2}$ mm. respectively; its prominence also was measured by 14 mm.; both corneae had had a bluish shimmer and were never transparent; the left eye now had very marked nystagmus; L. V. = finger counting at 4 feet; the left disc showed marked central excavation. II. 8, George H., aged 10, had been noticed soon after his birth to have opacities affecting his very large corneae; now the central part of each cornea was very protuberant, whitish, opaque and vascularised; the periphery of the right cornea was transparent over a narrow zone; the left eye had no transparent zone; there had been no history of ophthalmia neonatorum; not alone the cornea but the whole eyeball on each side was enlarged; the right lens showed an anterior capsular cataract; vision was reduced to perception of light; the sensibility of the corneae was normal; in the right eye horizontal and vertical corneal diameters measured 15 mm. and 19 mm. respectively, corresponding values for the left eye were 14 mm. and 17 mm.; prominence of the right eye was measured by 18 mm., of the left eye by 17 mm.; this patient had always been healthy, had a normal skull, good hearing and was a well-developed youth. II. 9, Pauline H., was seen aged 9 months; soon after birth she was noticed to have bilateral opacities in her very large corneae; the left cornea was very large and protuberant, the right cornea was only a little larger than normal but it was clear that the condition was progressing; the child died from some acute illness the same year. Two brothers and four sisters of this sibship were healthy and saw well; the father, aged 50, had some myopia but saw well; the mother had normal eyes. No consanguinity recorded. Bibl. No. 51.

Fig. 995. *Jungken's Case.* Buphthalmos in seven brothers of a Swedish family. The parents and two sisters had normal eyes. No consanguinity recorded. Bibl. No. 19.

Fig. 996. *Derby's Case.* Buphthalmos in three males and one female of a sibship of eight; two males and the female were blind; the disease in all cases came on in early childhood; the eyes rapidly enlarged and ultimately ruptured during some straining effort or from the effect of a blow. The parents were still living and were perfectly healthy; the disease had not been known to occur in the family before the affected sibship. No child of any member of the affected sibship, whether blind or seeing, had shown signs of any other form of eye disease. II. 3, seen aged 22, said the condition in his case had steadily increased since birth; the right eye was more markedly affected than the left and was operated on by an iridectomy two years ago; no improvement in vision followed this treatment; R. V. = ? p. l.; the eye was now very prominent; T. = + 2; anterior chamber was very deep; the corneal diameter was greatly enlarged; optic disc was not excavated. The left eye of II. 3 was less prominent; T. = + 2; corneal diameter was rather less enlarged; anterior chamber was deep; L. V. with − ¼ D. = $\frac{1}{3\frac{1}{2}}$ and vision was steadily failing; this eye showed a deep excavation of the optic disc; some temporary improvement followed an iridectomy. Seen at the age of 38 this man had L. V. = hand movements at 10 feet, his affected brothers and sister were blind before the age of 17; II. 3 had been able to read up to the age of 12 years. No consanguinity recorded. Bibl. No. 76.

Fig. 997. *Zahn's Case.* III. 2, Karl M., was seen at the age of 9 months when he had bilateral buphthalmos; the condition was first noticed shortly after birth; two older and two younger siblings of the patient were normal. The grandfather of III. 1 was reported to have become blind early in life following dropsy of the eyes. No consanguinity. Bibl. No. 168.

Fig. 998. *Zahn's Case.* Buphthalmos in four siblings and in their second cousin. II. 5, Paul F., was seen aged 8 weeks in 1891; both eyes were affected; the age of onset was not known. II. 6, Marie F., was seen at the age of 9 weeks in 1902; both eyes were said to have been affected at birth. The parents of these children were very distantly related; they had seven other children of whom two died in infancy without any defect in their eyes having been noticed; II. 2 and II. 3 had buphthalmos; II. 4 represents three healthy unaffected children. A cousin of the father, I. 2, of the affected sibship had a son II. 7, Friedrich T., who was seen aged 21 days (1891) with bilateral buphthalmos which was said to have been present at birth. The parents of II. 7 were third cousins. Consanguinity. Bibl. No. 168.

Fig. 999. *Johnson's Case.* I. 1, J. F., was not aware that any member of his or his wife's family had suffered from eye disease; when he was aged about 7 years his parents first noticed some disease affecting his left eye with which he had no perception of light; he thinks he never had vision with this eye and does not remember any inflammatory reaction in it; the left pupil was now dilated, the lens was calcareous and partially disintegrated; tension was not raised; R.V. = $\frac{2}{20}$, L V. = no p.l. This man, his wife and children had robust general health. Of the children, II. 1, 2, and 3 had no physical defect. II. 4, J. F., aged 7, had buphthalmos · her parents noticed at the age of 2 months that her eyes were increasing in size, lachrymation was constant and profuse, corneae were hazy, sight was dim; after 2 years' treatment with drops, operation was performed and no further increase in size had occurred; eyeballs were enormously enlarged, tension about + 1, corneae somewhat hazy with horizontal diameter of ½ inch, vertical diameter of $\frac{5}{8}$ inch; anterior chambers were of about the usual depth; right lens was opaque and fundus could not be seen; the left fundus showed retinal vessels diminished, the disc bluish white and considerably cupped; R.V. = no p.l., L.V. = finger counting at 2 feet. II. 5, M. F., aged 2 years, was noticed at the age of one month to have eyes which were increasing in size, they were photophobic, lachrymation was frequent, corneae were becoming hazy; at 2 months iridectomy was performed on the right eye, the iris was incarcerated and the pupil distorted; probably sclerotomy was performed on the left eye; now the right eye was larger than the left; the anterior chambers were of normal depth; tension in the right eye was slightly increased, in the left eye was normal; the father thought this child saw well but she would not allow examination; there was a large area of retino-choroidal imflammation below the macula; the discs were slightly pale but showed no cupping. II. 6 showed a gradual development of the disease; her eyeballs increased in size, the right more markedly than the left; corneae became hazy; pupils were slightly dilated and responded slowly to light; anterior chambers were somewhat shallow; tension was + 2; lachrymation and photophobia were present; double iridectomy upwards was performed. At a later date the parents said there was now no further trouble with the eyes; the right coloboma was satisfactory, in the left the iris had become incarcerated and the pupil distorted. No consanguinity recorded. Bibl. No. 136.

PLATE LXVII.   DESCRIPTIONS OF PEDIGREE PLATES   511

PLATE LXVII. Fig. 1000. *Mann's Case.* Buphthalmos in three children of a sibship of six. I. 1 and 2 say they have never had trouble with their eyes and have never attended at hospital for them; the mother of I. 2 once attended at hospital for some apparently trivial eye trouble of a temporary character and now (1931) sees very well; the brothers and sisters of I. 1 and 2 are all free from eye trouble and have between them 25 children, all of whom are believed to have normal eyes. Of the affected sibship, II. 1, Ernest C., born 1914, is at the Norwood College for the Blind; he had congenital buphthalmos for which the right eye has been excised; vision in the left eye is reduced to perception of light only. II. 2, aged 12, is buphthalmic and has undergone various operations; she has a good visual result in the right eye and attends an ordinary school, but is blind in the left eye. II. 3, aged 10, and II. 4, aged 8 years, have normal vision. II. 5, aged 3½ years, has bilateral buphthalmos and dislocated lenses; he is blind. II. 6, aged 1 year, is said by the mother to be normal. No consanguinity recorded. Hitherto unpublished.

Fig. 1001. *Fleischer's Case.* II. 3, Agnes P., aged 21, had had large eyes since birth; she now had raised tension and a glaucomatous contraction of the visual fields; V. = $\frac{5}{6}$; trepanation was followed by recovery. Two brothers of II. 1, and a cousin, had suffered from buphthalmos. No consanguinity recorded. Bibl. No. 224.

Fig. 1002. *Rampoldi's Case.* II. 5, seen aged 10 months, was born with bilateral buphthalmos and diffuse keratitis; nystagmus was noted. The mother, I. 2, had had five children of whom the first two had no eye affection but died early in life, the last three all had congenital keratitis and buphthalmos. No consanguinity recorded. Bibl. No. 81.

Fig. 1003. *Muralt's Case.* II. 2, Joseph Z., seen aged 8, was a well nourished, normally developed boy with marked photophobia and reddening of the conjunctiva bulbi; he had bilateral megalophthalmos more marked on the right side; the ophthalmoscope showed a deep pressure excavation of the papilla more extreme on the right side; the discs were pale; the intraocular pressure was much raised and the corneae were thin; visual acuity could not be determined because of the extreme photophobia; corneal horizontal diameters were 12—13 mm. in the left, 15 mm. in the right eye, the vertical diameters were similar; prominence of the eyeball was measured by 15 mm. in the right, 12 mm. on the left side; iridectomy was performed on both sides and subsequently R. V. = $\frac{1}{20}$, L. V. = about $\frac{1}{2}$. II. 1, Heinrich Z., aged 10, had horizontal corneal diameters of 15 mm. on the right, 17 mm. on the left side; prominence of the eyeball was measured by 18 mm. on the right and 16 mm. on the left; he had a high intraocular pressure, and deep pressure excavation of the disc on each side; there was a capsular cataract in the right lens; this boy went to school until three years ago and could read, but could no longer see even to count fingers. A brother and sister saw well; the parents saw well and knew of no similar eye disease amongst their relations. No consanguinity recorded. Bibl. No. 51.

Fig. 1004. *von Ammon's Case.* II. 1, seen aged 19, had megalophthalmos of a medium grade; she had exophthalmos and squinted at times; her corneae were very arched and half conical; the sclerae were normal posteriorly but towards the front they were thinned and bluish; some opacity of the lens was noted. The mother of II. 1 suffered from the same defect; the siblings of II. 1 were not affected. No further information is given; a coloured plate illustrates the condition. No consanguinity recorded. Bibl. No. 32.

Fig. 1005. *Dürr and Schlegtendal's Case.* II. 2, Annette E., seen aged 18, had seen badly from childhood; she had hydrophthalmos first in the right, later in the left eye; in other respects she was well developed if rather backward in growth. At the age of 14 it was noted that in the right eye the cornea was markedly arched; the anterior chamber was 9 mm. deep: the horizontal diameter of the cornea measured 15 mm., vertical diameter 15·3 mm.; the deep parts of the peripheral cornea were opaque; the sclera was ectatic in the region of the ciliary body and bluish in colour; the bulb was of stony hardness; cataract was present; V. = no p. l.; the left eye had markedly prominent cornea with diameters of 15·0 mm. horizontal, 14·7 mm. vertical; the papilla was deeply excavated; myopia of 8 D.; L. V. = $\frac{1}{12}$; field very contracted. The right eye was excised; iridectomy on the left eye led to V. = $\frac{1}{9}$ with − 8 D., but the tension remained very high. The right lens was not enlarged. The parents of II. 2 were first cousins; they had normal eyes and were healthy; two of their sons, August E., aged 20, and Karl C., aged 8, also suffered from hydrophthalmos; otherwise no hereditary disease was known to have occurred in the family. We are not told whether there were normal siblings between Annette, aged 18, and Karl, aged 8 years. Consanguinity. Bibl. No. 100.

Fig. 1006. *Angelucci's Case.* Buphthalmos in three brothers whose mother had exophthalmic goitre. No further information is given in the citation of the case by de Lapersonne. No consanguinity recorded. Bibl. No. 158.

Fig. 1007. *Reis's Case.* II. 3, Hans M. S., aged 5 weeks, the child of consanguineous parents, had a slightly opaque enlarged and bulging cornea in his right eye; the disc was not excavated; the left cornea was so opaque that the disc could not be seen, and the anterior chamber was much deeper than on the right side. The condition progressed so that at the age of 4 years the left lid could not be closed, the iris could not be seen through the opaque cornea, and the bulb was hard; the right disc could still be seen, but this eye was being irritated by the left eye which was now excised. The two brothers of this child were similarly affected. Consanguinity. Bibl. No. 170.

Fig. 1008. *Aurand's Case.* II. 2, aged 8 years, had both eyes normal at birth; the right eye commenced to enlarge at the end of two months, with some flow of tears but no signs of inflammation; the growth slowly increased, with pain occasionally, and complete blindness ensued; the vision of the left eye was normal, but the diameter of the cornea was abnormally large; there was no sign of hereditary syphilis; media in the affected eye were clear but there was very marked glaucomatous atrophy of the disc; fundus in the left eye was normal. II. 3, aged 6, was born with normal eyes, but at the age of 3 months he began to suffer from inflammatory reactions in the right eye; at about the age of one year the left eye began to increase in size; now the right eye was of normal size, but an opaque lens was luxated into the anterior chamber and the eye was blind; the left eye was buphthalmic to a less degree than the right eye of his brother; he had iridodonesis and subluxation of the lens upwards and inwards; tension was + 2; the disc was pale and the eye could only distinguish fingers. These brothers were the two youngest children of a sibship of seven; five siblings and the parents had normal vision; the parents were healthy; the mother had been well at the birth of the children and had no history of miscarriages. No consanguinity recorded. Bibl. No. 259.

Fig. 1009. *Muralt's Case.* Buphthalmos in two brothers. I. 1 said to be myopic, I. 2 said to be hypermetropic, probably no serious defect in either. II. 2 said to be a very high grade myope. II. 3, Theodor S., aged 4½ years, saw very little with the left eye and had a colossal keratoglobus; the cornea was opaque at the margin and the eyeball was of a stony hardness; the right eye showed similar but less severe defects; deep pressure excavation of the disc with kinking of the vessels was seen on ophthalmoscopic examination. II. 1, Emil S., aged 7, was noticed soon after birth to have abnormally large corneae; at that time the patient was dazzled by light and evidently had very defective vision; he was now totally blind; a year ago bilateral buphthalmos with complete blindness was reported, since then the right eye had ruptured and was lost. No consanguinity recorded. Bibl. No. 51.

Fig. 1010. *Zahn's Case.* II. 1, Marie W., aged 9 years, was seen to have bilateral buphthalmos which had been noticed in her first year of life. II. 3, Joseph W., aged 3, was similarly affected in the right eye only, the disease in his case was noted at birth. Other siblings were healthy. No consanguinity. Bibl. No. 168.

Fig. 1011. *Zahn's Case.* II. 1, Ursula U., was seen aged 10 years with bilateral buphthalmos; the disease first became noticeable in her second year of life. II. 3, seen aged 6 months, had during this month shown the same condition in both eyes. Three siblings were healthy and no further cases of eye disease had been known to occur in the family. No consanguinity. Bibl. No. 168.

Fig. 1012. *Peter's Case.* An Italian child aged 5 months was first seen aged one week, when both corneae were large, measuring 15 mm. in diameter and bluish in colour, with central opacities; the sclerae were bluish in colour; anterior chambers were very deep; pupils were large even under the influence of eserine; tension was raised; the child had good light perception and apparently good projection. A brother of the patient, aged 6 years, had a similar condition at birth; his left eye was removed at the age of one year, the right eye was now blind and in an irritable state. Consanguinity. Bibl. No. 225.

Fig. 1013. *Argyll Robertson's Case.* Buphthalmos in a mother and her three children; the mother showed the condition to the more marked degree; the condition was bilateral in one daughter and the son; a second daughter had one eye normal in all respects. The son, II. 2, was subject to recurrent attacks of inflammation with increased tension which were checked by the use of eserine. The diseased eye in II. 3 was enucleated, as it caused sympathetic irritation in the other eye. The father of the three affected children was blind from an accident to one eye, which led to sympathetic inflammation in the other, at an early period of life. No consanguinity recorded. Bibl. No. 106.

Fig. 1014. *Golomb's Case.* II. 3 was seen, aged 9½ years, with hydrophthalmos in the right eye, phthisis bulbi of the left; the patient had seen very badly as quite a small child; at the age of 2 years he became blind in the right eye, following some trauma, soon afterwards the left eye also was blind. One brother was said to have the same disease. No consanguinity. Bibl. No. 199.

Fig. 1015. *Zahn's Case.* II. 1, Emma S., was seen at the age of 8 years with bilateral buphthalmos; the time of onset of the disease was not known; a younger sister, who was mentally defective, was reported to have the same changes in her eyes. No consanguinity. Bibl. No. 168.

Fig. 1016. *Golomb's Case.* II. 3 was seen aged 9 months with bilateral buphthalmos; both eyes were enlarged and prominent, with very large opaque corneae; the child noticed a light; signs of rickets were observed; the mother said the enlargement of the eyes had been noticed some months before. II. 2 had the same disease; operation had been performed and vision was now ⅓. Bilateral iridectomy was performed on II 3. No consanguinity. Bibl. No. 199.

Plate LXVII.   DESCRIPTIONS OF PEDIGREE PLATES   513

Fig. 1017. *Golomb's Case.* Buphthalmos in the right eye, phthisis bulbi in the left was seen in Hugo N., aged 13 years; he was blind and did not know when he lost his sight; one brother had lost his sight from the same disease. No consanguinity. Bibl. No. 199.

Fig. 1018. *Golomb's Case.* II. 3, Rudolph G., was seen aged 13 years, with bilateral buphthalmos; he had been blind for eleven years; both bulbs were now enucleated. One brother was said to have the same disease. No consanguinity. Bibl. No. 199.

Fig. 1019. *Fleischer's Case.* II. 1 had an iridectomy performed at the age of 9 weeks for bilateral buphthalmos; he died aged 1 year. II. 2, Eugen L., aged 6 years, had had the right eye larger than the left for 4 weeks, also inflammation of the eyes; the left eye had a rather large cornea but was otherwise normal; the right eye showed a marked enlargement of the cornea, raised tension, diffuse opacity of the cornea, very deep anterior chamber; R. V. = finger counting at 1 m., L. V. = $\frac{4}{5}$; trepanation was resorted to twice, also iridectomy. Three years later there had been no recurrence of acute trouble; both corneae were large, R. = 13·5 mm. in diameter, L. = 12·5 mm., they were clear and shining; anterior chambers were deep; the papilla in the right eye was white, with a shallow temporal excavation. The child was robust in other respects. No other case of eye disease had been known to occur in the family. No consanguinity recorded. Bibl. No. 224.

Fig. 1020. *Streatfield's Case.* II. 3, Harriet H., aged six months (1882), had very large staring eyes; the condition had been noted at birth but had become more marked since; the irides were tremulous and thinned; no tears were noted in the corneae; anterior chambers were very shallow; tension in each eye was at least + 2. An elder sister of II. 3 had also been born with large eyes; a double iridectomy had been performed in this case with bad results so that the left eye had to be excised, the right eye had just perception of light. No consanguinity recorded. Bibl. No. 79.

Fig. 1021. *Venneman's Case.* Buphthalmos, unilateral in a mother, bilateral in her son, aged 2 months. The child had two voluminous eyes. At the age of 13 years the mother's left eye, up to this time voluminous but painless, gave trouble, and operative assistance was required; after operation all pain disappeared and the eye had since remained quiet; she is now aged 20 years. No consanguinity recorded. Bibl. No. 159.

Fig. 1022. *Vogt's Case.* Buphthalmos in rabbits. Three black and white one year old rabbits of one litter were seen with bilateral high grade buphthalmos; the condition had apparently been observed nine months before. Two of these rabbits were mated and there resulted a litter of three, all of which had bilateral high grade buphthalmos; the disease in these animals was not congenital but was first noticed a few weeks after birth. Bibl. No. 232.

GLAUCOMA

Fig. 1023. *Plocher's Case.* This very interesting pedigree is the most complete family history of glaucoma known to me; the disease has been traced through six generations, twenty members being affected and three others having had prodromal symptoms. The earlier history of the families was obtained by the recorder from the church registers where, on the one side it was traced back to Hans Räuber, born in 1681, all of whose descendants appeared to be normal; on the other side it was traced to Simon D., I. 3, born 1753, who was said by his great grandson, IV. 5, to have had very bad eyes and to have been blind. I. 3 died, aged 60, in 1814; he had ten children of whom the eldest, II. 2, normal herself, married a descendant of Hans Räuber and transmitted the disease to a large number of her descendants. The second child of I. 3 had three normal children and later a normal grandchild, IV. 11, who married her second cousin, the affected IV. 5; together they handed on the disease to all their four children. II. 5, II. 8 and II. 9, died in infancy. II. 6, herself normal, married and had six children of whom two were blind, also a grandchild in America, IV. 12, who was blind. II. 11, himself unaffected, had a blind daughter in America. II. 13 was blind; this was the only affected member in the family of Simon D. amongst those who lived long enough to develop the disease.

The eyes of the descendants of II. 1 and 2 are described by the recorder in great detail, any treatment they may have had and their progress being traced over a considerable period of time. It is only possible here to give a brief summary of the findings in the various cases.

II. 1 and 2 had three children. III. 2, born 1814, was operated on for glaucoma in 1859 and later became blind; III. 3 lived to be 87 years of age and had good sight; III. 4, born 1817, became blind from glaucoma in his 45th year. III. 1 and III. 5 had good sight.

IV. 1, born 1842, died aged 50; at the age of 41 she had raised tension, with a history of prodromal symptoms for several months; the eyes were free from inflammation but there was marked glaucomatous excavation; R. V. with − 1·25 D. = $\frac{2}{5}$, L. V. = $\frac{1}{100}$; iridectomy was done first on the left, later on the right eye; seven years later the tension was still raised; this patient was unmarried. IV. 2, born 1843, was able-bodied at the age of 73 and had good eyes; her three children and four grandchildren had no trouble with their eyes. IV. 4, born 1846, had been almost blind since her 28th year; for some years before this she had severe toothache and headache, and it was noticed that her visual acuity was gradually diminishing;

she was then aged 71, but had never consulted an oculist, and some unqualified person had treated her in such a way that it was not possible to say whether or no she had had glaucoma; this woman never married. IV. 5, born 1852, noticed the sight of both eyes failing when he was aged 37; he had been completely blind since 1896; this man was said to have always had red eyes and rainbow vision; when seen, at the age of 65, he was completely blind and had multiple opacities in the cornea. IV. 5 married his second cousin; all their four children had glaucoma. All the three children of III. 4 were affected; of them IV. 7, born 1845, had an iridectomy performed in 1878 for glaucoma simplex which first troubled her at the age of 31; she died aged 42. IV. 8, born 1849, sought treatment in 1906; he had first noticed trouble with his eyes three years before at the age of 54, since when he had had transient attacks of cloudy vision, especially in winter; this patient had no pain; the right eye had a steamy cornea with a rather shallow anterior chamber; fundus was difficult to see but no excavation of the papilla was identified; R. T. = + $\frac{1}{2}$, R. V. = $\frac{6}{20}$; in the left the cornea was dull, the anterior chamber rather shallow; the papilla was excavated and the field much narrowed. L. T. = + $\frac{1}{2}$; this eye was nearly blind. IV. 9 had good vision. IV. 10, born 1857, was under treatment for choroiditis in 1888 and 1891; she complained of headaches; the right papilla was deeply excavated in 1888 at the age of 31, but she made no complaint of failing vision until five years later when she said that her left vision had failed badly during the previous fortnight; she was found to have glaucomatous excavation, with arterial pulsation specially marked in the left eye: tension of + 2; this patient had myopia of − 8 D.

V. 6, born 1881, was wounded in the left eye in 1894; at the age of 25 he was first under treatment for glaucoma; he underwent repeated operations during about ten years, after which R. V. = fingers at $\frac{3}{4}$ m., L. V. = fingers at $\frac{1}{2}$—$\frac{3}{4}$ m. V. 7, born 1882, was seen at the age of 35, when she said that her eyes had never shown signs of inflammation, but that she had been seeing rainbows occasionally, particularly in the winter, for several years; she was liable to slight headaches; refraction was + 1·0 D.; externally and ophthalmoscopically her eyes were completely normal; two of the five children of V. 7, aged 11 and 10 respectively, VI. 7 and 8, were already seeing rainbows and one of them, VI. 8, had occasionally inflammatory symptoms in her eyes. V. 9, born 1888, first sought aid for symptoms of glaucoma simplex at the age of 27; for eighteen years before this she had been subject to bad headaches, and seen rainbows, but had good sight; this patient was excitable and readily got tachycardia; she was trephined and later R. V. = fingers at $\frac{1}{2}$ m., L. V. = $\frac{6}{60}$ with correction. V. 9 was married to V. 10 who saw well; they had four children, aged 10, 9, 7 and 2$\frac{1}{2}$ years respectively, who had not yet shown any signs of trouble. V. 11 born 1890, had seen rainbows for many years, especially in winter, she also suffered from severe headaches; the tension in each eye was raised, but her eyes, externally and ophthalmoscopically, were in other respects completely normal; R. V. = $\frac{4}{5}$, L. V. = $\frac{4}{5}$; the only child of V. 11 was aged 4 years. V. 13, born 1864, had bilateral chronic glaucoma at the age of 34; two years later an iridectomy was done; in 1902 this patient was seen, when marked contraction of visual fields, high tension, and bilateral atrophic glaucomatous excavation of the papilla were noted. V. 15, born 1869, was single but had two illegitimate twin daughters; she was examined at the age of 38 when R. V. with + 3·0 D. = $\frac{3}{20}$, L. V. = $\frac{6}{5}$; she showed no signs of glaucoma but had a central scotoma in the right field and a coloboma of the choroid in the left eye. The two children of V. 15 were healthy and saw well. V. 19, born 1877, first noticed a diminution in vision, with clouds before her eyes, at the age of 29; the left papilla was deeply excavated; L. V. with − 3·0 D. = $\frac{6}{60}$; the right papilla was also deeply excavated; R. V. = fingers at 5 m.; tension = + 1. The four children of V. 19 were healthy and saw well when examined at the ages of 13, 12, 9 and 7 years respectively. V. 21, born 1878, was seen with glaucoma simplex at the age of 26; tension = + 1; R. V. = $\frac{6}{8}$, L. V. with − 0·5 D. = $\frac{6}{8}$; total glaucomatous excavation was noted at this date and iridectomy was performed; severe symptoms persisted and further treatment is described; in 1917 there was a mature cataract in the left lens; at this time R. T. = 22 mm. Hg, L. T. = 35 mm. Hg. The only other affected member of generation V was V. 24, born 1890, who was seen with glaucoma in 1908; she stated that she had noticed a diminution in her right vision for two years, also a defect in the vision of her left eye for one year; she often had bad headaches and rainbow vision; she had deep glaucomatous excavation of the papillae, and other characteristic signs. Members of generation VI were all young at the date of publication; VI. 7 and 8 were the only two who had yet shown any signs of the disease. Consanguinity. Bibl. No. 226.

Fig. 1024. *Cridland's Case.* Chronic glaucoma in a brother and sister. II. 3, aged 20, complained that for a year her eyes had ached and felt weak; she noted occasional rainbows round the light at night; the patient's corneae appeared small and measured 10 mm. in each eye; anterior chambers were rather deep; discs showed well-marked cupping more of a physiological than a glaucomatous character; T. = 42 mm. Hg (Schiötz) in each eye; R. V. = L. V. = $\frac{4}{5}$; fields showed some contraction everywhere except below; operation was performed on both eyes. The brother of II. 3, aged 30 years, had been under treatment for glaucoma for two years. No consanguinity recorded. Bibl. No. 246.

Fig. 1025. *Kirkpatrick's Case.* I. 3, the daughter of a Jewish mother, developed glaucoma between the ages of 47 and 50 years, and died after an unsuccessful operation; she had four sons and three daughters, of whom II. 9 died, aged 26; three sons and two daughters were alive and healthy, one daughter, II. 3, was

Plate LXVII.   DESCRIPTIONS OF PEDIGREÉ PLATES   515

blind from glaucoma in both eyes. Two sons of II. 3 were attacked by glaucoma in one eye, at an interval of a year, at the ages of 45 and 47 years respectively; the younger son became first affected. II. 2, the father of the affected sons, III. 1 and 2, had a healthy family history. No cousins of III. 1 and 2 had developed the disease. No consanguinity recorded. Hitherto unpublished.

Fig. 1026. *James's Case.* I. 1, a country parson, the eldest of a family of eight, died over 60 years of age and so far as was known exhibited no signs or symptoms of glaucoma; the youngest brother of I. 1, also the wife of this brother, I. 6, were said by II. 2 to have chronic glaucoma; the other six siblings of I. 1 were evidently not known to have shown any signs of similar trouble. I. 5 and 6 were said to have children who had shown no signs of glaucoma. I. 2, wife of I. 1, accidentally discovered that the vision of her right eye was defective, she saw M.: Doyne who diagnosed glaucoma; vision was less than $\frac{6}{60}$, the disc was cupped, the field curtailed in an unusual way for glaucoma, tension was raised, pupils equal; the eye was trephined; I. 2 was aged 61 at this time; the eye did not do well and about two years later it was excised; the left eye had V. $= \frac{6}{9}$ and exhibited no signs of glaucoma up to the death of the patient at the age of 65. I. 2 was the eldest of a sibship of four; so far as was known no other member of her family showed signs of glaucoma. I. 1 and 2 had nine children, of whom II. 1, aged 60 years, had shown no signs of the disease. II. 2, aged 58, complained of no symptoms of glaucoma; R. V. with − 5·5 D. sph. − 1·0 D. cyl. axis 50° in, $= \frac{6}{5}$, L. V. with − 5·5 D. sph. − 0·5 D. cyl. axis 50° in, $= \frac{6}{5}$: the tension was normal in the left, slightly raised in the right eye; the left field was normal; the right field showed a defect characteristic of chronic glaucoma, up and in, and slight general enlargement of the blind spot; the patient was under observation for a time after which the diagnosis was confirmed and the right eye was trephined, with a small basal iridectomy. II. 3 was seen, aged 56, in 1925, by Mr Foster Moore, when R. V. = L. V. $= \frac{6}{5}$; tension was raised in each eye, discs were cupped and arterial pulsation was present; practically the whole of the upper part of the left field was absent, the right field showed a defect typical of chronic glaucoma; after consultation both eyes were trephined: this patient had first noticed trouble with her eyes in 1923; when seen in 1926: R. V. = L. V. $= \frac{6}{5}$, with + 2·0 D. sph. II. 4, aged 54, had noticed some trouble with her eyes for six months when she consulted Sir John Parsons; tension was normal in the right, slightly raised in the left eye; R. V. $= \frac{6}{5}$, L. V. $= \frac{6}{5}$ partly, with + 1·0 D. sph. $= \frac{6}{5}$; each disc was deeply cupped; left field was contracted almost to the fixation point, right field showed the usual defect in the nasal area; both eyes were trephined and when discharged from hospital central vision was good, both fields were contracted almost to the fixation point, in the up-in direction. II. 5, aged 53 (1926), had noticed halos since 1918, and had a history of very bad vision, without pain, in the left eye during the last two years; the right eye was now also showing signs of failure; R. V. $= \frac{6}{5}$ partly, L. V. = faint perception of light; tension was normal in the right, slightly raised in the left eye: on the right the disc was pale with some disturbance of vessels, there was a steep edge to the not very deep cup, the field showed a typical contraction; the left disc showed a typical glaucoma cup, and was very pale, arterial pulsation was noted and there was a small retinal haemorrhage below the disc; the case was watched for a month when iridectomy was performed and the right eye trephined; when last seen in 1926 R. V. with − 0·5 D. sph. $= \frac{6}{5}$; tension was soft in this eye, and the field showed some slight improvement. II. 5 had two sons who have apparently shown no signs of defect (1931). II. 7 was examined at the age of 50; she complained of no symptoms, but was anxious on account of the family history; no abnormalities were found. II. 8 was examined at the age of 48 in 1924 when her central vision and fields were normal. II. 9, aged 46, had good vision and no symptoms but sought reassurance; the left field and blind spot were normal; the right field showed a slight defect up and in reaching to within 30° of the fixation point; the blind spot also showed a very slight general increase; fundi showed no abnormality; R. V. = L. V. $= \frac{6}{5}$ with slight correction; physiological cups were noted; there was definite increase of tension in the right eye; seen later a diagnosis of threatening glaucoma in the right eye was confirmed; a small iridectomy was done, also a trephine operation. Later information (March 1931) notes some suspicion of glaucoma in the left eye of this patient. II. 10 was examined at the age of 42; he was found then to be normal and has remained so up to the present (1931). No consanguinity recorded. Bibl. No. 274, with additional notes from the recorder.

Fig. 1027. *Rudin's Case.* Glaucoma was observed in two brothers at the ages of 27 and 20 years respectively; their father and paternal grandmother had become blind at the age of 30 years, probably also from glaucoma. No consanguinity recorded. Bibl. No. 226.

Fig. 1028. *Cantonnet's Case.* I. 1 developed chronic glaucoma at the age of 77 years; he had nine children, of whom one daughter, II. 2, became affected with glaucoma. II. 2 had eight children of whom two were glaucomatous. No details of cases are given. No consanguinity. Bibl. No. 254.

Fig. 1029. *Klein's Case.* III. 1 became affected with glaucoma at the age of 26 years; her mother had become similarly affected between the ages of 30 and 40; also her grandmother developed symptoms of glaucoma between the ages of 40 and 50 years. No consanguinity recorded. Bibl. No. 75.

Plate LXVIII. Fig. 1030. *Jacobson's Case.* I. 1, aged 70, was almost blind in both eyes from glaucoma simplex; iridectomy was performed and some vision was retained. II. 1, aged 45, and II. 2, at the age of 40, became affected also with glaucoma simplex; iridectomy was performed in each case. No consanguinity recorded. Bibl. No. 90A.

Fig. 1031. *Mules's Case.* I. 1, aged 49, was found to have R. V. = $\frac{6}{18}$, T. = + 1; the field was uniformly contracted to about half its normal size; well marked excavation of the optic disc was noted; refraction was myopic, but glasses led to no improvement in vision; the left eye of I. 1 was normal at this date. II. 1, aged 18, had R. V. = $\frac{6}{9}$, T. = + 1; the field was slightly contracted; no excavation of the disc; L. V. = shadows only, T. = + 1; the disc was deeply excavated. II. 2, aged 16$\frac{1}{2}$, had R. V. = shadows only, T = + 1; the disc was excavated; left eye was normal. II. 3 had slight myopia, − 0·75 D., in each eye, V. = $\frac{6}{9}$; tension was slightly raised; there was no excavation of the discs and the fields were normal. None of these cases presented any corneal lesion or sign of inflammatory change; no pain or difficulty was complained of except the failure of sight. No consanguinity recorded. Bibl. No. 80.

Fig. 1032. *Mooren's Case.* Bilateral glaucoma in three siblings and in a cousin. No consanguinity recorded. Bibl. No. 49A.

Fig. 1033. *Lawford's Case.* I. 1 died aged 68; she became blind at the age of 60, evidently from glaucoma, from the description by her daughter who was a trained nurse. II. 1 had a painless rapidly progressing bilateral glaucoma at the age of 58; double iridectomy was performed. II. 2 was operated on for acute glaucoma at the age of 47 and recovered her sight. II. 3, at the age of 60, had a chronic painless bilateral glaucoma; symptoms had been noticed for twelve months; the condition was in an advanced stage in the left eye, well marked in the right; six months after seeking assistance she was blind; six months later she died. Five living siblings of II. 1—3 were said to have good sight. No consanguinity recorded. Bibl. Nos. 180, 200.

Fig. 1034. *Kummer's Case.* Two brothers and two sisters of a sibship of six had glaucoma simplex; the sisters and one brother were blind; one brother was operated on and still retained some vision. The six siblings had between them sixteen children, of whom four males and one female had glaucoma; some of the unaffected members of this generation were still young. One member developed the disease at the age of 19; two were between the ages of 40 and 50; one was over 50; the remaining cases developed between the ages of 20 and 30. Two cases were complicated by cataract. No consanguinity recorded. Bibl. No. 53.

Fig. 1035. *Nettleship's Case.* I. 1 had glaucoma which developed at the age of 60; with the aid of operation he retained a little sight till his death at the age of 91. II. 1 had chronic glaucoma, signs of which were noticed before the age of 40; sclerotomy was performed; he still had some vision at the age of 63. II. 2 was said to be liable to attacks of pain and redness of the eyes which were believed to be due to gout. II. 4, aged 55, had both eyes operated on for glaucoma. II. 5, aged 54$\frac{1}{2}$, had her right eye operated on for glaucoma a few months ago; trouble was now commencing in the left eye. II. 6 had undergone an iridectomy which may have been only a precautionary measure. No consanguinity recorded. Bibl. No. 174.

Fig. 1036. *Lawford's Case.* Eight cases of glaucoma in three generations. I. 1 was blind for some years before his death at the age of 85; the disease was called amaurosis and the pupils were dilated; information from his two daughters left little doubt that their father had suffered from glaucoma; of his thirteen children II. 1, 3 and 8 died in infancy; II. 5 and 10 died at an adult age from "accident and paralysis"; eight of this sibship lived to an age at which glaucoma might have developed; II. 9 and 12 were living and free from symptoms at the ages of 77 and 71 years respectively. II. 6 had bilateral quiet glaucoma which developed at the age of 66, operation was performed; at the age of 71 this patient died from cerebral haemorrhage. II. 14 was normal when seen in 1907, but later was found to be suffering from bilateral subacute glaucoma, the onset of which was first noted at the age of 61; this man was alcoholic; he died, aged 65, from heart failure. III. 5 and 7 were operated on for well-marked glaucoma simplex developing at the ages of 47 and 39 years respectively. III. 6 and 8 had chronic painless glaucoma, the onset of which occurred at the ages of 55 and 47 years respectively; each had one eye operated on, and in each the other eye was seen at a later date to be showing signs of the disease. III. 3 became affected at the age of 52 and underwent a bilateral operation. III. 2 and 9 were free from symptoms of the disease at the ages of 61 and 44 years respectively. No case of disease had appeared in generation IV at a time when the eldest member was aged 29. Corneal diameters of III. 5 and III. 6 measured 12 mm., those of III. 8 measured 12·5 mm. No consanguinity recorded. Bibl. Nos. 180, 200.

Fig. 1037. *Fleischer's Case.* This pedigree was originally published in 1907; later information was communicated by the recorder to Plocher, who published it in 1919. IV. 4 became affected with chronic glaucoma at the age of 25; her four siblings were not yet affected. The mother, III. 1, the only child of her parents, became similarly affected at the age of 20 and in spite of operative treatments was blind in both eyes at the age of 36. The grandfather, II. 2, was also blind from glaucoma at the age of 24; he had three sisters of whom two were free from the disease, one was operated on for glaucoma. The great-grandfather, I. 2, was operated on in Würzburg and became blind in the fourth decade of life; his sister, I. 3, had glaucoma; I. 4 remained unaffected. No consanguinity recorded. Bibl. Nos. 178, 226.

Plate LXVIII. DESCRIPTIONS OF PEDIGREE PLATES 517

Fig. 1038. *Harlan's Case.* Glaucoma in five generations, V. 3, aged 17, had complained of failing sight for about a month; several nights she had seen coloured haloes round the lamp; she had a sense of discomfort; eyeballs were prominent and pupils slightly dilated; R. V. = L. V. = $\frac{20}{100}$; T = + 1; on ophthalmoscopic examination it was found that the optic disc was whitish and deeply excavated; vessels were numerous, the veins dilated and tortuous; no pulsation was visible except on slight pressure. The mother, IV. 6, aged 49, was absolutely blind, both anterior chambers were obliterated; at the age of 19 her "eyesight began to gradually waste away," she saw haloes and had attacks of inflammation, but never much pain. The maternal grandfather, III. 2, lost his sight in the same way, the trouble beginning at the age of 18. The maternal great grandmother and great-great grandfather were said to have been similarly affected. The maternal uncle, IV. 5, at the age of 35, had pain in his eyes and head; three years later he was absolutely blind. The maternal aunt, IV. 4, saw perfectly till the age of 18 when she became suddenly blind; she died three years later. Two uncles and an aunt over the age of 55 saw well. One cousin, now at a blind asylum, began to lose her sight at the age of 16; another cousin had been operated on at Baltimore, one eye was excised and an iridectomy was done for the other. A double iridectomy was performed on the patient, V. 3, with improvement in vision and removal of all discomfort. No consanguinity recorded. Bibl. No. 85.

Fig. 1039. *Rogman's Case.* II. 2, aged 62, had an attack of acute inflammatory glaucoma, after several weeks in bed suffering from rheumatism: she had bilateral iridectomy performed. The mother of II. 2 became suddenly blind in both eyes at the age of 83 years; immediate operation was performed; I. 2 died two years later with no recovery of vision. II. 2 had seven sons and four daughters of whom three sons had glaucoma. III. 1, aged 44, had had symptoms of chronic glaucoma for some time; now acute symptoms threatened, and bilateral operation became necessary. III. 2, aged 33, had a similar history. III. 3, aged 38, had had symptoms of chronic glaucoma for at least ten years, and was treated by injections of pilocarpine. No consanguinity recorded. Bibl. No. 144.

Fig. 1040. *Calhoun's Case.* II. 1 said that his parents and other near relatives had good sight; he had been a railroad and farm worker; at the age of 29 he first complained of his sight, and was found to have bilateral glaucoma; iridectomy was done on the left eye; later the right eye was enucleated on account of pain; at 59 L. V. = perception of light; media were clear; the disc was cupped and white; vessels were narrowed; the iris was grey and atrophic; T. = + 2; the horizontal diameter of the cornea was 12 mm. II. 1 had five children, of whom III. 1 first noticed defective vision in her right eye at the age of 12; three years later bilateral iridectomy was performed; at the age of 41, R. V. = 0, L. V. = $\frac{5}{200}$; the horizontal corneal diameter measured 11 mm. in each eye; R. T. = + 3, L. T = + 1; anterior chambers were very deep; media were clear; nerves were atrophic and cupped; vessels were narrowed; irides were brown. IV. 1, aged 18, became affected at the age of 17; in 1909 R. V. = $\frac{20}{100}$, L. V. = $\frac{20}{30}$; five years later, after a number of operations, R. V. = $\frac{4}{200}$, L. V. = $\frac{20}{100}$; anterior chambers were deep; irides were brown; corneal diameters measured 11·5 mm.; fields were markedly contracted on the nasal side. IV. 2, at the age of 13 had had failing vision for about three months; he had always had good health; R. V. = L. V. = $\frac{20}{50}$; anterior chambers were deep; T. = + 1; fundi were normal; fields showed slight contraction for form, marked narrowing for colours; irides were brown; corneal diameters measured 11·5 mm.; various operations were performed and latest records of vision were $\frac{20}{100}$ in the right, $\frac{20}{70}$ in the left. IV. 3 became affected at the age of 13; at 14 R. V. = $\frac{20}{50}$, L. V. = $\frac{20}{70}$; R. T. = normal, L. T. = + 1; fields were contracted and colour vision was much disturbed; corneal diameters measured 11·5 mm. on the right, 12·0 mm. on the left; a number of operations left the patient with R. V. = $\frac{20}{40}$, L. V. = $\frac{20}{50}$; anterior chambers were deep. III. 3, aged 39, saw haloes at the age of 11 years and was unable to see well; the left eye had became inflamed at the age of 3 and had since been blind; now R. V. = $\frac{20}{70}$; R. T. = 17 mm. Hg; anterior chamber was deep; optic atrophy was noted but there was little cupping of the disc and vessels were of normal calibre; the field was very contracted; the right eye had been operated on at the age of 12; the left eye was aphakic; irides were blue; corneal diameter measured 11 mm. III. 8 became affected at the age of 21; two years later R. V. = p.l., L. V. = $\frac{20}{70}$; anterior chambers were very deep; R. T. = + 2, L. T. = + 1; the left field was markedly contracted on the nasal side; irides were brown; corneal diameters measured 11·5 mm.; operation was performed and subsequent observations were recorded; at the age of 32 R. V. = p.l., L. V. = $\frac{4}{200}$; R. T. = 24 mm. Hg, L. T. = 33 mm. Hg. IV. 4, aged 14, had R. V. = $\frac{20}{70}$, L. V. = $\frac{20}{40}$; anterior chambers were very deep; fundi were normal; corneal diameters measured 12 mm.; fields were decidedly contracted and perception of colours was much disturbed; operations were performed; at the age of 17 R. V. = $\frac{20}{50}$, L. V. = $\frac{20}{30}$. The recorder considered that this case was suspicious but he could not definitely diagnose glaucoma; tension was normal at the first examination; irides were blue. III. 4, aged 38, and IV. 5, aged 4 years, had amblyopia which was possibly of glaucomatous origin. IV. 1 and IV. 3 suffered from tuberculosis. The refraction in this family was emmetropic or slightly hypermetropic. No consanguinity recorded. Bibl. No. 205.

Fig. 1041. *Nettleship's Case.* Glaucoma in three generations. Large physiological cups were noted in III. 2 at the age of 21; six years later the condition was unchanged; refraction was low myopia. III. 4, emmetropic, had very large physiological cups when first seen at the age of 20; three years later she had bilateral chronic glaucoma. The mother of III. 2 and 4, seen aged 42, with hypermetropia of about 3 D., had deep bowl-like excavation of the discs; vision was full and there were no symptoms of glaucoma; at the age of 45 she had chronic glaucoma. The grandfather, I. 6, had advanced chronic glaucoma in both eyes at the age of 72, which had first been noted about a year previously. These three cases were benefited by operation. Further details of the pedigree were given by Lawford in 1907 (Bibl. No. 180), showing that the disease had occurred also in the grandmother's family. It has not been possible to obtain more recent information of generation IV. No consanguinity recorded. Bibl. Nos. 98, 174.

Fig. 1042. *Vogt's Case.* Glaucoma in seven members of three generations; details of cases are not given, nor are we told the age at onset of the disease. In 1923 I. 1 was aged 74; II. 2, 4, 5 and 6 were aged 49, 47, 45 and 43 respectively; III. 1—5 were aged 21, 16, 15, 13 and 4 years respectively. The glaucoma was bilateral in each case. No consanguinity recorded. Bibl. No. 253.

Fig. 1043. *Somya's Case.* II. 2 had his left eye enucleated for severe signs of glaucoma at the age of 47; the right eye was also affected and an iridectomy was performed on it; this man was myopic; when seen, aged 53, the tension was + 1; there was enormous excavation of the disc; R. V. with − 10 D. = fingers at 15 feet; the field was markedly contracted, upwards and inwards; occasional pain in the right eye had never been so severe as in the left before its removal. II. 2 had three wives; of two children from the first marriage, III. 1 saw well; III. 2 had bilateral chronic glaucoma at the age of 26, when she complained of pain in her eyes and of bad vision at times; she had excavated papillae, raised tension, fields markedly contracted upwards and inwards; refraction was myopic; double iridectomy was performed, after which R. V. = fingers at 6 ins., R. T. = still somewhat raised; in the left eye tension was now normal. By his second wife II. 2 had no children. By his third wife II. 2 had two children, of whom III. 3, aged 15, had high myopia and prodromal signs of glaucoma. III. 4, aged 13, complained of pain in his eyes and cloudy vision; there was some excavation of the papillae and slightly raised tension with slight contraction of the upper field; bilateral iridectomy was performed, after which symptoms cleared up; this boy also had high myopia. The third wife, II. 4, had high myopia and cataract in her left lens, but showed no sign of glaucoma. II. 2 had healthy parents who had been free from eye disease; he knew of no other cases of eye disease in his family. No consanguinity recorded. Bibl. No. 113.

Fig. 1044. *Priestley Smith's Case.* Primary glaucoma in father and daughter. I. 1, Jabez B., aged 52, had a history of acute glaucoma in the left eye ten years ago, resulting in blindness; this eye now showed absolute primary glaucoma, V. = 0; T. = + 3, refraction indeterminate; horizontal diameter of cornea 10·5 mm. The patient now reported a gradual failure of sight in his right eye during a year, with acute symptoms and blindness for seven weeks; there was absolute primary glaucoma, V. = 0; hypermetropia of 2·5 D.; horizontal diameter of cornea measured 10·5 mm. II. 1, aged 20, had a history of acute, or subacute, glaucoma in the right eye, preceded by rainbow vision about a year ago; five months later the eye was blind and was subsequently excised on a recurrence of pain; the left eye showed primary chronic glaucoma; hypermetropia of about + 6 D.; T. = + 2; the disc was cupped; media were clear; V. = perception of hand movements; horizontal diameter of cornea measured 10 mm.; the patient gave a history of failing sight in this eye for three months; iridectomy was performed and marked improvement followed. The excised eye of II. 1 was very small, with corneal diameter of 10 mm.; horizontal diameter of globe 22 mm., vertical diameter 21 mm., diameter from pole to pole 21·75 mm.; the lens was relatively large; complete closure of the filtration angle was noted; the optic nerve showed deep excavation. No consanguinity recorded. Bibl. No. 121.

Fig. 1045. *Howe's Case.* I. 4 had good vision until about 40 years of age, when he developed an inflammatory type of glaucoma; in about six months the sight of one eye was lost, and within three years the other eye was also nearly blind; the siblings of I. 4 were normal and had normal descendants. II. 2 lost his right eye by an accident in childhood; at the age of 28 he noticed a failure in the sight of his left eye; a year later iridectomy for glaucoma led to no improvement and the man became blind. II. 5 first noticed a defect in her sight at the age of 25; she became totally blind four years later. III. 2 had pain in her left eye at the age of 28; this increased, with all the characteristics of glaucoma, and the eye became blind; she was found to have chronic glaucoma in the right eye also; iridectomy led to no improvement and she became practically blind. III. 4, seen in 1884, had perfect vision in one eye, V. = $\frac{20}{40}$ in the other, with excavation of the disc and slight contraction of the visual field. III. 6, aged 17, had noticed a failing vision for three months; the disease advanced rapidly and now R. V. = p. l., L. V. = fingers at 3 feet 10 ins.; some improvement followed a double iridectomy. III. 7, aged 29, noticed some failure in sight at the age of 19; he had now slight ciliary injection, the veins in the sclerotic were dilated; pupils were wide and immoveable; discs showed deep excavation; T. = + 3; V. = 0. III. 9, aged 25, said his sight began to fail six years ago; now the left eye showed chronic glaucoma with V. = p. l.; the right eye showed symptoms of glaucoma with typical excavation of the nerve and V. = $\frac{20}{70}$; iridectomy on the right eye led to marked improvement. No consanguinity recorded. Bibl. No. 94.

Plate LXVIII.   DESCRIPTIONS OF PEDIGREE PLATES   519

Fig. 1046. *Rampoldi's Case.* Glaucoma in a female who had four blind relations. III. 1, aged 62 years, had absolute glaucoma in the right eye and acute inflammatory glaucoma in the left; her brother and sister had no trouble with their eyes. I. 2 died, aged 60 years, with paralysis agitans. II. 2, the mother of III. 1, became affected with bilateral cataract at the age of 75; operation was performed with good result, but she later became blind, and it was not known from what cause. II. 3 became blind at the age of 70, it was not known whether the cause was glaucoma, cataract or optic atrophy. III. 4, the son of II. 3 and a doctor of medicine, became blind from optic atrophy; he afterwards, at about the age of 40, had an apoplectic attack; he died some years later leaving two healthy sons. III. 6, a goldsmith, became blind at the age of about 50, apparently from optic atrophy; he died a year later leaving two healthy sons and one daughter. There is no indication in the account of this family as to whether the optic atrophy in III. 4 and 6 was or was not secondary to glaucoma though the ages of onset are rather unusually late for a primary hereditary optic atrophy. III. 1 was twice married but had no children. No consanguinity recorded. Bibl. No. 84.

Fig. 1047. *Holland's Case.* Glaucoma in a woman of the Reki tribe on the Baluch-Persian frontier; all her four sons and one of her grandsons lost their sight from the same cause. I. 1 became blind, at about the age of 60, in both eyes, from glaucoma. II. 2 lost the sight of both eyes at the age of 60; he had had an iridectomy done with no improvement; his son and two daughters were alive and free from eye symptoms. II. 3 lost the sight of both eyes at about the age of 60; one of his two sons, aged 30, had completely lost the sight of one eye from glaucoma, the other eye could only distinguish hand movements; some improvement followed an iridectomy, but the patient was still unable to see to count fingers; the second son of II. 3 and his three daughters were free from eye symptoms. II. 5 lost the sight of both eyes at the age of 55; he had one son and two daughters who were free from eye symptoms. II. 7 lost the sight of both eyes at the age of 50. All the cases were seen and photographed, except I. 1; in none had the onset been acute but had been characterised by pain in the temples with gradual loss of vision.

The family attributed their blindness to the effects of swearing falsely on the *Quran!* No consanguinity recorded. Bibl. No. 257.

Fig. 1048. *Frank-Kamenetzki's Case.* II. 1, Wassili M., aged 37, a peasant in Irkutsk, had noticed a year before a marked diminution in his vision; he had polycoria, one nearly circular pupil was displaced a little inwards, a second oval pupil was situated upwards and outwards in the iris; he had marked bilateral glaucomatous excavation; R. T. = 43 mm. Hg, L. T. = 53 mm. Hg (Schiötz); R. V. = hand movements, L. V. = fingers at 2 m.; iridectomy was performed and the iris was noticed to be very thin and disintegrated; later a traumatic cataract developed and the lens was extracted. II. 3, Peter A., cousin of II. 1, also a peasant in Irkutsk, aged 27, had absolute glaucoma of the right eye, chronic glaucoma simplex in the left; R. V. = 0, L. V. = 0·05. No consanguinity recorded. Bibl. No. 260.

Fig. 1049. *Ray's Case.* The recorder had under treatment a man suffering from glaucoma in both eyes, whose father had been blind for a number of years from an eye disease which "gave rise to frequent attacks of neuralgia." No consanguinity recorded. Bibl. No. 112.

Fig. 1050. *Singleton's Case.* The recorder writes that a family was known to him in which a woman, whose father was blind, had a husband blind from glaucoma; two of her children, who had reached adult age, also had glaucoma. No consanguinity recorded. Bibl. No. 190, p. 42.

Fig. 1051. *Schenkl's Case.* I. 1 became blind in her left eye at the age of 60 years; she had had a heavy cold and severe headache; general treatment was unavailing; twenty-one years later her right eye became blind in the night; operation was refused, the woman remained blind and suffered from severe pain in the eyes. I. 1 had four children of whom II. 1 had no trouble with her eyes. II. 2, aged 60 (1876), had severe pain in the left side of his head one night and became blind in his left eye; he had been quite well a few hours before; when seen, the left eyeball was stony, with tension of + 3; anterior chamber was shallow; vision was reduced to perception of light; symptoms subsided after an iridectomy had been performed; a year later the patient had been able to return to his work as a hairdresser. In 1879, II. 4, aged 60, had a sudden almost acute onset of acute pain in her left eye following some emotional disturbance; the next night the pain became almost unbearable and in the morning aid was sought; all symptoms of acute glaucoma were present and vision was reduced to perception of light; iridectomy was performed; symptoms subsided, and vision slowly improved as in the case of II. 2. II. 3 became similarly affected in the left eye at the age of 62; the condition was complicated in her case by a severe bronchial catarrh with respiratory difficulty; this patient refused operation; eserin was given and the acute pain subsided, but the pupil remained somewhat dilated, the anterior chamber was shallower than normal, and the tension was raised; no recurrence of acute pain had been reported at the time of publication. No consanguinity recorded. Bibl. No. 103.

Fig. 1052. *Pflüger's Case.* II. 2, aged 20, reported that for more than two years his vision in both eyes had been slowly diminishing, he had had no pain; fields were markedly contracted; R. V. = $\frac{1}{200}$, L. V. = $\frac{8}{200}$; marked excavation of the nerve was noted; chronic glaucoma was diagnosed. A similar condition was found in the eyes of a brother one year older, whose vision also was slowly diminishing; for II. 1 R. V. = $\frac{20}{200}$, L. V. = $\frac{15}{200}$. The condition was typical and progressive in each; the father refused operation for his sons. Other siblings were said to see well. No consanguinity recorded. Bibl. No. 59.

Fig. 1053. Lawford's Case. I. 2 and I. 9, two males in a sibship of ten, were, from the accounts of relations, very probably subjects of glaucoma; I. 2 lost his sight late in life; he died aged 78. I. 9 lost his sight at about the age of 50 and died shortly afterwards. II. 5, 6, 7 and 8 developed a quiet painless type of glaucoma rather late in life; the age of onset is not given but these brothers were aged 77, 72, 67 and 66 at the time they were under observation. The children of I1. 8 had none of them yet shown signs of disease. No consanguinity recorded. Bibl. No. 180.

Plate LXIX. *Fig. 1054. Arlt's Case.* Glaucoma in a mother and daughter. No consanguinity recorded. Bibl. No. 37.

Fig. 1055. Benedict's Case. I. 1 was an extremely gouty old General whose son, II. 1, also suffered from this disease. II. 2 and 3 became blind from glaucoma. The son who remained free from glaucoma had blue eyes, whereas both his sisters had dark eyes. No consanguinity recorded. Bibl. No. 27.

Fig. 1056. Bowman's Case. I. 2, aged 60—70, had been blind in one eye for 20 years, in the other eye for 15 years, probably from acute glaucoma in each case. II. 1, aged 43, had always had imperfect sight; both lenses showed fine opacities. II. 2, aged 38, had always had imperfect sight; she had juvenile nuclear cataracts in each lens. II. 3, aged 33, had absolute glaucoma in both eyes; the right eye failed gradually twelve years ago; the left, also gradually, six years ago; she had had no perception of light for three years; both lenses were clear, but were displaced, up and in, so that only a quarter of each was visible in the dilated pupil. No consanguinity recorded. Bibl. No. 48.

Fig. 1057. Arlt's Case. Glaucoma in a father and his three sons. No consanguinity recorded. Bibl. No. 37.

Fig. 1058. Stellwag von Carion's Case. Acute glaucoma in II. 1 and in her uncle, I. 3; the mother, I. 2, was blind from glaucoma which had developed without any pain. I. 2 and 3 also had cataract. No consanguinity recorded. Bibl. No. 38.

Fig. 1059. Lawford's Case. Two cases of glaucoma in the offspring of normal parents. II. 1 had painless double glaucoma at the age of 60 years; operation was followed by good results. II. 2 had a quiet glaucoma, which developed at an earlier age than in her brother; operation on both eyes was successful in one case and failed in the other. II. 3 was diabetic. No consanguinity recorded. Bibl. No. 180.

Fig. 1060. Pagenstecher's Case. Glaucoma in a mother and her three sons; the mother was blind; the two elder sons became affected at the ages of 59 and 49 years respectively. No consanguinity recorded. Bibl. No. 44A.

Fig. 1061. Lawford's Case. Three cases of glaucoma in the offspring of unaffected parents. II. 1 had an attack of acute glaucoma from which she recovered after operation. II. 2 had chronic painless glaucoma when aged about 42; she had an operation on both eyes about six years ago and still retains some vision. II. 3 also had chronic glaucoma developing at the age of 42; operation on both eyes was unsuccessful. II. 2 and 3 had myopia of 6 to 7 D. No consanguinity recorded. Bibl. No. 180.

Fig. 1062. Pagenstecher's Case. II. 1 was operated on for subacute glaucoma at the age of 45 years; his father had been under treatment five years previously for acute glaucoma. No consanguinity recorded. Bibl. No. 44A.

Fig. 1063. Arlt's Case. A mother and two daughters were blind from glaucoma. No consanguinity recorded. Bibl. No. 37.

Fig. 1064. Ray's Case. The recorder had under observation two sisters both of whom were blind in one eye from acute inflammatory glaucoma; their mother was said to have become blind in old age, most probably from the same trouble. No consanguinity recorded. Bibl. No. 112.

Fig. 1065. Muller-Kannberg's Case. Chronic glaucoma simplex in father and daughter. I. 1, seen aged 52, had had a bilateral iridectomy done eight years before for glaucoma; the right eye was now blind though its vision had been good up to the time that glaucoma had developed; the left eye, which had never seen so well as the right, still retained some vision; the tension of both globes was still high; the right papilla was excavated; a coloboma of the left optic nerve was noted. II. 1, aged 26, had suffered from chronic glaucoma for three years; two years before bilateral iridectomy was performed; the right eye was now blind; the left field was contracted and L. V. = fingers at 6 feet. Two younger siblings of II. 1 were very short-sighted and had very high ocular tension. No consanguinity recorded. Bibl. No. 117.

Fig. 1066. Nolte's Case. Glaucoma simplex in two brothers; they and their unaffected sister, I. 3, had marked nervous symptoms. The right eye was first affected in I. 1 and 2 at the ages of about 40 and 30 years respectively; the left eyes became affected later. A son of one of the affected brothers had hare-lip. I. 1, 2, 3 and II. 1 were all melancholic. No consanguinity recorded. Bibl. No. 128A.

Fig. 1067. Werner's Case. I. 1, aged 53, knew of no eye disease in her family except in herself and her three children; at the age of 29 years she had headaches for 3½ months with cloudy vision occasionally; she sought advice and a bilateral iridectomy was performed; now she was quite blind; tension was + 1 in each eye; anterior chambers were deeper than normal; the right lens was opaque; the papillae showed glaucomatous excavation; refraction in the left was myopic, about 1·0 D.

PLATE LXIX.   DESCRIPTIONS OF PEDIGREE PLATES   521

II. 1 died young. II. 2, aged 21, had noticed coloured rings and diminishing vision at the age of 17 years, when R. V. = fingers at 2 m., T. = 60 mm. Hg; anterior chamber was much deeper than normal, the pupil was dilated and reacted slowly; media were clear; the papilla showed a deep exeavation; the eye was trephined after miotics had failed to reduce the tension; three years later R. V. = fingers at 2·5 m., T. = 10 mm. Hg; the left eye had a similar history; an iridectomy and anterior sclerotomy were performed on it; three years later L. V. = fingers at 1·5 m., T. = 25 mm. Hg. II. 3 had headaches for six months and noticed a diminution of vision of the age of 19 years; R. V. = fingers at 1—2 m., field was markedly contracted, T. = 60 mm. Hg; anterior chamber was deeper than normal; pupils reacted sluggishly; media were clear; the papilla was deeply excavated; this eye was trephined and three months later T. = 26 mm. Hg; V. = fingers at $\frac{3}{4}$ m.; the patient had been taking pilocarpine during this time; the state of the left eye was similar to the right though V. with – 1·5 D. = $\frac{5}{15}$; iridectomy with the use of pilocarpine led, after three months, to V. = $\frac{5}{30}$, T. = 18 mm. Hg. II. 4 noticed cloudy vision and coloured rings at the age of 15; now, aged 17, R. V. = $\frac{6}{8}$ = L. V.; R. T. = 33 mm. Hg, L. T. = 36 mm. Hg; anterior chambers were of normal depth, pupils reacted sluggishly; the papillae were slightly excavated and there was perhaps some slight contraction of the fields. II. 5, 6 and 7, aged 15, 11 and 9 years respectively, had not yet shown signs of trouble with their eyes. No consanguinity recorded. Bibl. No. 281.

Fig. 1068. *Wright and Nayar's Case.* II. 3, a Hindoo, aged 26, complained of dimness of vision and headaches during three years; R. V. = $\frac{6}{36}$, L. V. = $\frac{6}{24}$; pupils were sluggish and moderately dilated; anterior chambers deep; corneae large, 14 mm. horizontal diameter, 13 mm. vertical; the corneae were clear, showing no tears in Descemet's membrane; glaucomatous cupping was noted on each side, R. tension = L. tension = 80 (McLean); the right eye was trephined, the left eye treated with miotics; four years later R. V. with – 3·0 D. sph. – 1·0 D. cyl. axis vert. = $\frac{6}{9}$, L. V. = no perception of light. II. 4, aged 24, had had defective sight for six years; R. V. = L. V. = no perception of light; right tension = 60, left tension = 80 (McLean); corneae were large, with horizontal diameters of 14 mm., and presented a bluish haze, with linear opacities on the right side; the anterior chambers were deep, the pupils, excentric upwards, were dilated and inactive; there was complete cupping of the discs; four years later the lenses showed cataractous changes and there were marked opacites in the deeper layers of the cornese. II. 5, aged 19, had R. V. = L. V. = $\frac{6}{5}$; his corneae were clear and about normal in size; he had some fine opaque lens deposits; four years later the condition remained unchanged and this patient showed no signs of glaucoma. II. 6, aged 15, had R. V. = L. V. = $\frac{6}{5}$; his corneae were large with horizontal diameters of 14 mm.; fields were full and the corneal microscope revealed no opacities, but there was deep central cupping of both nerve heads; the right eye was trephined; four years later the trephined eye was in a much better state than the left eye which was now trephined also.

These four brothers had two sisters who refused examination but there seemed little doubt that they, and their parents, had perfectly good vision; the brothers knew of no instance of similar trouble amongst their relatives. No consanguinity recorded. Bibl. No. 294.

Fig. 1069. *Courtney and Hill's Case.* Glaucoma in seventeen cases of five generations. I. 2 originally came from Scotland and emigrated to America where he married I. 1. When I. 1 was aged about 30 and was pregnant with her third child, she first noticed that her vision was failing; she became blind before the child was born; of her six children four were believed to have had glaucoma; one son and one daughter retained good vision; II. 1 was married but had no children; II. 7 visited many European clinics, about 1840, in search of a cure for glaucoma; she apparently received drastic treatment and finally became insane. II. 3 married and had six children, of whom one son, III. 3, was drowned at the age of 15 without having shown symptoms of eye trouble; three daughters, III. 2, 7 and 8, had good vision throughout life, but two of them had affected sons. III. 4 became blind before the end of her third decade, having an iridectomy performed on each eye when she was already practically blind. III. 6 noticed that her vision was failing at about 20 years of age; she had a double iridectomy performed at Will's Hospital, Philadelphia, at the age of 22, in 1877; she is said still to have some vision, but lives in an almost inaccessible mountain district and could not be seen. III. 2 had one son, IV. 1, III. 8 had two sons, IV. 13 and 14, all of whom had glaucoma; all three retained a useful measure of vision following operation. III. 4 had six children of whom one male and two females presented no signs of glaucoma. IV. 7, J. W., aged 45, first noticed a failure of vision at the age of 19; three years later he had double iridectomy performed, but the visual defect progressed and pain was troublesome; a double trephine was done four years later when he was aged 26; in March, 1931, he was seen to have R. V. = hand movements, L. V. = $\frac{6}{200}$, excentric; his corneae each measured 11 mm. in horizontal and vertical diameters; anterior chambers were of normal depth; discs were deeply cupped and atrophic. IV. 5 and IV. 9 were diagnosed as having glaucoma between the ages of 20—25 years; both sisters have undergone bilateral iridectomy and retain useful vision.

IV. 7 has five children, of whom a son, H. C., V. 5, aged 23, has had failing vision for seven or eight months; in 1930 R. V. = $\frac{5}{30}$, L. V. = $\frac{5}{30}$, T. = 60 mm. Hg (Schiötz) in each; immediate operation was advised but the patient delayed a month, during which the condition progressed, and then agreed to a double Lagrange operation. V. 6, aged 17, had normal vision and normal tension; her corneae measured 11 mm.

in both diameters; anterior chambers were of normal depth. V. 7, W. H., aged 15, had noticed some failure in the left eye three months before, also more recently the right eye had been failing; now R. V. = $\frac{5}{15}$, L. V = $\frac{5}{22}$; R. T. = L. T. = 42 mm. Hg (Schiötz); each cornea measured 11 mm. in both diameters; anterior chambers were of normal depth; iridectomy and trephine operations were performed; ultimate vision was hand movements in the right, $\frac{5}{30}$ in the left eye. V. 8, aged 15, had normal vision; anterior chambers were of normal depth and corneae measured 11 mm. in each diameter; tension was raised and some contraction of the nasal field was noted; operation was advised but had not yet been performed. V. 9, aged 5 years, was examined but showed no symptoms yet.

V. 1, aged 16, the eldest of her sibship, was said by the family to have characteristic symptoms of the disease but she has not been examined by the recorders. Of the children of IV. 11 none has yet shown symptoms of glaucoma; the eldest, V. 10, was aged 17 years.

This family was of above the average intelligence. I. 2 by a second marriage had entirely normal descendants. No consanguinity. Bibl. No. 289.

Fig. 1070. *Shumway's Case.* I. 1 became entirely blind from glaucoma at the age of 20 years; no operation was performed. This woman married and had five children of whom two sons, still living, had good vision after a correction of considerable degree for myopia. II. 1 developed glaucoma at the age of 17; she was operated on sixty years ago but did not see after the operation; she was still living; both eyes showed advanced phthisis bulbi. II. 3 began to lose sight at the age of 13; double iridectomy was performed; twenty-three years later R. V. = perception of light, L. V. = $\frac{2}{30}$ with correction; the nerves were atrophic and deeply cupped. II. 5 began to lose sight at the age of 14; a year later the right eye was blind; the left eye was operated on, but also became blind; thirty-two years ago the right eye was removed; the left eye now showed phthisis bulbi. II. 3 was married and had one daughter in whom glaucomatous symptoms appeared at the age of 15; both nerves were cupped and tension was raised; operation was refused; at the age of 22 both eyes were blind; a year ago double enucleation was necessary to relieve pain and discomfort. This patient married and had one daughter, now aged 16, who shows marked symptoms of the disease. No consanguinity recorded. Bibl. No. 289.

Fig. 1071. *Kauffmann's Case.* Glaucoma in six members of four generations. I. 2 and 4 had glaucoma; I. 4 married and had one daughter, who died young, and was at this time free from eye disease. I. 2 had four children, of whom II. 1 became affected with glaucoma at about the age of 24; there were five from eye disease; no signs of glaucoma had appeared in their seven children, or eight grandchildren, up to the present time. II. 4 was blind from glaucoma at about the age of 24 years; his daughter, III. 3, also became blind from glaucoma between the ages of 25 and 30 years. III. 3 had six children, of whom the eldest daughter, aged 24 years, was affected with glaucoma. No consanguinity recorded. Bibl. No. 179.

Fig. 1072. *James's Case.* II. 1, A. G., aged 41, had tension raised in each eye; he was fat and unhealthy, a good deal worried, and had noticed a fogginess in the vision of the left eye during an attack of influenza a year before; this had mended and was associated with no haloes; two weeks later the left eye became inflamed and painful and the vision in both eyes became so bad that he had to be led about; now there was a subsiding stage of acute glaucoma in each eye; the anterior chambers were somewhat shallow, pupils semi-dilated and oval, tension = + 1, V. = hand movements, fields fairly full; iridectomy was performed in the right eye, the left was trephined; after three days the right eye was the best; a year later R. V. = $\frac{6}{12}$ with − 2·0 sph. + 3·0 cyl., L. V. < $\frac{6}{60}$. Several years later the mother of A. G., aged 72, was seen with signs of chronic glaucoma in the right eye; eserine controlled the tension, the disc was only slightly cupped; V. = $\frac{6}{12} - \frac{6}{6}$; at a subsequent date the blind spot showed slight enlargement but there had been no further deterioration. No consanguinity recorded. Bibl. No. 220. With notes from the recorder.

Fig. 1073. *Schnabel's Case.* II. 1, a delicate very nervous woman, aged 36, very suddenly became blind in the left eye from glaucoma; her mother had become affected with glaucoma twenty years previously. No consanguinity recorded. Bibl. No. 63.

Fig. 1074. *Schweigger's Case.* II. 1, aged 15 (1883), had noticed rainbow vision for six months; L. V. = $\frac{5}{5}$, R. V. with − 0·75 D. = $\frac{5}{5}$; fields were full; there was a bilateral deep and precipitous physiological excavation of the disc; rainbow vision persisted, and visual acuity diminished. Three years later R. V. = L. V. = $\frac{5}{5}$, but there was a contraction of the upper part of the field in each eye almost to the fixation point; corneae were clear, pupils not dilated; iridectomy was performed upwards but rainbow vision persisted. The recorder had operated on the father and uncle of II. 1 for glaucoma. No consanguinity recorded. Bibl. No. 108.

Fig. 1075. *Snell's Case.* I. 1 first noticed his failing vision at the age of 50, when glaucoma was diagnosed; for several years he was treated with miotics, in 1910 iridectomy was performed; in 1912 R. V. = $\frac{6}{9}$, L. V. = $\frac{1}{100}$; fields were contracted; a trephine was carried out in 1912 which permanently lowered the tension to or below normal, and was now (1923) reduced to ability to count fingers; discs in 1912 were both very white with deep excavations. II. 1, aged 35 (1923), had in 1921 R. T. = 50 mm. Hg, L. T. = 46 mm. Hg (Schiötz); fields were much contracted; iridectomy was performed on the right eye in 1922; there was a shallow excavation; colour of the discs was good; the fundi

PLATE LXIX.   DESCRIPTIONS OF PEDIGREE PLATES   523

were normal in other respects; corneal horizontal diameters measured 11 mm. II. 1 had one brother with normal eyes. No consanguinity recorded. Bibl. No. 251.

Fig. 1076. *Sattler's Case.* II. 1, not yet aged 11 years, had had failing vision during ten months; anterior chambers were deep, pupils perhaps a little dilated though response to light was prompt; the ophthalmoscope revealed an enormous excavation of the nerve and the vessels dipping into it were numerically increased; refraction was myopic; with -4 D., R. V. $= \frac{8}{10}$, L. V. $= \frac{8}{30}$; T. $= +2$; bilateral iridectomy upwards was performed with an apparent arrest of the failure in sight several weeks after the operation. The mother, I. 1, had simple glaucoma with complete loss of vision at the age of 17 years; no further cases of the disease were known to have occurred in the family. No consanguinity recorded. Bibl. No. 171.

Fig. 1077. *Löhlein's Case.* I. 1 and 2 were healthy, had not suffered from glaucoma and were not short-sighted; of their children, II. 1, at the age of 15, noticed rainbow vision and defective vision; she had simple chronic glaucoma with no signs of inflammation; anterior chambers were deepened; excavation of the nerve was noted; iridectomy was performed. II. 2 became affected with chronic glaucoma simplex at the age of 17; she had no pain or inflammatory symptoms; refraction was hypermetropic, 1·5 D.; a persistent hyaloid artery was noted. II. 3 became affected at the age of 10 years with the same disease. II. 4 had marked congenital hydrophthalmos. No consanguinity. Bibl. No. 201.

Fig. 1078. *Bartel's Case.* II. 1, aged 45, had bilateral glaucoma simplex at the time of the climacteric; one sister also had intraocular pressure raised to 60 mm. Hg, in an eye which was free from signs of inflammation. The mother, and three maternal aunts of II. 1, also had glaucoma at the time of the climacteric and gradually became blind. A bilateral iridectomy was performed for II. 1 but the relief was only transitory. No consanguinity recorded. Bibl. No. 245.

Fig. 1079. *Story's Case.* II. 1, aged 30, had chronic inflammatory glaucoma; his mother had noticed his left pupil enlarge at times when his sight became dim; he saw no coloured haloes, had a very shallow anterior chamber, and small eyes with corneal diameters of 11 mm. in each; tension was not raised and fundi were normal; two weeks later he was seen when the left pupil was wider than the right and tension was $+2$; the left fundus showed venous and arterial pulsation; pilocarpine reduced the frequency of attacks. The patient's mother had one eye blinded from glaucoma, chronic inflammatory glaucoma in the other eye. No consanguinity recorded. Bibl. No. 114.

Fig. 1080. *Derby's Case.* II. I, H. C., seen aged 20, had noticed a diminution of vision for several months; he had been able to teach in a school up to this time; now R. V. $=$ L. V. $= \frac{1}{10}$; he had had rainbow vision; each cornea was large and each anterior chamber was abnormally deep; tension was raised in the right eye, normal in the left; glaucomatous excavation and arterial pulse were noted on each side; each field of vision was contracted especially down and in; there was no corneal anaesthesia; iridectomy was performed on the right and later on the left eye; two years later R. V. $=$ L. V. $= \frac{14}{200}$, and the condition was unchanged when seen again after an interval of nine years. There would seem to be no doubt that this case was one of juvenile glaucoma. II. 2 on accompanying the patient above described was seen to present "the usual signs of hydrophthalmos" in her right eye; the left eye was atrophied, having previously ruptured. II. 3 had in one eye a cataract and no perception of light; in the other eye she had a partial cataract and complete atrophy of the optic nerve. The father of these children, I. 1, became blind at the age of 25; he had eleven children of whom four were blind; the vision of these children generally began to fail at about the age of 14, the first symptom being blurred vision, followed by watering, rainbow vision and gradual loss of sight without pain. No consanguinity recorded. Bibl. No. 76.

Fig. 1081. *Grimsdale's Case.* Chronic glaucoma in a brother and two sisters, becoming evident in each case at the age of about 70 years; no information was available of the parents or of normal members of the sibship; the three patients are now (1931) dead. No consanguinity recorded. Hitherto unpublished.

Fig. 1082. *Ring's Case.* The recorder saw a male student with glaucoma; the mother of the patient and one or two of her siblings were similarly affected. No consanguinity recorded. Bibl. No. 171.

Fig. 1083. *Snell's Case.* Glaucoma in a mother and her three children. I. 1 had glaucoma which was diagnosed at the age of 16; she became blind at 30 and died from paralysis at the age of 50 years; she had always been short-sighted. II. 1, aged 16 (1918), had had failing vision since the age of 10, following an attack of measles; he had worn glasses for short sight for six years; his corneae measured 11·5 mm. in diameter; anterior chambers were shallow; R. T. $=$ L. T. $= 56$ mm. Hg (Schiötz); R. V. with $-3·50$ D. sph. $-1·00$ D. cyl. ax. $75° = \frac{20}{40}$, L. V. $=$ perception of light in a small area of the field only; in the right eye the field was contracted on the nasal side, above and below to $30°$, outwards to $55°$; pupils reacted to light; media were clear; the optic discs were two or three times larger than normal, the disc having a very deep central excavation surrounded by a halo-like ring; in 1918 a Lagrange operation was performed on the right eye, iridectomy on the left; tension remained down until 1921, though R. V. was never, after the

67—2

operation, better than $\frac{20}{100}$ and was now as low as $\frac{2}{300}$; left eye was blind; after a trephine in 1921 R. V. $= \frac{1}{300}$, T. $= 37$ mm. Hg. II. 2, aged 15 (1918), had never had a serious illness, but he was very nervous, with a peculiar twitching of his head and shuffling gait, also constant blinking; pupils reacted to light; corneae measured 11 mm. in diameter; T. $= +2$; R. V. with -4.50 D. sph. $= \frac{20}{40}$, L. V. with -4.0 D. sph. $= \frac{20}{50}$; fields were contracted on the temporal side to 15°, on the nasal side to 10°; media were clear; optic discs were almost exactly similar to those of his brother; in 1920 T. $= 60$ to 70 mm. Hg; R. V. with glasses $= \frac{20}{40}$, L. V. $=$ nil; a double trephine was carried out after which the eyes were soft and V. with glasses was $\frac{20}{40}$. II. 3, aged 13, had corneae of 12 mm. in diameter; R. V. with -4.00 D. sph $= \frac{20}{25}$, L. V. with -3.00 D. sph. $= \frac{20}{25}$; fields were slightly contracted; media clear; a whitish area surrounding the disc was suggestive of a persistent nerve sheath; this patient was very nervous; a diagnosis of glaucoma was made at a later date and a trephine was carried out in 1923. All three children were myopic to nearly the same degree. No consanguinity recorded. Bibl. No. 251.

Fig. 1084. *Löhlein's Case*. II. 1 had normal vision up to the age of 28 years, when absolute glaucoma rapidly developed in the left eye; the right eye showed glaucoma simplex and myopia of 5 D. The father of the patient, aged 64, was almost blind from glaucoma simplex; it is not stated when symptoms were first noted in the father. No consanguinity recorded. Bibl. No. 201.

Fig. 1085. *James's Case*. I. 2, aged 87, had noticed failing vision for some months; the right eye was very defective; both chambers were very deep, the pupils small and reacting slowly to light; R. V. $= < \frac{6}{60}$, L. V. $= \frac{6}{12}$; there were some fine striae in each lens; the right disc was cavally cupped and nearly the whole of the upper part of each field was lost, the nasal sides also were contracted; the condition worsened under eserine and chronic glaucoma was diagnosed; the right eye was trephined, the left had a small basal iridectomy. This man has one son, who is known to the recorder and is believed not to have shown symptoms of glaucoma, but a nephew of I. 2, aged about 54—56, has a "peculiar glaucoma" in each eye. No consanguinity recorded. Bibl. No. 220, with notes from the recorder.

Fig 1086. *Cross's Case*. I. 1 became blind from glaucoma at the age of 30 years. II. 1, aged 21, had had failing sight in the right eye for nine months; R. V. $= \frac{6}{6}$; the field was much narrowed on the nasal and upper sides; cornea was "full"; a deep white cup was noted and a pulsating artery in the fundus; T. $= +2$; in the left eye V. $= \frac{6}{6}$, field was slightly narrowed on the nasal side, T. $= +1$; the disc was pink and not distinctly cupped, but was surrounded by a white edge. No measurements were taken on the corneae in this boy, but they were described as "full" and suggested to the recorder some extension of the globe in association with unquestionable glaucoma in both eyes. No consanguinity recorded. Bibl. No. 106.

Fig. 1087. *Usher's Case*. Glaucoma in two, probably in three, generations. I. 1 was known to have been blind before he died; of his children, II. 2 was operated on for glaucoma by Sir George Berry; the onset of the disease had occurred at the age of 46 years. II. 3, aged 70, had glaucoma at the age of 65; operation was performed in Aberdeen. II. 6 became blind in America; no details of his affection were available. II. 2 had seven children, of whom III. 1 showed symptoms of glaucoma at the age of 38; operation was performed on both eyes. Information of the family history was provided by III. 3. No consanguinity recorded. Hitherto unpublished.

Fig. 1088. *Wallenberg's Case*. A patient, aged 25, was seen who one year before had had a double iridectomy for glaucoma; the vision in the right eye was almost normal; in the left eye bleeding in the retina had followed iridectomy, vision was only $\frac{1}{12}$ of the normal, and the field was contracted on the nasal side to the fixation point. Members of this family were liable to a virulent form of glaucoma with rapid blinding of both eyes occurring at 20 to 24 years of age; apparently the paternal grandmother, one paternal uncle, two sisters and one brother had all been blinded by this disease. Macro-cornea was noted in the patient and his affected siblings. The father, uncle and brother had all been imprisoned for violence in fits of temper; the two sisters were prostitutes; all members of the family reacted to slight amounts of alcohol. No consanguinity recorded. Bibl. No. 182.

Fig. 1089. *Dérer's Case*. Glaucoma in a father and his four sons; three daughters were healthy and unaffected. I. 1 became blind from glaucoma at the age of 34; three of his sons had been blinded from the same cause at the ages of 22, 19 and 16 respectively; all cases had very deep anterior chambers, atrophic irides, fixed semi-dilated pupils and excavation of the optic nerve. A fourth son had sought treatment two years ago, when he was aged 28, for bilateral, not inflammatory, glaucoma; tension was raised; anterior chambers were deep; total excavation of the nerve head was noted; V. $= \frac{6}{8}$ and $\frac{6}{12}$ in the two eyes respectively; the condition progressed, and now V. $= \frac{6}{24}$ and $\frac{6}{30}$. No consanguinity recorded. Bibl. No. 284.

Fig. 1090. *Axenfeld's Case*. Three siblings became affected with glaucoma between the ages of 20 and 40 years, a sister who was younger than these siblings had not yet become affected but she was noted to have a congenital "Luckenbildung" in the lamina cribrosa of one eye. There was a history of blindness in earlier generations, but the nature of its cause was only known in one uncle to the siblings, who had also chronic glaucoma with occasional acute attacks. No consanguinity recorded. Bibl. No. 173.

Plate LXX.   DESCRIPTIONS OF PEDIGREE PLATES   525

ANIRIDIA

Plate LXX. Fig. 1091. *Benson's Case.* Aniridia in mother and son. II. 1, aged 9, had a total absence of iris in both eyes; the globes of the eyes were somewhat small and the corneae imperfectly developed in that they appeared to have the same curvature as the surrounding sclerotic; lenses were shrivelled and opaque; V. = fingers at 18 inches and had apparently never been better; nystagmus was marked. I. 2 had good sight. I. 1 had the same kind of eyes as her son. No consanguinity recorded. Bibl. No. 64.

Fig. 1092. *Juler's Case.* Aniridia in mother and daughter. I. 1, aged 59, showed complete absence of iris and opacity of the lens in the left eye; vision was less than $\frac{6}{80}$; tension was normal; the right eye had been removed following an injury; this eye showed a narrow band of iris varying greatly in width and at one part entirely absent; the edge of the lens was irregular and opaque. II. 1 lost her right eye from glaucoma; the left eye showed complete absence of iris, the lens was opaque and dislocated upwards; tension was raised and the patient complained of occasional pain. No consanguinity recorded. Bibl. No. 157.

Fig. 1093. *Licsko's Case.* I. 1, aged 42, had the greater part of the iris missing in both eyes; she had glaucoma; of her two children II. 2, aged 21 months, had bilateral coloboma iridis; II. 1, aged 4 years, was noted to have atrophic anterior layers of the iris. No consanguinity recorded. Bibl. No. 275.

Fig. 1094. *Bergmeister's Case.* Aniridia in a father and his two sons; his only daughter had completely normal eyes. I. 1, aged 34 (1904), had bilateral nystagmus; no iris could be seen in either eye, the border of the lens being clearly visible; he had in the right eye a central anterior capsular cataract as well as some anterior and posterior cortical cataract; fundus was not visible; tension was + 1 in both; vision of the left eye was reduced to finger counting at 2 m. and the field was much contracted; the patient had seen badly from birth; the right eye became suddenly blind at the age of 19 years. An uncle of I. 1 was reported to have suffered from eye disease but no details of his condition were known. I. 1 had three children, of whom the two younger, aged 4½ years and 3 weeks respectively, had complete bilateral absence of iris and anterior polar cataract. The right eye of I. 1 was enucleated, when the iris was found to be present as a slight rudiment throughout the circumference. No consanguinity recorded. Bibl. No. 164.

Fig. 1095. *Theobald's Case.* I. 1 had an atypical coloboma iridis in each eye; the right coloboma was large and directed upwards, on the left side the defect was smaller, directed upwards and outwards; the choroid was normal. II. 2, aged 18 months, was seen to have a complete absence of each iris; lenses were clear and vision seemed to be fairly good; he had a congenital squint in the left eye. The mother, I. 1, said that the eyes of an older child than II. 2 presented a similar appearance. No consanguinity recorded. Bibl. No. 99.

Fig. 1096. *Blair and Potter's Case.* I. 1, Thomas P., aged 37, had a large coloboma of his left iris, down and in, with slight notching of the lens and also fine dotted opacities at the anterior surface of the lens; in his right eye there was a peculiar discoloration of that portion of the iris corresponding to the coloboma in the left eye, which was inactive and unaffected by a mydriatic whilst the rest of the iris dilated freely. II. 1, Florence P., aged 14, had in her right eye no iris excepting a narrow strip internally; her choroid was defective below and internal to the disc; in her left eye there was no iris excepting some remnants visible on the inner side, the left choroid was normal; lenses were clear; R. V. with $\dfrac{-10\ \text{D. sph.}}{-1\ \text{D. cyl. ax. hor.}} = \dfrac{6}{12}$;

L. V. with $\dfrac{-8\cdot5\ \text{D. sph.}}{-1\ \text{D. cyl. ax. } 10°} = \dfrac{6}{12}$. II. 2, George P., aged 11, had no demonstrable iris in his right eye; in his left eye some slight tags of iris could be seen up and in; this boy had anterior pyramidal cataract in both lenses; marked cupping of each disc with normal tension was noted; R. V. with correction = $\frac{6}{60}$; L. V. with $\dfrac{-7\ \text{D. sph.}}{-6\ \text{D. cyl. ax. } 160°} = \dfrac{6}{18}$. No consanguinity recorded. Bibl. No. 160.

Fig. 1097. *Polte's Case.* Coloboma iridis in two brothers; almost complete absence of iris in their mother. I. 1, aged 47, had a few slight opacities of both corneae; iris was a barely perceptible ring of tissue at the limbus in each; lenses were opaque and displaced upwards; nystagmus was noted; R. V. with + 12 D. = $\frac{12}{60}$, L. V. with + 12 D. = $\frac{2}{36}$. II. 1, aged 12, had bilateral congenital coloboma iridis, downwards and inwards, reaching in the right eye as far as the ciliary body; in the lower outer part of the right iris there was a small cleft, also two small slits were seen on either side of the coloboma and parallel to it; posterior cortical cataract was present. R. V. = $\frac{2}{36}$, not improved by glasses. In the left eye the coloboma did not reach to the ciliary body; posterior cortical cataract was present; L. V. = fingers at 1½ m. This boy had horizontal nystagmus; pupils did not react to light but dilated under the influence of atropin. II. 2, aged 10, had bilateral coloboma iridis downwards and inwards; posterior cortical cataracts were noted, also nystagmus. II. 1 and 2 were mentally somewhat defective. II. 2 had cryptorchidism. No consanguinity recorded. Bibl. No. 185.

Fig. 1098. *Moissonnier and Pouchet's Case.* Aniridia in a mother and two daughters. I. 1, aged 42, had never had good vision, she now had bilateral corneal opacities from a former keratitis; she had double congenital aniridia; the lens was in position, but showed some fine opacities; refraction was hypermetropic, about 5 D.; nystagmus was present; she was a woman of slight intelligence. II. 1, with good eyes, died young. II. 3, aged 19, was completely blind; her corneae were slightly opaque at the centre; she had complete bilateral aniridia; lenses were displaced upwards; this patient could see up to the age of 14, and then became rapidly blind; the recorder believed that the subluxation of the lenses occurred during life and that the observed sclero-choroiditis was due to movements of the lens. II. 3 was badly developed and showed signs of rickets; teeth were normal; she was mentally more degenerate than her mother. II. 4, aged 15, was also badly developed and showed signs of rickets; she had complete bilateral aniridia; corneae were transparent but the right lens showed several opacities and the left lens was opaque; the papillae were small, pale and ill defined. No consanguinity recorded. Bibl. No. 162.

Fig. 1099. *Stephenson's Case.* I. 1 had normal eyes, clubbed feet. I. 2 had opacities of the corneae and lenses, strabismus in the left eye, and nystagmus; all these defects had been present since birth; there was no history of eye defects in earlier generations. These parents had three children with irideremia. II. 1, John M., aged 12, was normal mentally; he had nystagmus; slight convergence was noted; the corneal transverse diameter measured 10 mm.; irregular opacities radiated from the sclero-corneal junction containing fine vessels; the irides were absent excepting a narrow rim not more than 0·5 mm. in width; the equator of the lens was visible; lenses were clear; fundi showed an incomplete coloboma of each optic disc; R. V. with $\dfrac{-6 \cdot 0\,\text{D. sph.}}{-1 \cdot 0\,\text{D. axis }180°} = \dfrac{6}{36} = \text{L. V.}$, with similar correction. II. 2, Michael M., aged 10, a small ill-developed and mentally very dull child, was slightly deaf and had double talipes varus; his eyes showed nystagmus; transverse diameter of corneae was 10 mm. only; marginal opacities of the cornea were noted; the iris consisted of a narrow rim about 0·5 mm. in width; the equator of the lens was visible; opacities were noted in each lens; fundi showed an incomplete coloboma of each optic disc; refraction was myopic; the child had not yet learned to read. Both these brothers had defect in the enamel of their incisors. II. 3, Maggie M., died aged 18 months of whooping cough; her eyes were said to be like those of the two brothers. No consanguinity. Bibl. No. 129.

Fig. 1100. *Schroter's Case.* II. 1, aged 42, had during school age been able to see quite well to read small print and do fine work, lately her sight had failed; she was found to have no iris; she had nystagmus and strabismus, also cataract of both lenses. The parents of II. 1 and all relations of their generation had normal eyes; the mother, I. 2, attributed the defect in her child to the fact that when she was pregnant, she had seen a blind old man at a Communion service, who was unable to find the altar. II. 1 had two children, the eldest of whom had bilateral aniridia; this child, III. 1, had also bilateral cataract; she was myopic and further had nystagmus and strabismus. The second child of II. 1 had normal eyes. No consanguinity. Bibl. No. 49.

Fig. 1101. *Focachon's Case.* Aniridia in father and son. II. 2, Victor L., aged 35, had complete bilateral absence of iris; his sclerotics were bluish and he had cataract in the left lens; his parents had well formed eyes. At this time II. 2 had two children, of whom III. 1 had well formed eyes; III. 2 had complete bilateral absence of iris. The globes in father and son were perhaps smaller than is normal. Writing at a later date Cornaz (Bibl. No. 35, p. 16) reports that II. 2 had had nine children; only the one son mentioned above had aniridia, and he was dead; no post mortem examination was made. No consanguinity recorded. Bibl. No. 26.

Fig. 1102. *Galezowski's Case.* II. 2, aged 29 (1904), had a total bilateral absence of iris; her lenses were opaque; nystagmus was noted; she had never seen well enough to learn to read and for two years had been unable to go about alone. Of the two children of II. 2, a daughter had normal eyes; a son, aged 7, had bilateral not quite complete aniridia. III. 2, the son, had also opacities in both lenses and nystagmus; he was born at 8 months and had a hernia at the age of 3 weeks; his teeth were defective. The parents of II. 2, and her sister, II. 3, had normal eyes. No consanguinity recorded. Bibl. No. 165.

Fig. 1103. *Galezowski's Case.* Aniridia in every known descendant of I. 2 who was herself affected. I. 2 had eleven children, all of whom were born without irides; eight of these children were dead; of the three living daughters, the eldest, II. 1, was known to have several children with aniridia, but she was out of touch with her sisters, and it was not known how many children she had or whether any of them were normal. II. 4 had twelve children, of whom only two were living; all were said to have been born without irides. II. 5, aged 48 (1878), had a narrow scarcely appreciable segment of iris in the inward and upper region; she had cataract in both lenses. II. 5 had two sons who both had the same anomaly; neither were living. No consanguinity recorded. Bibl. No. 71.

Fig. 1104. *de Beck's Case.* An interesting history of aniridia and coloboma iridis in three generations. I. 2, John K., with bilateral aniridia, died past middle life, having suffered no marked impairment of vision.

Plate LXX.   DESCRIPTIONS OF PEDIGREE PLATES   527

I. 1 had normal eyes. I. 3, William K., aged 62, had bilateral coloboma iridis; he had lately become blind owing to double cataract. I. 2 had nineteen children, of whom II. 1, now dead, had normal eyes. II. 2, twin to II. 1, had normal eyes. II. 4, aged 42, a miner, had double aniridia, not quite complete at the upper margin, where there remained in each eye a very narrow strip of iris, clearly shown by oblique illumination; no nystagmus; vision had always been rather poor; both lenses showed glistening white nuclear cataracts, nearly or quite mature. II. 6 had normal eyes. II. 7, twin to II. 6, aged 36, a miner, had bilateral coloboma iridis directed downwards and slightly inwards, extending to the margin of the cornea; irides grey; pupils showed some little response to light; both eyes presented well-marked white nuclear cataracts. II. 4 and II. 7 gave no history of pain or inflammatory trouble in the eyes; both were operated on for cataract. II. 9 had normal eyes. Thirteen siblings died young, with apparently normal eyes. II. 12, the son of I. 3, aged 28, had bilateral aniridia with fair vision. III. 5 and III. 9, now dead, had eyes "just like their father's." III. 6, aged 9, had bilateral aniridia with fair vision. III. 14, the daughter of II. 7, aged 4, had bilateral aniridia with fair vision. No consanguinity recorded. Bibl. No. 130.

Fig. 1105. *Cunningham's Case.* Aniridia in eight members of four generations; only one member of the family was examined; the history was provided by the mother, III. 8, of this patient. IV. 5, seen aged 10, complained of bad sight; she was found to have R. V. = L. V. = $\frac{6}{24}$, with correction; her iris consisted of some tissue in the upper and inner segment of each eye, more extensive in the right than in the left eye; some dotted opacities on the anterior lens capsule were more marked on the right than on the left side. No consanguinity recorded. Bibl. No. 189.

Fig. 1106. *Page's Case.* Aniridia, microphthalmos and nystagmus in four members of three generations. III. 6, aged 15, had almost total absence of iris, smallness of globes and corneae, and constant nystagmus, generally rotatory, occasionally horizontal; in the left eye there was some trace of iris throughout the circumference, more definite in the lower than in the upper segment; on the right, the iris was absent in the upper and only just visible in the lower segment; some displacement of the lens was noted in the right eye, the lower margin being tilted forwards; there was difficulty in examining the fundus, owing to nystagmus, but the vessels appeared to be smaller than normal and the choroid showed some patches of atrophy. The mother, II. 2, one sister, III. 2, and a niece, IV. 1, were said to be similarly affected. No consanguinity recorded. Bibl. No. 58.

Fig. 1107. *Gutbier's Case.* (Taken from Beger.) This history of aniridia in eight males and two females of four generations is of considerable historic interest and has been widely quoted; the original account has proved inaccessible but Beger described the case in *von Ammon's Journal* shortly after the original publication. II. 8, Christian K., was the son of healthy parents, and was, so far as the family knew, the first member of the family to be affected with the anomaly; his seven brothers were free from the defect; he was dazzled by a bright light. II. 8 had eight children of whom three sons were similarly affected; the eldest son, III. 2, with a healthy wife had four sons, still living, all of whom had no iris except the second son, IV. 4, in whom a trace of iris was present. III. 3 had one son whose eyes, like those of his children V. 7, were normally developed. III. 5 died a few days after birth. Of the four affected sons of III. 2, IV. 2 had a completely healthy son. IV. 4 had a normally developed son, and a daughter without irides who could see well in a dim light. IV. 6 married an epileptic wife and had two children, of whom a daughter was without irides and suffered from nystagmus; the other child was deformed. IV. 7 had a healthy son. No consanguinity recorded. Bibl. No. 21.

Fig. 1108. *Laskiewicz-Friedensfeld's Case.* Four cases of aniridia in three generations. III. 1, aged 28, was healthy and for the most part well developed, but she had no trace of iris in either eye, and had bilateral cataract; she had never seen so well as other people. III. 2, aged 23, also had complete congenital aniridia and posterior polar cataract in each eye. III. 1 stated that her father and her paternal grandfather also had aniridia and cataract. No consanguinity recorded. Bibl. No. 61.

Fig. 1109. *Lang's Case.* II. 1 had bilateral aniridia, lamellar cataract and nystagmus; she had three children, of whom III. 1 had normal eyes; III. 2 was said to have had the same eye defects as his mother; III. 3 had bilateral aniridia, striae in each lens, and nystagmus. No similar defects were known to have occurred in other members of the family. No consanguinity recorded. Bibl. No. 86.

Fig. 1110. *Mohr's Case.* Aniridia in a mother and her three sons. II. 1, seen aged 24, was an illegitimate child; according to the statement of her mother, her father had normal eyes; her mother, I. 1, also had normal eyes. The patient had always been healthy, but complained now of attacks of inflammation in her left eye; she was found to have total absence of iris, cataractous lenses, horizontal nystagmus, and convergent strabismus; sight was very poor, not improved by glasses. III. 1, aged 2 years, had horizontal nystagmus; on focal illumination, a narrow rim of iris could be seen, not more than 1·5 mm. in width at its broadest upper part and absent altogether at the lower part; signs of a persistent pupillary membrane were noted; sclerotics were bluish; both lenses showed cataractous changes; fundi were slightly deficient in pigment. III. 2, aged 28 weeks, had horizontal nystagmus and bluish sclerotics; both irides were lacking excepting a narrow rim of tissue at the outer side; anterior cortical cataract was noted in both lenses. At a later date a third son of II. 1 was described by Hopf (Bibl. No. 148), who was born with apparently no iris; the child died and the eye was subsequently examined. No consanguinity recorded. Bibl. No. 123.

Fig. 1111. *Carra's Case.* Aniridia in mother and son. II. 2 was seen aged 41; she was a healthy woman and presented no other developmental anomaly; neither her parents nor any of her collaterals had suffered from defects of the eye; she was married at the age of 24 and had two children, a son, III. 1, who died aged 7 months and was reported to have had congenital aniridia, and a daughter, III. 2, who died aged 7 years and had perfectly normal eyes. No consanguinity recorded. Bibl. No. 142.

Fig. 1112. *Stoeber's Case.* Absence of iris in father and son. III. 1, aged 2 months, had bilateral aniridia; the child had no other defect and did not appear to be dazzled by a light; he was the first born child of his parents. II. 2, aged 29, had had feeble vision since infancy; he had bilateral aniridia and posterior capsular cataract; nystagmus was present, also double convergent strabismus; the parents and five siblings of II. 2 had well formed eyes. No consanguinity recorded. Bibl. No. 31.

Fig. 1113. *Henzschel's Case.* Aniridia in a father and in three of his children. I. 1, aged 51, had only a rudiment of brownish iris visible at the lower margin of the cornea; he saw badly and suffered from photophobia. I. 2 had normally developed eyes. II. 1, aged 28, had no iris; she saw badly and had severe photophobia. II. 2, aged 21, had no iris and suffered from photophobia; her sclerotic was very thin and in many places the choroid could be seen through it; she had a gerontoxon. II. 3, aged 13, was also without an iris. Two living members of this sibship had normal eyes; seven siblings had died and no information is given concerning them. No consanguinity recorded. Bibl. No. 17.

Fig. 1114. *Herrnheiser's Case.* Complete absence of iris seen in twin boys aged 15 years; in each case the foetal ring, at the corneo-scleral margin, had persisted; there were opacities in the lenses of all the four eyes; the lenses were in their normal position; in only one of the four eyes could the papilla be seen, in this case it appeared to be smaller than the normal. Before the birth of these boys the mother had suffered, for a long period, from some inflammatory eye disease; the nature of her trouble was vague but her vision recovered. No consanguinity recorded. Bibl. No. 101.

Fig. 1115. *Holm's Case.* Aniridia in a father and in his two children. I. 2 had bilateral aniridia; he had strabismus and nystagmus and said he had always seen badly; R. V. = L. V. $< \frac{6}{60}$; it was noted that both bulbs were small; the corneae also were small, with slight opacities at the limbus but clear central areas; the anterior chambers were very shallow; the lenses were proportional to the size of the eyes, but had a marked forward curvature and showed anterior and posterior polar cataracts. II. 2, aged 19 months, had complete bilateral aniridia; corneae were normal; lenses were clear; fundi were not examined; nystagmus was present. This child died and a post mortem examination of the eye was made a day after death; a well-developed bulb was found but abnormally small lenses were noted; the lenses were clear; the ciliary body was normally developed; the main interest of the case was the absence of a fovea centralis in the retina. II. 1, aged 5 years, was reported by Dr Schou to have eyes similar to those of her brother. No consanguinity recorded. Bibl. No. 240.

Fig. 1116. *Hamilton's Case.* Irideremia in a father and in three of his children; his fourth child had coloboma iridis. II. 1, H. J., aged 36 (1905), had always had defective vision; no iris was visible in either eye; bilateral ptosis and microphthalmos were present; in the right eye there were numerous opacities of the vitreous, the disc was small with ill-defined margins and the retinal vessels small; in the left eye opacities of the lens prevented any view of the fundus; the right field showed concentric contraction for all colours, more marked on the temporal side; bilateral nystagmus was present. III. 3 was dead but was said to have had defective eyes like his father's. III. 2, aged 16 (1905), had always had defective vision; she had bilateral ptosis and nystagmus; her right iris consisted of a small peripheral rim on the outer side only, the left showed a somewhat wider rim on the inner side with undulations here and there; lenses were both slightly dislocated upwards; several small opacities showed on the anterior part of the right lens; fields showed a marked concentric contraction for all colours. III. 4, aged 13 (1905), had always had bad sight; she had very little if any ptosis; slight nystagmus was present; no iris was visible; lenses were both dislocated upwards; several small opacities were present on the anterior surface of each lens; fields showed concentric contraction for all colours. III. 2 and 4 had no photophobia. III. 5 had a right coloboma iridis, nearly straight inwards, with a base equal to about one-fifth of the corneal margin; the left showed a coloboma of about the same size and shape, with a narrow rim of iris at the base; lenses showed several dot opacities on the anterior surface; no nystagmus was present. All these cases had small and ill-developed globes, also high arched palates and asymmetrical upper jaws; III. 2 and 4 had defective dental enamel. II. 5, aged 28 (1905), had normally developed eyes. II. 5 knew of no consanguinity in the parents of previous generations and of no further cases of defective vision in the stock. No consanguinity. Bibl. No. 169, with additional information obtained from Drs T. K. and C. W. Hamilton, through Dr Rischbieth.

Fig. 1117. *Croll's Case.* Aniridia in seven and probably in eleven members of three generations. III. 2, aged 38, had apparently a complete absence of iris in both eyes; R. V. = L. V. = $\frac{6}{200}$; she had no knowledge of her grandparents but reported that her mother, II. 2, had "queer eyes" and cataract with poor vision; the three brothers of II. 2 had also "queer eyes" and poor vision. II. 2, 3, 4 and 5 had been examined by a physician at their homes, who said that they were all born with peculiar eyes. II. 1, the father of III. 2, saw well. III. 3, aged 22, was not seen, but from her sister's account the recorder concluded that she had bilateral aniridia with poor vision. III. 4, aged 17, had bilateral aniridia and R. V. = L. V. = $\frac{20}{100}$. III. 1, aged 42, an Italian, saw well and so far as he knew there was no abnormality in the eyes of any member of his stock.

III. 1 and 2 had five children of whom IV. 1, Frank, aged 10, had bilateral aniridia and R. V. = L. V = $\frac{10}{200}$; he was backward at school. IV. 2, George, aged 8, had bilateral aniridia and R. V. = L. V. = $\frac{20}{200}$; these two boys were unable to go to school alone and had to be taught in special classes on account of their bad sight. IV. 3, John, aged 6, had bilateral aniridia and R. V. = L. V. = $\frac{20}{200}$. IV. 4, Stella, aged 3 years, had bilateral aniridia and R. V. = L. V. = $\frac{20}{100}$. IV. 5, Atilla, a boy, aged 5 months, showed no abnormalities in his eyes. No consanguinity recorded. Bibl. No. 280.

PLATE LXXI. Fig. 1118. *Clausen's Case.* Aniridia in four generations. III. 2, Minna K., aged 53, had bilateral aniridia, excepting a slight rudimentary tag of iris tissue in the upper sector of the right eye; both lenses showed cataract, the right lens was subluxated up and out; bilateral operation for cataract was performed, and some vision was retained. IV. 1, Karl K., son of III. 2, aged 22, had bilateral aniridia, also cataract and subluxated lenses, up and out, in each eye; after extraction of both lenses R. V. with + 8·0 D. sph. = $\frac{6}{40}$, L. V. with + 8·0 D. sph. = $\frac{6}{40}$. III. 1, Friedrich M., aged 54, had R. V. = fingers in front of eyes, L. V. = hand movements; the irides of this man were imperfectly developed, oval lacunae are described in which the stroma is absent and the pigment layer is exposed; both lenses showed cataract; anterior chambers were very deep. III. 4, Anna T., had bilateral coloboma iridis downwards; cataracts were noted in both lenses. III. 5, Maria St., had bilateral aniridia, with a slight tag of iris tissue, up and in, showing in both eyes; she had posterior cortical cataract in both eyes. The paternal grandfather, I. 2, also his brother, I. 1, had aniridia. I. 2 had two daughters free from the anomaly and one son, II. 2, who inherited the defect. II. 2 transmitted defect to four of his six daughters and to one of his three sons. No consanguinity recorded. Bibl. No. 238.

Fig. 1119. *Ulianitsky's Case.* Aniridia in four generations. III. 4 was the patient, but other affected members appear to have been seen. The father, grandfather, two sisters and son of III. 4 were all affected; one of his sister's children had a narrow tag of iris above and on the temporal side about 0·5 mm. wide; all the affected members, except those of the last generation, had marked opacities of the anterior capsule of the lens; all were said to have subluxated lenses; no case had nystagmus; all had corneae normal in size and transparency. The abstract of this history makes no mention of normal members of the stock. No consanguinity recorded. Bibl. No. 292.

Fig. 1120. *Lewis's Case.* Aniridia in four generations. H. B., aged 16, was examined; it is not clear whether this refers to IV. 1 or to IV. 4; he had bilateral aniridia and horizontal nystagmus, his refraction was + 6 D. in the right, + 7 D. in the left, eye. The mother of H. B,. III. 2 or III. 4, had bilateral aniridia, vertical nystagmus and definite diffuse lens opacities in both eyes; her father and paternal grandfather, also her sister and brother were similarly affected; the sister had had both lenses removed for cataract, with a disastrous result in the left eye. IV. 2 had coloboma iridis. No consanguinity recorded. Bibl. No. 270.

Fig. 1121. *Gand's Case.* II. 2 had bilateral aniridia, also congenital dislocation of the lenses; his parents and his eight siblings were free from the anomalies; his four children however all presented exactly the same anomalies as their father; one of the four children, a daughter, was married and had a child who presented the same anomalies. No further information is given in the abstract from which this account is taken. No consanguinity. Bibl. No. 89.

Fig. 1122. *White's Case.* b m iridis in a mother, aniridia in her three children and one grandchild. II. 2, aged 54, had R. V. = $\frac{2}{10}$, L. V. $\frac{20}{100}$; she had bilateral coloboma iridis; in the right eye the cleft was complete, directed upwards and outwards, in the left eye it was partial, downwards and outwards; she had no coloboma of the choroid; both lenses showed slight opacities. II. 2 reported that her father had good eyes, her mother became blind with cataract at the age of 72; one of her sisters had bad eyes. III. 2, aged 26 (1917), had R. V. = $\frac{20}{100}$, with correction of − 4·5 D. sph. = $\frac{2}{10}$; her left eye was almost blind; the right eye had only a slight fringe of iris at the lower border, the lens was slightly ectopic and showed some opacities; there was no iris in the left eye, the lens was full of small opacities and was ectopic, its lower margin being several millimetres above the lower edge of the cornea. III. 3, aged 20, was a cretin, she had no irides, her lenses were ectopic and she had nystagmus. III. 4, aged 18, had no irides; both lenses were ectopic, the upper edges being nearly level with the centre of the cornea; the right eye had a clouded cornea, the left cornea was clear; L. V. = $\frac{20}{100}$ with + 10 D. sph. III. 2 had a daughter, aged 15 months, who had no irides and whose right lens was very slightly displaced upwards. Other members of this family were said to have similar defects but they had not been seen by the recorder. No consanguinity recorded. Bibl. No. 223.

Fig. 1123. *Drinkwater's Case.* This history was originally described at a meeting of the North Wales Branch of the British Medical Association in 1907; in 1923 the recorder, with some difficulty, kindly traced the mother, II. 3, of the affected sibship, III. 3—13, and obtained further information of the family. II. 3, with aniridia, had normal parents and was the only member of her sibship to show the anomaly; she had two normal daughters by her first husband, II. 2, who was 17 years her senior; by her second husband she has had eleven children, of whom eight have aniridia. III. 6 and III. 9 are said to be practically blind; they were in a blind school to which III. 11 was also shortly to be admitted. The husband, II. 4, was in an asylum for two years before his death in 1923. No further details of cases are given. No consanguinity recorded. From notes kindly provided by the recorder.

Fig. 1124. *D'Ewart's Case.* Attention was first called to the aniridia in this family by Dr D'Ewart who noted the condition in his patient, III. 10, suffering from gastro-enteritis, and in the mother of this child. Dr D'Ewart kindly put me in touch with Dr Nora Smith of the Public Health Office in Manchester, to whom I am greatly indebted for further details of the family.

II. 6 first visited the Royal Eye Hospital, Manchester, when she was aged 6 weeks; her mother was told that she had "absent iris"; she can now just see shapes and distinguish colours; she says that her defect arose in answer to her mother's prayer that her husband, I. 1, should have a great shock, to lead him to bring his conduct into line with her requirements. The father of II. 6 had good sight; he drank, and died, aged 49, of pneumonia. The mother of II. 6 had good sight and died, aged 59, from bronchitis. I. 1 and 2 had seven children, of whom II. 2, Agnes, aged 43 (1931), has good sight; she is married and has normal children. II. 3, Thomas, aged 40 (1931), sees well and has normal children. II. 6 is not very intelligent; she has been twice married; by her first husband she had two children, of whom III. 3, Jessie G., aged 15, is in Henshaw's Institution for the Blind; she is suffering from congenital absence of the iris in both eyes, and has marked nystagmus; R. V. $= \frac{6}{60}$, with $- 1$ D. sph. $- 2 \cdot 5$ D. cyl. $= \frac{6}{24}$, L. V. $= \frac{6}{60}$, with $- 2$ D. cyl. $= \frac{6}{24}$. III. 4, Thomas G., was examined by the school medical officer and found to have no defect. By her second husband, II. 6 has had six children, of whom III. 5 and 6 were examined and found to have no abnormality of the eyes and no refractive error. III. 7, aged 5, is in a sunshine home for blind babies at Southport; a report, sent by the courtesy of the ophthalmic surgeon, states that bilateral aniridia is associated with coloboma of the lens and with a large coloboma of the choroid; this child can see objects but the prospects of amelioration are poor. III. 8, William B., aged 3, is in the same home as his brother, III. 7; he also has bilateral aniridia but has normal lenses and no choroidal defect; from the ophthalmic surgeon's report the vision of this boy should be fairly good in each eye; his fundi are said to be of the normal myopic type with pale discs. III. 9, Frederick B., aged 2 years, is said to have normal sight. III. 10, Florence B., seen aged 8 months, was said by Dr D'Ewart to be in a pitiable condition, even the subdued light of the ward causing acute discomfort; this child died before admission to one of the homes for blind babies.

Other siblings of Mrs B., II. 6, include II. 8 who was still-born; II. 2 states that this boy's eyes were examined at birth and he was found to be suffering from the same defect as Mrs B. II. 9, Joseph, is said to have had normal sight; he was killed during the War at the age of 18 years. II. 10 died, aged 1 year, from whooping cough; his eyes are said to have had the same defect as those of Mrs B. II. 11, James, aged 27, is said to have normal eyesight; he is married and has normal children. No consanguinity recorded. Bibl. No. 290, with additional information through Dr Nora Smith and the Secretary-General to the National Institute for the Blind.

Fig. 1125. *Gutfreund's Case.* II. 2, aged 30, had seen badly since his youth; he now saw very badly owing probably to vascularised opacities in each cornea; the right eye showed a complete absence of iris, the left eye had a small tag of iris in a position upwards and outwards. No similar affection had been known to occur in the antecedents of II. 2. The daughter of II. 2, aged 11 months, had a complete absence of iris in the right eye, the left eye showed a small rudiment of iris in the outward direction; she had horizontal nystagmus; corneae were clear; lenses were normal; vision was not demonstrably lowered. No consanguinity recorded. Bibl. No. 183.

Fig. 1126. *Cross's Case.* II. 2, aged 48, had no trace of iris tissue; she had always been practically blind; her eyeballs were normal in size; both lenses were cataractous. There was no history of eye trouble in the parents of this patient but two of her three children showed inherited defect. III. 1, aged 8½ years, had R. V. = L. V. $= \frac{6}{60}$; her left iris had a large coloboma outwards; the right eye showed "a peculiar absence of the choroidal portion of the iris, so that the exposed uvea looked as if it were a portion of a peculiar shaped pupil"; the second child, II. 2, had normal eyes. II. 3 had very imperfect irides completely wanting below; any iris present elsewhere was so narrow that the edges of the lenses could easily be traced; the child was practically blind. No consanguinity recorded. Bibl. No. 122.

PLATE LXXI.   DESCRIPTION OF PEDIGREE PLATES   531

Fig. 1127. *Gifford's Case.* II. 1, aged 34, had congenital aniridia; both lenses showed anterior and posterior cortical opacities; vision had failed rapidly during the last year. No information is given of the parents of II. 1; we are told however that one sister, one half sister, one half brother and one niece were affected by the same condition. No consanguinity recorded. Bibl. No. 267.

Fig. 1128. *Lindberg's Case.* 1. 1 and 2 are reported to have had no eye or other anomalies; their son, II. 2, seen aged 44, had phthisis bulbi in the right eye; the left eye presented a segment of ill-developed iris to the upper and inner sides, in which a rudimentary pupil, up and in, could be seen; a congenital anterior polar cataract was noted, also punctiform opacities diffusely scattered in the lenses; L. V. = finger counting at 2·5 m.; this patient had nystagmus; no fovea centralis could be detected; no yellow colour at the macula could be seen by red free light. A brother, II. 3, aged 36, with strabismus, had clear lenses and no defect of the iris or retina; he had however a cleft palate. II. 2 had four children, of whom III. 1, aged 14, had bilateral complete aniridia; he had congenital cataract in both lenses together with punctate diffuse opacities; fundi could not be seen; divergent strabismus, nystagmus on fixation, ptosis and embryontoxon are also noted. III. 2, aged 13, had bilateral complete aniridia; the fovea centralis was absent in each eye; lenses were similar to those of III. 1 but less severely affected; R. V. = L. V. = $\frac{5}{80}$; nystagmus, ptosis and embryontoxon are noted; this girl further had a cleft palate and a gross systolic cardiac bruit. III. 3, aged 10, had R. V. = L. V. = $\frac{6}{5}$ and appeared to be completely normal. III. 4, aged 9, had bilateral congenital cataract; R. V. = $\frac{4}{5}$, L. V. = $\frac{5}{80}$; slight nystagmus was noted; corneae, sclerae, anterior chambers, fields and tension were normal; the irides were mal-developed in that the anterior layers were absent; the right pupil was somewhat larger than the left, both reacted well to light and convergence; normal discs and an absence of the fovea centralis were noted in each eye.

The mother, II. 1, aged 45, was normal with R. V. = L. V. = $\frac{5}{4}$. No consanguinity recorded. Bibl. No. 250.

Fig. 1129. *Bernard's Case.* II. 1, aged 7 years, was seen to have bilateral not quite complete aniridia; peripheral opacities were noted in both lenses, also an anterior polar cataract in the left eye only; R. V. = $\frac{2}{10}$, L. V. = $\frac{1}{10}$; only the right fundus could be seen, it was normal though the disc was a little pale; nystagmus was not present; teeth were normal and the child was healthy and intelligent. III. 1 was the only child of her mother, II. 2, who had complete bilateral aniridia. II. 2 had had an operation for cataract on both eyes; R. V. = $\frac{5}{10}$ with + 14 D., L. V. = $\frac{5}{10}$ with + 12 D.; fundi were normal; nystagmus was not present; this woman was healthy and of normal intelligence. The parents of II. 2 had good sight; she had one brother and one sister with normal eyes; one brother, II. 5, was still-born. No consanguinity recorded. Bibl. No. 265.

Fig. 1130. *Prichard's Case.* III. 1 had bilateral aniridia; the child was very ill and probably died; the mother was a servant in the house of the father and the child was illegitimate; the father's mother and two of his brothers had very defective sight and the child's mother stated that their eyes exactly resembled those of the child; she said that the father had dark but perfect eyes; the mother, II. 1, was healthy with blue eyes. The history must be regarded as rather uncertain. No consanguinity recorded. Bibl. No. 34.

Fig. 1131. *Pflugk's Case.* II. 2, a female with congenital aniridia, had four children, of whom the first and third had the same anomaly but were now dead; the second child was living and had aniridia; the fourth child had normal eyes. The parents of II. 2 had normal eyes. No consanguinity recorded. Bibl. No. 190.

Fig. 1132. *Caudron's Case.* Aniridia in four generations. III. 2 sought aid for cataract; in the right eye she had corneal opacities, no trace of iris, the lens completely opaque and ocular tension raised to + 2; she had no perception of light; the left eye had corneal opacities, a slight trace of iris was visible on the nasal and on the temporal side, the lens was completely opaque, tension was normal; the patient said she had always had very bad vision; she had slowly lost the sight of the left eye during recent years. III. 2 had two children who died soon after birth; she had no knowledge regarding their eyes. III. 3 had normal eyes. III. 4 had aniridia; she had had ten children, of whom six had died young and nothing was known of their eyes; of the four surviving children, three had no iris. The mother and maternal grandfather of III. 2—4 also had aniridia. No consanguinity recorded. Bibl. No. 91.

Fig. 1133. *Dwyer's Case.* Fifteen cases of aniridia in five generations. The recorder appears to have seen perhaps nine of these cases, but gives no detailed account of the condition in individuals; he states that on casual inspection there appeared to be a total absence of iris but that probably tags of the structure were present; photophobia and nystagmus were marked in the cases seen and vision was evidently defective, for one child was in a school for the blind, two other children were attending school with little benefit; all the adult cases had corneal opacities. No consanguinity recorded. Bibl. No. 255.

Fig. 1134. *Nunneley's Case.* II. 3, aged 8 years, was seen to have total absence of iris; corneae and lenses were clear and sight at this time was good; twelve months later the right lens had become opaque. The eyes of II. 1 were small, soft and ill developed; her irides were thin, dull, and reacted sluggishly; the pupils were displaced considerably from the centre towards the nasal side. II. 2 presented anomalies similar to those of II. 1, to a less remarkable extent. The eyes of the parents were healthy; there was no history of defective eyesight in other relations. No consanguinity recorded. Bibl. No. 62.

Fig. 1135. *Bernard's Case.* II. 3, aged 9 years, had bilateral aniridia; he had slight posterior cortical opacities in his lenses; fundi were normal though the discs were very pale; horizontal nystagmus was noted. Two siblings of II. 3 had normal eyes, two had aniridia; his mother had had one miscarriage. The father of II. 3 was normal; the mother, I. 2, had aniridia, posterior cortical cataracts and some peripheral opacity of the corneae; the fundi of I. 2 were normal though the discs were a little pale; she had slight horizontal nystagmus. No consanguinity recorded. Bibl. No. 265.

Fig. 1136. *Van Duyse's Case.* Aniridia in a mother and in two of her three children. I. 1, aged 37, had so far as one could see complete aniridia; there was a slight opaque pericorneal area; anterior polar cataracts were present in the lenses, also some equatorial cortical opacities; fundi were normal; nystagmus was noted. II. 1, aged 10, is described as "simple" and is said to have been the same as her mother in this respect; apparently her eyes were normal. II. 2 died, aged 14 months, in convulsions; he had a total absence of iris. II. 3 died, aged 9 months, of gastro-enteritis; he had tags of iris here and there, unequally developed and containing no sphincter or dilator muscles. No consanguinity recorded. Bibl. No. 177.

Fig. 1137. *Lewis's Case.* A child, aged 11 months, had bilateral aniridia with lowered vision and photophobia; the father of the child had a congenital bilateral coloboma iridis on the nasal side. The child was well developed in other respects. No consanguinity recorded. Bibl. No. 216.

Fig. 1138. *De Benedetti's Case.* Three siblings all had bilateral congenital aniridia; all three saw very badly; in the six eyes the lenses were luxated upwards and secondary glaucoma had occurred; a fourth brother had good vision and normal eyes except for a coloboma iridis. The father of this sibship had been blind for many years and had the same structural anomalies. No consanguinity recorded. Bibl. No. 92.

Fig. 1139. *Dumont's Case.* II. 4, aged 21, had bilateral complete aniridia and congenital luxation of the lenses; the same affection was presented by his father and by three of his six siblings. No consanguinity recorded. Bibl. No. 93.

Fig. 1140. *Velhagen's Case.* I. 1, aged 49, had a congenital coloboma iridis in the right eye, directed inwards and upwards; there was a small rudiment of iris tissue at the corneal margin of the cleft; the pupil reacted normally; the left eye showed a notch at the pupillary margin of the iris in a position corresponding to that of the coloboma in the right eye. II. 1, an imbecile daughter of I. 1, aged 17, had in each eye a small tag of iris only, situated at the outermost periphery; her lenses, normal in size, had anterior polar cataracts. R. V. $= \frac{2}{15}$, L. V. $= \frac{2}{50}$; nystagmus was very marked. II. 2, aged 9, had no demonstrable trace of iris; he also had anterior polar cataracts which were less developed than those of his sister; R. V. with correction $= \frac{1}{50}$, L. V. $= \frac{1}{12}$. No consanguinity recorded. Bibl. No. 252.

Fig. 1141. *Treacher Collins's Case.* David B., aged 7 months, had a congenital absence of both irides, also anterior polar opacities in both lenses; the child saw light but took no notice of objects. The mother of the child had congenital absence of both irides; she had a leucoma of the right cornea following ulceration and a staphylomatous condition of the sclerotic; her right eye was excised. No consanguinity recorded. Bibl. No. 111.

Fig. 1142. *Waardenburg's Case.* Aniridia in a father and his two children. I. 1, aged 37, had aniridia; his vision was very poor owing to opaque ectopic lenses which moreover were small; nystagmus was noted. II. 1, aged 9, had aniridia in the left eye, coloboma iridis in the right; she had congenital cataract in the left lens; nystagmus was present. II. 2, aged 6, with bilateral aniridia had congenital cataract and nystagmus. No consanguinity. Bibl. No. 233.

Fig. 1143. *Cunha's Case.* II. 1, aged 6 years, had congenital bilateral aniridia, strabismus, opacities in the lenses and bad vision; her mother, I. 1, presented the same conditions. No consanguinity recorded. Bibl. No. 281A.

Fig. 1144. *Prichard's Case.* A mother, with good sight and normal iris in the left eye, had coloboma iridis downwards in the right eye; her child had a coloboma iridis horizontally outwards in the right eye, in which the internal side of the cornea was opaque; in the left eye the child had aniridia and a large central opacity in the cornea. No consanguinity recorded. Bibl. No. 34.

Fig. 1145. *Juler and Batten's Case.* II. 1, aged 21, had no trace of iris in either eye; her lenses were displaced upwards and only the lower half of each lens could be seen; the right lens was opaque and the left partially so; in the right eye T. $= + 1$, there was no perception of light; in the left eye T. $= + 2$, V. $=$ perception of light; the patient had never seen with the right eye but could see to go about with the left eye until the age of 13; she had four siblings who were free from congenital defects; operation was performed for glaucoma.

I. 1, at the age of 59, complained of severe pain in her right eye; the eye was removed for panophthalmitis and glaucoma following an injury three weeks before the record; the right eye had a narrow band of iris bordered by pigment, varying in width and at one point almost completely absent; the edge of the lens, which was opaque, was slightly irregular; in the left eye there appeared to be a complete absence of iris and considerable opacity of the lens, partly of the anterior polar variety and partly deep seated; V. was less than $\frac{6}{60}$; T. = normal. There was no history of bad vision in any other member of the family; the eyes of the only grandchild of I. 1 had normal irides. No consanguinity recorded. Bibl. Nos. 146, 156.

Fig. 1146. *Knape's Case.* Bilateral congenital aniridia in father and son; the condition was incomplete in the father, complete in the son; lenticular opacities were present in both cases. No consanguinity recorded. Bibl. No. 166.

COLOBOMA IRIDIS

Fig. 1147. *Ridley's Case.* I. 1 had normal eyes. I. 2 had in the right eye a partial coloboma iridis and opacities in the lens; in the left eye she had a coloboma iridis upwards and outwards, a large posterior polar cataract and an excentric pupil. I. 1 and 2 had a child, aged 1 year 8 months, who had normally formed lids but only tiny constantly moving rudimentary stumps in both orbits; when first seen, a month earlier, though the lids were normal, no sign of even a rudimentary eye was present in either orbit. No consanguinity recorded. Bibl. No. 163.

Fig. 1148. *von Hoffmann's Case.* II. 1 had a complete coloboma in both eyes, affecting presumably choroid and iris; his sister on the other hand had coloboma of the choroid with a normally developed iris in each eye. No consanguinity recorded. Bibl. No. 52.

Fig. 1149. *Ring's Case.* Microphthalmos, coloboma iridis and posterior polar cataract in a mother and two children. The mother, I. 1, was aged 35; in one eye she had a definite coloboma iridis, the other iris showed a pronounced notch below and in; a child who had died a month previous to the record had shown a precisely similar appearance; a second child exhibited a definite notching in each iris; in all three cases opacities in the lens prevented any examination of the fundus. No further information is given in the abstracts of the paper. No consanguinity recorded. Bibl. Nos. 222, 223.

PLATE LXXII. Fig. 1150. *Attlee's Case.* Coloboma iridis in a mother and her child; in the mother the cleft was directly upwards; in the child it was upwards and outwards in each eye, more directly upwards in one eye than in the other. No consanguinity recorded. Bibl. No. 213.

Fig. 1151. *Fichte's Case.* Unilateral coloboma iridis, downwards and slightly inwards, in the left eye of a female aged 16 years; one of her siblings was said to be similarly affected, but was not seen, and it is not clear whether the defect was also unilateral in this case; no information is given of the parents. No consanguinity recorded. Bibl. No. 36.

Fig. 1152. *Bloc's Case.* (Taken from Pellier de Quengsy.) Coloboma iridis in a man and in two of his five children. I. 1 was seen to have elongated and almost immobile pupils; one of his sons had also oblong pupils; one of his daughters had only one oblong pupil; three of his children were free from the anomaly. "Plusieurs parents de cet homme ont le même vice de conformation." No consanguinity recorded. Bibl. No. 12, p. 436.

Fig. 1153. *Gescheidt's Case.* Coloboma iridis in a father and in the youngest of his five children, a female aged 6 months. No consanguinity recorded. Bibl. No. 23.

Fig. 1154. *Erdmann's Case.* Coloboma iridis in a father and in two of his six children; the family consisted of four boys, of whom two were affected, and two girls who were unaffected. No consanguinity recorded. Bibl. No. 14A.

Fig. 1155. *Hessin's Case.* Coloboma iridis in five members of a sibship of ten; the parents had normal eyes; no eye anomaly was known to have occurred in earlier generations. II. 1 was dead; he had been normal so far as was known. II. 2 had colobomata of the left iris and choroid only; irides were brown. II. 3, with light irides, had bilateral colobomata of the iris and choroid. II. 4, 6, 9 and 10 had normally developed eyes. II. 5 was dead; he had bilateral coloboma of the iris. II. 7 with brown irides had coloboma iridis on the right side only. II. 8 with light irides had bilateral colobomata of the iris and choroid. No consanguinity recorded. Bibl. No. 207.

Fig. 1156. *De Beck's Case.* Coloboma iridis in six females and three males of four generations. I. 1, a clergyman, had good eyes; his wife lived to over 90 years of age and saw well; these parents had eight children, of whom five had coloboma iridis. II. 10, Jeremiah P., seen aged 80, had bilateral coloboma iridis, directed down and slightly in, about as wide as an ordinary pupil, with the sides parallel and reaching to the corneal margin; pupils reacted to light rather sluggishly; vision had always been extremely poor and was now practically nil; corneal diameters measured 10 mm.; in the right eye tension was low, the iris atrophic and adherent to the remnant of a shrunken cataractous lens; the left eye was in a state of phthisis bulbi.

II. 2 had normal eyes. II. 4 had coloboma iridis, down and in, in both eyes, also a probable dislocation of the lens; pupils reacted to light; vision had been better than that of II. 10, but was apparently not good. II. 6 had eyes almost identical with those of II. 10. II. 8 and II. 12 had good sight. II. 13 died aged 20; she was said to have had very bad sight, with nystagmus, and to have had eyes very like those of II. 10. II. 14 had bilateral coloboma iridis downwards, not reaching quite to the corneal margin; she died aged 6, and appears to have had good vision.

The normal son, III. 1, of II. 2, married a normal daughter of II. 4; these first cousins had four normal children, of whom IV. 4, the second born, had a child, V. 6, with coloboma iridis; the defect thus reappearing after two generations of normal individuals.

II. 6 had two children, of whom III. 6 had bilateral coloboma iridis similar to that of her mother. II. 8 had five children with normal eyes, of whom four died in childhood. III. 9 died young. III. 10 had bilateral coloboma iridis, down and in; in the left eye the cleft was complete, in the right it did not extend quite to the periphery; vision was very good; irides brown; pupils, slightly displaced downwards, reacted well. III. 10 had one child, IV. 8, aged 15, who had the same defect as his mother; he had good health in other respects. Consanguinity. Bibl. Nos. 88, 115.

Fig. 1157. *Snell's Case.* Coloboma iridis in five generations; aniridia in two individuals of the stock. In all cases the coloboma was confined to the iris, the choroid remaining unaffected; the position of the cleft was similar in all cases but the extent of the defect varied considerably. The recorder had examined most of the affected members of the pedigree also many of their normal relations. Two affected sisters, I. 4 and 6, had three normal brothers. I. 4 had three sons and a daughter, of whom only the daughter, II. 5, showed the defect. II. 5 was twice married; by her first husband she had one son, III. 2, who had a large coloboma iridis in each eye, that in the right eye being the larger and involving nearly a third of the iris; the situation of the cleft in each eye was outwards and downwards. By her second husband II. 5 had five children, of whom two sons and one daughter had coloboma iridis; one affected son, III. 5, had three normal sons and one daughter with aniridia; the affected daughter, III. 7, had one normal son. III. 2 had six children, of whom two sons and one daughter were affected; of these IV. 1, aged 35, had a defect which was larger in the left than in the right eye; she had no children. IV. 3, aged 27, had one daughter who had complete bilateral aniridia. IV. 5, aged 24, had a daughter, aged 3 months, with coloboma iridis. IV. 7, 9 and 10 were normal and two of them had normal children. III. 3 died aged 3 years. III. 9 and 10, normal children of II. 2, had unaffected offspring. No consanguinity recorded. Bibl. No. 187.

Fig. 1158. *Shannon's Case.* III. 2, Ella T., aged 8, had small pear-shaped corneae measuring about 8 mm. by 10 mm., with apex down and in; she had complete bilateral coloboma iridis; R. V. = L. V. = $\frac{1}{10}$; marked horizontal nystagmus was noted; media were clear; the fundi showed large oval colobomata of the choroid, involving the optic nerve; the site of the disc was indeterminate; in other respects this child was normal. III. 3, Emma T., aged 7, had R. V. = fingers at 6 feet, L. V. = $\frac{20}{30}$; the right eyeball was small, the cornea pear-shaped, with apex down and in, measuring 8 mm. by 10 mm.; the left eyeball was of normal size; both eyes had a coloboma iridis, directed down and in, reaching to the corneal periphery; iris markings were indistinct; the right eye was convergent; the R. fundus showed an extensive coloboma, involving the retina, choroid and optic nerve; the L. fundus showed a less extensive coloboma of the choroid, not involving the optic nerve. III. 4, Mary T., aged 6, had eyes of normal size and no squint; R. V. = fingers at 3·5 feet; L. V. = $\frac{20}{30}$; she had bilateral coloboma iridis, of key-hole type, reaching to the corneal margin; the R. fundus showed an extensive coloboma of the choroid involving the white disc; coloboma of the L. choroid extended to the lower margin of the disc. III. 5, Hazel T., aged 4, had R. V. = L. V. = $\frac{20}{30}$; she had bilateral coloboma iridis; on the right side a narrow bridge of iris tissue stretched across the lower third of the coloboma, which was of key-hole type and complete; on the left side, the coloboma was pear-shaped, complete, and pointed directly downwards; bilateral coloboma of the choroid did not involve the disc. III. 6, Charlotte, aged 15 months, was a healthy child with no ocular defects. II. 5, Charles T., aged 30, the father of III. 2—6, was a farmer, with excellent general health but defective vision; R. V. = $\frac{20}{30}$ and the right eye was of normal development; L. V. = fingers at two feet; the left eye was convergent, normal in size, showing a partial coloboma iridis directed downwards and inwards; the cleft reached half way to the corneal margin; the fundus showed a typical glistening white coloboma, of oval form, reaching up to and very slightly involving the lower border of the papilla; the disc was otherwise normal. II. 8 had normal eyes; no history of abnormality of the eyes could be traced in her family. II. 1, William T., aged 47, had both eyes normal. II. 2, George T., aged 42, had a normal right eye; his left eye had perception of light only; the eyeball was very small with a pear-shaped cornea measuring 8 mm. by 10 mm.; there was an incomplete coloboma iridis of the key-hole type; a posterior polar cataract prevented a view of the fundus. II. 2 had one child whose eyes were normal. II. 4, Alexander T., aged 40, had normal eyes. II. 6, Violet K., aged 24, had normal eyes; she had two children, of whom the eldest had normal eyes; the second child, Mary K., aged 7 months, had both eyeballs microphthalmic, the corneae were "gothic" in form and complete pear-shaped coloboma of the irides extended through the choroid, involving the papillae; double nystagmus was noted; the right eye was convergent.

Plate LXXII.   DESCRIPTIONS OF PEDIGREE PLATES   535

I. 1, Patton T., aged 70, the father of II. 5, had normal eyes; he said that his wife, now dead, had had no difficulty with her eyes and he did not think any member of her family had suffered from eye trouble; he could not recall any evidence of ocular defects in his parents or grandparents. No consanguinity recorded. Bibl. No. 223.

Fig. 1159. *Bloch's Case.* Bilateral coloboma iridis in a father, I. 3, and in his son, II. 4; his daughter, II. 5, had the same affection in one eye only. I. 2 had normal pupils; his son, II. 2, had unilateral coloboma iridis. The children of II. 2 were said to have bilateral coloboma iridis. No consanguinity recorded. Bibl. No. 10.

Fig. 1160. *Streatfield's Case.* Coloboma iridis in seven individuals; only males are affected but a normal mother, II. 2, transmits the defect to three of her four sons. III. 2 had a moderate sized cleft of both irides, directed downwards. III. 1 had a similar defect in both eyes. III. 3 had a similar defect in one eye and some symmetrical indication of the deformity in the other. The mother's father, I. 2, his brother, I. 3, and the eldest brother of II. 2 were said to have a similar defect in both eyes. III. 8, the eldest son of II. 3, had in his right iris an indication of coloboma vertically downwards, the incomplete fissure only extending about half way through the width of the iris; in the left iris he had a double incomplete coloboma, one of which corresponded in position with the furrow in the right iris and the other was to its outer side; the irides in this case were rather deficient in the usual markings. II. 2 had perfectly natural pupils and four of her children, a boy and three girls, were also unaffected. The vision of the defective eyes was good and all the individuals were healthy. No consanguinity recorded. Bibl. No. 42.

Fig. 1161. *Selz's Case.* Coloboma of the choroid associated with a number of other anomalies of the eye in seven members of three generations. II. 2, aged 60 (1900), was healthy and mentally normal; his parents and two siblings had normal eyes; he complained of bad sight and was found to have bilateral coloboma of the iris and choroid, also bilateral cataract; the patient further had bilateral microphthalmos and a small coloboma of the right lens; corneae were circular; irides were light brown, the cleft in each being downwards and inwards; the sides of the clefts were parallel. II. 4, aged 56, had a coloboma in the left iris; she was mentally weak, in an asylum, and would not allow examination. II. 2 had five children, of whom III. 3, 4 and 6 had normal eyes. III. 2, aged 31 (1900), complained of bad vision; his eyes were of normal size; corneae and irides were normal; media were clear; the right fundus was normal; the left disc was anomalous and below it there was a coloboma of the choroid; a detailed description of the anomaly is given by the recorder. III. 5, aged 23 (1900), had a very prominent upper jaw and a high arched palate; her right eye was normal, her left eye had a convergent strabismus and was small; the L. cornea was clear with horizontal and vertical diameters of 8 mm. and 9 mm. respectively; the L. iris was yellowish, lighter than on the other side, and had a complete coloboma downwards; zonular cataract was noted in the L. lens; III. 5 also had a widespread defect of the L. choroid; retinitis pigmentosa was present in all parts of the fundus free from the coloboma; L. V. = hand movements at $\frac{1}{4}$ m.

III. 2 had three children, of whom IV. 1, aged 11 (1900), had markedly small eyes with nystagmus; corneae were small and somewhat oval; irides were almost lemon colour with colobomata downwards; a widespread coloboma of the choroid extended over the area of the disc in each eye. IV. 2, aged 10 (1900), had a normal right eye with corneal diameter of 12 mm.; her left eye was smaller with a corneal diameter of 10 mm.; the right iris was blue grey in colour, the left iris was light brown; coloboma of the left iris had converging sides, and was directed downwards and inwards; media were clear; a widespread coloboma of the left choroid and an anomalous distribution of the vessels is described by the recorder. IV. 3 had a completely normal left eye; his right eye was of the same size and light brown colour as the left, but had a coloboma iridis, down and in; a coloboma of the choroid and anomalous distribution of the vessels were noted. IV. 1, 2 and 3 were healthy, but had very highly arched palates. No consanguinity recorded. Bibl. No. 150.

Fig. 1162. *Halbertsma's Case.* Coloboma iridis, with other anomalies, in three generations. II. 1, aged 54, had a complete coloboma iridis in the right eye only, downwards and slightly inwards; irides were blue grey, the right a little lighter than the left; the anterior layers of the iris stroma showed some diffuse atrophy, more marked on the right side; pupillary reaction was sluggish in the right eye; the right anterior chamber was shallower than the left; the right cornea was flattened; eye movements were good; fundi normal; with correction R. V. = $\frac{6}{24}$, L. V. = $\frac{6}{6}$. II. 1 had seven children, of whom III. 1, aged 28, had slight diffuse atrophy of the iris stroma; irides were blue-grey; pupils were normal; fundi normal. III. 2, aged 27, had greyish green irides with circular pupils; in the left iris there was an atrophic streak, about 1—2 mm. in width, in the anterior stroma layer, directed downwards; the right iris was normal; R. V. = L. V. = $\frac{2}{5}$, with correction; the right disc was pale, the left was normal. III. 3, aged 26, had normal eyes. III. 4, aged 25, had bilateral complete coloboma iridis; on the left side some atrophy of the iris stroma was noted; lenses were clear and fundi normal; R. V. with slight correction = $\frac{10}{10}$, L. V. with − 10 D. sph. = $\frac{1}{10}$. III. 5, aged 22, had always had weak eyes; he had fair hair and blue eyes; in the right iris a radial strip, about 1—2 mm. in breadth, upwards and slightly outwards, was less well developed than elsewhere; the left iris showed a strip 2 mm. in breadth, downwards, in which the anterior stroma layers were atrophic; pupils reacted to light and accommodation; R. V. = L. V. = $\frac{6}{8}$; fundi were normal. III. 6, aged 21, saw well as a child, now R. V. = L. V. = $\frac{6}{9}$ with − 2·5 D. sph.; pupils were normal; the right iris was normal, the left showed slight diffuse atrophy of the stroma, with ill-defined markings; irides were light blue; fundi normal. III. 7, aged 20, had bilateral key-hole shaped coloboma iridis, downwards; lens and media were clear; fundi normal; R. V. = L. V. = $\frac{10}{10}$ with − 2·5 D. sph.

I. 1 was seen, from a photograph, to have a left pupil of oval shape directed up and in; her right pupil was slit shaped, directed down and in; she died soon after the birth of her only child. No other hereditary defect was known to have occurred in the family. No member of the affected sibship, III. 1—7, had married. No consanguinity. Bibl. No. 277.

Fig. 1163. *Weyert's Case.* Coloboma of the optic nerve in three generations. I. 1, Carl M., aged 70, had, in the left eye only, a partial coloboma of the optic nerve; his wife, aged 65, had normal eyes; of their five children II. 2, Elisabeth T., aged 36, had coloboma of both discs; II. 4, Olga J., aged 34, had bilateral coloboma of the disc; II. 6, Eugenie, aged 25, had normal eyes and her three children also were free of the anomaly; II. 7, Alexander M., aged 18, had bilateral coloboma of the disc; II. 8, aged 15, had normal eyes. II. 2 had five children of whom III. 1, Alexandra T., aged 7, had bilateral coloboma of the disc; III. 2, Marie T., aged 4, had coloboma of the right disc only; three younger children were normal. II. 4 had three children, of whom III. 4, Nicolai J., aged 8, had coloboma of the iris; two young daughters were normal. No consanguinity recorded. Bibl. No. 105.

Fig. 1164. *Harman's Case.* I. 1 and 2 represent two healthy parents; they had three children, of whom II. 1 had marked epicanthus; she died, aged 5½ years, from morbus cordis, probably of congenital origin. II. 2, aged 5, was healthy and normal. II. 3, aged 5 months, was a robust and lively baby; her right pupil was large and irregular looking as though a broad iridectomy had been performed up and out; the pupil was immobile; the left eye had a smaller and better shaped pupil but, as in the right eye, it was devoid of any pigmented border; in shape this pupil was an irregular oval, widest from above downwards; some dilatation of the left pupil was demonstrable; media and fundi were normal and the child had excellent vision. The recorder concludes that the case exhibited a complete absence of the sphincter of the iris in the right eye and its partial absence in the left. No consanguinity recorded. Bibl. No. 219.

Fig. 1165. *Zahn's Case.* I. 2 had a small coloboma iridis in the left eye only; her sister had a bilateral congenital coloboma of the iris and choroid; two sisters, I. 4 and 5, had normal eyes. I. 2 had a son, Karl K., who was seen aged 6 months with a hydrophthalmic right eye; his defect was first noticed at the age of 3 months. No consanguinity. Bibl. No. 168.

Fig. 1166. *Maynard's Case.* I. 1, aged 35, a Mussulmani of Dorunda, had been blind for ten years; in her right eye the iris was completely divided into two portions by two large broad colobomata, one down and out, the other up and in; the bases of the colobomata were very wide so that over a considerable area no iris was visible; the pupillary area was black, the upper portion of the iris bulged forwards; the cornea was hazy and bulging; media were hazy and there was only a dim reflex from the fundus; in the left eye I. 1 had a large open shaped coloboma of the iris upwards; the pupil was very large and the iris narrow; the lens was yellow and opaque; the cornea was less bulging than in the right eye. II. 4, aged 10, the son of I. 1, was a healthy looking boy who saw well until five years of age, when both eyes became inflamed and sight diminished; the right iris had two excentric pupils, one of which, situated up and in close to the margin of the cornea, had the remains of a pupillary membrane running across it; both pupils reacted to light but not perceptibly to accommodation; the iris was atrophic, without any pattern; media were clear; there was no choroidal cleft or persistent hyaline artery; there was a marginal leucoma of the cornea internally; the left eye had a very large triangular coloboma of the iris with a wide base; in other respects the iris appeared to be normal, it reacted to light and accommodation; media were clear and there was no choroidal cleft; the cornea showed signs of an old keratitis; R. V. = $\frac{6}{9}$, with + 2·5 D. sph. = $\frac{6}{5}$, L. V. = $\frac{6}{18}$, with + 4·0 D. sph. = $\frac{6}{8}$; each of the three pupils in this boy responded to atropine. The father of II. 4 had normal eyes; three brothers, II. 1—3, and one sister, II. 5, were stated to have good sight; it was unfortunately not possible to examine them. No consanguinity recorded. Bibl. No. 132.

Fig. 1167. *Spencer and La Rue's Case.* Defects of lens and iris in two boys and in their mother. I. 20, aged 35, said that the vision of her right eye had always been very poor; now R. V. = $\frac{2}{20}$, L. V. = $\frac{2}{10}$, improved to $\frac{6}{12}$ and $\frac{6}{5}$ respectively; in the right eye there was a coloboma of the iris at the position of 3 o'clock, reactions of the pupil were very slight; the pupil of the left eye was slightly oval, being elongated towards the position of 9 o'clock, the reactions were less active than normal; there was a coloboma of the lens corresponding to that of the iris; an opacity in the right lens was noted, also a very delicate central opacity of the left lens. I. 2 had three children, of whom II. 1, a son aged 13, had normal eyes. II. 2, a son aged 9, had R. V. = $\frac{4}{20}$, L. V. = $\frac{6}{20}$, with marked nystagmus; his iris consisted of an irregular rim at the ciliary border; the pupils were irregularly oval and had no reactions; there was a rather dense central opacity in the right lens and a fainter one in the left; a coloboma of the ciliary body and choroid involving the optic nerve was noted in each eye. II. 3, a son aged 2 years, had opacities of both lenses which prevented a satisfactory view of the fundus, but there was a strong suspicion of a coloboma involving all the uveal structures in each eye; this child had a narrow margin of light grey iris at the ciliary border, with irregularly oval pupils which showed no reaction. The father, I. 3, had normal eyes. I. 2 had eleven siblings; she knew of no other case of ocular defect in her family. No consanguinity recorded. Bibl. No. 264.

Fig. 1168. *Rosas's Case.* I. 1 had bilateral coloboma iridis; she had five children, of whom one had the same bilateral affection; one had unilateral affection; three were normal. No consanguinity recorded. Bibl. No. 16.

Fig. 1169. *Gleitsmann's Case.* II. 2, Lina B., aged 22 years, had bilateral coloboma iridis; her father had had very good vision all his life; her mother was short-sighted and had coloboma iridis in the right eye only; no similar anomaly had occurred in the sister of II. 2, or in any other member of the family so far as was known. The defect in II. 2 was noticed whilst she was in hospital at the time of the birth of III. 1, who showed no abnormality of the iris. Examination of II. 2 was not easy owing to her slight intelligence, inability to read, and unwillingness, but ophthalmoscopic examination revealed a coloboma of the choroid and some slight opacity of the lens in both eyes. No consanguinity recorded. Bibl. No. 54.

Fig. 1170. *Pfannmüller's Case.* Structural anomalies in the eyes of three sisters; no information is given of the parents. II. 1, E. S., aged 18 (1894), had R. V. = $\frac{2}{3}$, L. V. = finger counting at $2\frac{1}{2}$ m.; she had in the left eye a convergent strabismus; on examination a bilateral coloboma of the optic nerve was noted. II. 2, L. S., aged 16, had a normal right eye, excepting a bundle of opaque nerve fibres in the region of the upper papillary margin; her left eye showed congenital microphthalmos, the cornea measured vertically 3—4 mm.; she had also a coloboma iridis downwards; the fundus could not be seen. II. 3, P. S., aged 13, had always seen badly with the right eye and had never seen with the left; there was slight microphthalmos of the right eye, also a coloboma iridis downwards with converging sides; opacities were noted at the posterior surface of the lens; a choroidal coloboma could be identified; the left eye of II. 3 was rudimentary. II. 4, a boy aged 11 years, had completely normal eyes. No consanguinity recorded. Bibl. No. 119.

Fig. 1171. *Conradi's Case.* This case is of interest as being one of the early published accounts of inherited coloboma iridis. The recorder knew a man who had the defect and whose daughter and granddaughter were similarly affected; their sight was little interfered with. No consanguinity recorded. Bibl. No. 14.

Fig. 1172. *Streatfield's Case.* Coloboma iridis in a brother and sister; their grandfather and two cousins were said to be similarly affected. III. 1 had a bilateral cleft, directed downwards and inwards and extending to the margin of the cornea; his irides had the usual markings and were brown in colour; his vision was in all respects good; no other defect was associated with the coloboma. No consanguinity recorded. Bibl. No. 42.

Fig. 1173. *Ourgaud's Case.* Consanguineous parents had two children with mal-developed eyes, of whom III. 1 had bilateral coloboma of the iris and choroid; III. 3 had a congenital absence of globes with normal eyelids and annexes; no trace of globe could be found in the orbit. The maternal grandfather had coloboma iridis. Two paternal aunts had retinitis pigmentosa associated with deafness and with defective intelligence. Consanguinity. Bibl. No. 249.

ECTOPIA LENTIS

PLATE LXXIII. Fig. 1174. *Usher's Case.* Four cases of congenital symmetrical dislocation of the lens in three generations. V. 24, Catherine S., aged 14 (1908), does not see well, far or near; she is third born in a sibship of three; had measles when 7 years old, otherwise has been very healthy. Pupils equal, contract to light; R. V. = L. V. = $\frac{6}{24}$ with correction; refraction hypermetropia, 8 D. in both; both lenses opaque and displaced down-out; iridodonesis; fundi normal. The patient is nervous and excitable; is not very well nourished; palate high and narrow; fingers long, thin and blue in colour; heart, lungs and digestive system normal; nothing abnormal found in nervous system; urine amber, acid, 1016, no albumen, no sugar. Some twenty-three years later (March 28th, 1931) both lenses were white and lying in lower part of vitreous; pupils equal, contracted to light; irides bluish, with brown pigment in stroma; R. V. with + 7·5 D. sph. = $\frac{6}{12}$ = L. V. with + 7 D. sph., not fully; with + 11 D. sph., R. eye reads 1 J., L. eye reads 2 J.; tension normal; anterior chambers deep; iridodonesis of whole of iris in each eye. The weight of V. 24 is 8 st. 11 lbs., height 5' $8\frac{1}{4}''$ in boots; she is married and has two children, VI. 8 and 9.

V. 20, Isabella S., aged 16 (1902), first born in sibship, has been unable to see well since birth; has had no pain in the eyes, except occasional attacks of neuralgia, which extended to the eyes, usually from the right side of face; has never been strong; measles at age of 13; some time after this was troubled with cramps in the hands, which came on at irregular intervals, once or twice a week; she said that during the attack the arm flexed at the elbow, the hand flexed at the wrist, the fingers became flexed at the metocarpophalangeal joints, the fingers themselves remained straight; the thumb was pressed against the fingers; the cramps lasted for about two hours and were very painful; feet were not affected; no history of fits, vomiting or gastric trouble; palate much vaulted; chest pigeon-shaped; heart and lungs normal; urine amber, acid, 1010, a trace of albumen, no sugar. Upper central incisors were decayed, lower incisors had deficient enamel. R. V. = $\frac{6}{60}$, with − 33 D. sph. = $\frac{6}{20}$, 1 J. at 2″, L. V. < $\frac{6}{60}$, with − 33 D. sph. = $\frac{4}{60}$, 1 J. at 2″; the whole of the iris was tremulous; pupils equal, contract to light, are quite central; anterior chambers of uniform depth; both lenses small and dislocated downwards; in the R. lens capsule is a triangular area of grey granular opacity; myopic crescents in both fundi. In 1905 R. V. = L. V. = $\frac{6}{60}$ with − 25 D. sph. Both these cases were patients in the Aberdeen Royal Infirmary.

Writing from Canada, March 1931, V. 20 says "I have only been married four years. I had one miscarriage. I lost the sight of my left eye completely in 1918; a specialist told me the inner lining of left eye had dropped completely away, rendering further sight impossible. Dr Galloway needled my right eye five times. I just see well enough to manage my housework. The eye weakness was entirely on father's side, although neither his father nor mother had eye trouble, nor any of his brothers or sisters." The father, IV. 7, died of "apoplexy" at the age of 47; he was seen six years before when R. V. = $\frac{6}{60}$, with + 3·5 D. sph. = $\frac{6}{12}$, with + 8·5 D. sph., reads 1 J. at 9″; L. V. = $\frac{6}{60}$, with + 5 D. sph. = $\frac{6}{12}$ partly, with + 9 D. sph. reads 1 J. at 9″; irides tremulous; myopic crescent in each eye; both lenses were opaque and were in the lower part of the vitreous chamber.

VI. 9, Patricia S., aged 8 (1931), a healthy schoolgirl with fair hair and blue irides; height 4′ 4¾″ with boots on, weight 4 stone; is wearing − 10·5 D. sph. in R., − 9 D. sph. in L.; pupils equal, contract to light; irides tremulous at outer parts; horizontal diameter of cornea 10 mm.; eye movements full; both anterior chambers deeper at outer than inner parts; lens grey, outer edge clearly seen in each eye; tension normal; fundi normal; R. V. < $\frac{6}{60}$ with − 13 D. sph. = $\frac{6}{60}$, reads 1 J. at 2½″ with a glass; L. V. < $\frac{6}{60}$, with − 9 D. sph. = $\frac{6}{60}$, reads words of 1 J. at 3″ with a + 12 D. sph.; sits near blackboard at school where she is 21st in a class of 40. V. 22 and his two children, VI. 6 and VI. 7, are abroad and have good vision. III. 4, farmer, had good vision and was mentally normal, died aged 88. His wife, III. 7, had good vision and was clear mentally, died aged 86. II. 1 and II. 2 both lived longer than 70 years, had good vision and no mental trouble. II. 4, a farmer with good vision and mentally sound, married twice, first wife (II. 3) died in 1859, a leg had been amputated; his second wife was II. 5. There were ten children from the first marriage and seven from the second marriage; none of these, excepting III. 7, has descendants who are known to have dislocated lenses or any malformation of the eye and none have defective vision. III. 13 had a daughter, an only child, IV. 27, from her marriage with III. 12, who was silly, but had good vision, and died aged 19; III. 13 had previously a healthy illegitimate son by III. 14. III. 17 had a grand-daughter, V. 42, who has been in a mental home since the birth of her daughter, VI. 12. A considerable number of the members of the pedigree live abroad, such as all the descendants of III. 8, namely IV. 24 and V. 26, who are in Canada, but they keep in touch with their relatives in this country by writing and occasional visits, so that poor vision, or other defect, in any of them would be known to those in this country. No consanguinity. Hitherto unpublished.

Fig. 1175. *Usher's Case.* Congenital dislocation of the lens in five males and two females of three generations; in each case the affection was bilateral. I. 1, a millwright, married at the age of 29 and died, aged 59, from cancer of the stomach; he and all his known relatives, other than his descendants from I. 2, had good sight; his father was killed at the age of 70; his mother, who died aged 91, always had good vision; he had three sisters and five brothers. I. 2 had good vision and showed no evidence of dislocation of either lens; she was married at 16; when pregnant with II. 5, at the age of 17, was weak and unwell; at the age of 79 she was healthy and active, and the fundus was normal in each eye. I. 2 had seven children and two miscarriages; only one of her children was affected.

II. 5, John O., aged 33 (1899), carter, was born at full time; he stated that he had had dislocated lenses as long as he could remember; his left eye had troubled him for two days and had been red off and on since it was injured with a stone two years previously; L. V. counts fingers at 9″; T. = +1; lens partially dislocated into anterior chamber, inner part of lens lies in front of iris; eye much congested. R. V. = $\frac{6}{60}$, with + 10 D. sph. = $\frac{6}{60}$; iridodonesis; pupil small, circular, contracts to light; lens dislocated outwards, its inner edge being visible at centre of pupil; tension normal; fundus normal excepting a congenital crescent below the disc; the original position of the left lens was not known as no examination was made until after the injury. The right eye also was injured at a later date (1910), at this time L. V. = hand movements only, R. V. = $\frac{6}{24}$, with + 9 D. sph.; he had been a healthy man and was well nourished; urine acid, 1024, no albumen, no sugar; in 1913 he died from cancer of the stomach.

III. 10, James O., aged 19 (1910), labourer, said he never had good sight; R. V. = < $\frac{6}{60}$, or with + 10 D. sph. and + 3 D. cyl. = $\frac{6}{18}$, L. V. = $\frac{2}{60}$ not improved by glasses; on each cornea at its upper and inner part was a nebulous opacity extending from near the centre of the cornea to the periphery, these occupied about

Plate LXXIII.   DESCRIPTIONS OF PEDIGREE PLATES   539

a quarter of the cornea and merged into the sclerotic, at other parts the edge of the opacity was well defined; pigmented bands passed forwards from the iris surface to the opacity; iris stroma in each eye appeared to have been partially separated from the posterior layers and pulled forwards towards the corneal opacity; pupils circular, contracted to light; iridodonesis; lenses dislocated inwards, edge of lens visible at centre of pupil; no fundus details were seen. III. 12, William O., aged 15 (1908), comb maker, had never seen well; R. V. with + 9 D. sph. = $\frac{6}{60}$, L. V. with + 13 D. sph. = $\frac{6}{36}$; pupils circular; iridodonesis in each eye; lenses displaced inwards; some fine floating vitreous opacities in each eye; fundi normal; left eye diverges upwards and outwards. III. 14, George O., aged 15 (1910), ropemaker; R. V. with + 11 D. sph. = $\frac{6}{36}$, L. V. with + 13 D. sph. = $\frac{6}{60}$; R. lens dislocated outwards, edge of lens visible at centre of pupil; iridodonesis; fundus normal; a bluish grey opacity with well-defined upper margin was present on the lower third of cornea, thick pigmented bands passed to it from the circulus iridis minor, none of the bands were attached to the margin of the pupil; upper part of iris was brown with a smooth surface, whilst lower part was a bluish grey colour, with a rough surface and some large crypts; pupil slightly pear-shaped with narrow end downwards, contracted readily to light; left eye had an opacity in upper third of cornea, to which extensive bands passed from the anterior surface of the iris; the iris appeared to be connected with the whole extent of the corneal opacity and was much thinned; pupil almost circular, contracted well to light; lens was dislocated upwards and slightly inwards; no clear view of fundus was obtained. III. 15, Bella O., died aged 7 years; she had dislocated lenses. III. 17, Lizzie O., aged 13 (1910); lenses were dislocated outwards, inner edge of each lens passed across the pupil about its centre; fundi were normal; iridodonesis in each; refraction hypermetropia, 7 D.; III. 17 died, aged 15, with a history of discharge from an ear and head trouble.

IV. 4, James O., aged 4 (1921), illegitimate child of III. 12, had corneae of normal size; pupils equal, central, contract to light; anterior chamber shallower at inner parts; iridodonesis in each eye; lenses, dislocated inwards and tilted backwards at outer parts, occupy rather more than half the pupils; retinoscopy showed myopia 20 D. in each eye; fundi normal; palate high.

III. 11 and 16, brothers of the affected siblings, had both been married for about two years but had no offspring; the former was myopic and had choroidal atrophy around the left optic disc. III. 16 had a small upper jaw; V. = $\frac{6}{6}$ in each; fundi normal. III. 18 and 19 died in infancy.

Many other members of the family were examined but no further case of anomaly was discovered, excepting the case of III. 30 whose pupils were somewhat ectopic inwards. No consanguinity. Bibl. No. 258.

Fig. 1176. *Vogt's Case.* Ectopia lentis in many members of four generations. I. 2, E. P. X., became blind in 1797, at the age of 47, but he carried on his work as a clergyman until 1817; the cause of his blindness was unknown. I. 2 was twice married; by his first wife he had a son and a daughter, of whom II. 2., E. F. X. (1780—1844), had defective vision and was believed to have had ectopia lentis. By his second wife, I. 2 had six children, of whom II. 7 was blind in old age, II. 6 was operated on for cataract, and had a son with ectopia lentis and cataract. There would appear to be little doubt that I. 2 is responsible for the eye disease in his descendants.

II. 2 had thirteen children, of whom III. 5, T. X., had bilateral spontaneous dislocation of the lens, complicated by cataract; in 1874 it was reported that acute glaucoma in the left eye had caused loss of vision and the eye was enucleated; this patient, seen in 1881, had eight children who had shown no signs of ectopia lentis. III. 7, J. X., had no history of inflammation in his eyes; after the age of 60 a diminution of vision was noted and a spontaneous dislocation of the lens occurred; cataract also was present; at an earlier age the patient had seen well; at the age of 85, tension was normal; pupils were central, not quite round, reacting normally; the irides showed a marked tremor; the right lens was opaque and displaced downwards, so that its upper margin crossed the middle of the pupil; the left eye showed the total luxation of an opaque lens; fundi were normal. III. 7 had three children living, of whom IV. 6, L. X., had bilateral ectopia lentis and cataract; this patient was a myope; at the age of 45 she was reported to have had iritis in the left eye followed by double vision, with a history of similar trouble in the right eye a few years later; at 54 both eyes were free from inflammation, pupils were circular, central and reacted promptly; irides were tremulous, the right lens was subluxated downwards, and moved when the eye was moved; the left lens was completely luxated into the vitreous, it was cataractous and freely moveable with movements of the eye; tension was slightly raised; the patient had frequent headaches. III. 9, G. X., had bilateral spontaneous luxation of the lens reported to have occurred at the age of 45 years; at that time the patient had myopia of 4 D.; at the age of 66 both fields showed some concentric contraction, colour vision was normal; both irides were tremulous; the pupil was not quite round and presented a persistent pupillary membrane; lenses were displaced downwards; both discs were greyish white with some excavation; tension = + 2, the patient died five years later from apoplexy. III. 9 had seven children, of whom IV. 9, S. B. X., had markedly tremulous irides with no demonstrable dislocation of the lens at the time she was seen. IV. 10, J. X., was myopic from his youth; there was no history of inflammatory eye trouble; at 53 markedly tremulous irides were noted; pupils were central, not quite circular, reacting normally; both lenses were dislocated downwards and moved with the slightest movement of the eye; rainbows were seen, believed to be due to refraction at the border of the lens; lenses were clear; tension was normal; fundi were normal. IV. 11, G. X., lived abroad and details of his case were not available, but he was known to have had spontaneous luxation of the lens. IV. 12, J. X., had a bilateral spontaneous luxation of the lens at about the age of 32; he was subject to frequent headaches. IV. 13, L. X., had a bilateral marked tremor of the irides which had been noted during the last few years.

III. 11, A. X., 1823—1891, had spontaneous lens luxation, associated with cataract; this man had no children. III. 12, E. X., had bilateral complete luxation of the lens; this man had lived abroad for a long time; no detailed statement of his condition was available; nothing was known of the eyes of his nine children. III. 18, C. X., 1832—1896, was short-sighted from childhood; at the age of 48 commencing bilateral lens luxation was noted; at 55 both lenses were displaced downwards and the upper parts of the pupils were free; the lenses were clear. III. 18 had eight children, of whom IV. 27, O. X., born 1861, first noticed, at the age of 25, that his vision was diminishing; at 43 his eyes were free from inflammation; tension was somewhat raised in each eye; pupils were circular and central; irides were tremulous; both lenses were luxated downwards; the discs were slightly atrophic; the fields showed some contraction on the nasal side; double vision was complained of. IV. 28, P. X., was myopic, both lenses were displaced downwards; he complained of haloes; at the age of 35 a cataract extraction with iridectomy was performed.

III. 22, R. X., born 1842, saw quite well up to the age of about 45 from which time his vision gradually diminished; he had bilateral complete luxation of the lens, complicated by cataract; two children of this patient were short-sighted but showed no pathological eye changes. One sister of III. 22 was very short-sighted; she died aged 55. No consanguinity recorded. Bibl. No. 172.

Fig. 1177. *Strebel's Case*. Ectopia lentis and ectopia pupillae in seven males and seven females of four generations; the anomaly was associated with myopia and with heart disease in most cases. I. 2 and 3 were not seen, but the author judged from reports that they very probably had ectopia lentis, ectopia pupillae and myopia; they were not known to have suffered from heart disease. I. 2, married to I. 1, who exhibited no anomaly, had eight children, of whom II. 3 died, aged 16, from heart failure; she had ectopia lentis and pupillae and probably myopia. II. 4 died, aged 25, from heart failure; he also had ectopia lentis and pupillae and probably myopia. II. 5 exhibited all the defects and died from heart failure at the age of 42; she was the second wife of II. 2, who had normal children and grandchildren by two other wives, and whose relations were free from heart disease and saw well; of the three children of II. 2 and 5, the eldest, III. 7, died, aged 2 years, from an unknown cause; III. 8 and 9 showed all the defects to which the family was liable; III. 8 had mitral incompetence; III. 9 had mitral incompetence, aortic incompetence and aortic stenosis. II. 6 showed all the defects and died, aged 47 years, from heart failure; she had mitral incompetence and stenosis. II. 8 suffered from all the family defects and died, aged 50 years, from heart failure. II. 9 was the only child of I. 1 and 2 who was free from the family defects but two of her three children, III. 14 and 15, had ectopia lentis and pupillae and suffered from heart disease; they were not myopic. II. 11 and 12 had ectopia lentis and pupillae and died early from heart disease, but had no myopia. III. 9 married a woman who had the same surname as I. 3, we are not told however that they were related; they had five children, of whom the eldest, aged 16, had ectopia lentis and pupillae, myopia and heart disease, the latter leading to mitral incompetence and stenosis; IV. 16—19, aged 14, 12, 10 and 8 years respectively, were free from anomaly, or heart disease.

Few details are given of the individual cases in this pedigree but III. 9 and IV. 15 had glaucoma, following the luxation of lenses into the anterior chamber; the lenses were removed by operation. The heart affections were not congenital or due to structural anomalies but mostly had an infectious basis and appear to suggest an inherited liability to endocarditis in the presence of infection. No consanguinity recorded. Bibl. No. 202.

Fig. 1178. *Cameron's Case*. Ectopia lentis in thirteen females and one male of four generations; in each case both lenses were dislocated and vision was very seriously affected. I. 2 was said to be the only member of a sibship of seven to be affected; her only child, II. 1, was similarly affected. II. 1 had six children, of whom four were affected and each of these transmitted the defect to their children. III. 2 had to be trained in an institution for the blind. III. 4 with dislocated lenses had pin point pupils, which did not dilate under atropine, so that examination was difficult; iridodonesis was present; R. V. = L. V. = $\frac{3}{60}$, improved by + 11 D. sph. in each. IV. 6, aged 13, had both lenses partially dislocated upwards; R. V. = L. V. = $\frac{4}{60}$ or with + 12 D. sph. V. = $\frac{3}{60}$ in each; fundi normal. IV. 8, aged 11, had both lenses partially dislocated upwards; R. V. = L. V. = $\frac{3}{60}$, not improved by glasses, fundi normal. IV. 9, aged 6; R. V. = finger counting at 8″, L. V. = $\frac{1}{60}$; right lens was much displaced outwards, leaving most of the pupil free so that vision was improved by + 11 D. sph.; in the left eye, the lower margin of lens was across the centre of the pupil; fundi were normal. No further cases in this family were examined. No consanguinity recorded. Bibl. No. 266.

Fig. 1179. *Clark's Case*. A history of ectopia lentis associated with coloboma lentis in two generations. I. 2, David H., was blind for thirty years before his death; he was supposed to have had cataract; he had two sisters and one brother, of whom no information is given. II. 2, Samuel H., was blind for ten years before his death. Of the nine children of II. 2, the three eldest, aged 70, 68 and 64 years respectively, had normal

Plate LXXIII.   DESCRIPTIONS OF PEDIGREE PLATES   541

eyes but III. 2 had one child, IV. 1, a daughter aged 26, Bertha A., with bilateral coloboma lentis. III. 5, Tillie H. M., aged 63, had bilateral coloboma lentis and cataract. III. 6, aged 61, had normal eyes. III. 7, M. R. H., aged 59, had both lenses dislocated downwards; he had been under observation for nineteen years and had excellent vision. III. 8, J. O. H., aged 55, had a small semicircular coloboma of the lower border of the right lens associated with a dislocation upwards; he had a rather advanced cataract. III. 10, aged 53, had (?) cataract. III. 12, aged 51, had normal eyes.

Of the three children of III. 8, one son was normal; IV. 4, J. H., aged 23, had coloboma lentis in the left eye; IV. 3, Millie H., aged 25, had a large coloboma in both lenses. IV. 5, Kenneth A., aged 30, had bilateral dislocation of the lenses upwards. IV. 1 and 4 had been under observation for some years and had practically normal vision when corrected. No consanguinity recorded. Bibl. No. 229.

Fig. 1180. *Rötth's Case.* Ectopia lentis, associated with heart disease and with high myopia. I. 1—3 had normal eyes; I. 2 was married twice and had a daughter by each husband; II. 2 had normal eyes, II. 1 had weak eyes and was believed by the recorder to have probably had ectopia lentis, she also had at the age of 50 years an enlarged heart with the apex almost in the axillary line. II. 2 married a myope and had two children, a daughter, III. 2, who had ectopia lentis, myopia, and myocardial degeneration, and a son, III. 3, who was normal. III. 2 had seven children, of whom IV. 1, aged 26, was normal; IV. 2 was said to have died suddenly from heart disease at the age of 21 days; IV. 3, aged 23, was normal; IV. 4, aged 20, had ectopia lentis and high myopia; IV. 5 died, aged 16, and was believed to have probably had ectopia lentis; IV. 6, aged 15, had ectopia lentis, high myopia, and mitral disease; IV. 7 died, aged 7½ years, from heart disease. No consanguinity recorded. Bibl. No. 263.

Fig. 1181. *Bresgen's Case.* Ectopia lentis in ten members of a small pedigree. Fritz S., IV. 1, complained of difficulty in seeing; he was found to have bilateral congenital ectopia lentis, both lenses being displaced upwards and inwards; his mother had also seen badly since her youth and it was found that the same anomaly occurred in her and in her other five children. The paternal grandmother of III. 2 had been very short-sighted since her childhood, but could always do fine work; the recorder considered that she also with great probability had ectopia lentis. The father of III. 2 had very good vision; he was the only child of his parents. III. 2 had two siblings, a sister with ectopia lentis and a brother with good vision, whose son had bilateral ectopia lentis. No other abnormality was found in association with the anomaly. No consanguinity recorded. Bibl. No. 66.

Fig. 1182. *Fecht's Case.* Ectopia lentis in four members of a sibship of ten. II. 2, Johann J., aged 46 (1927), had always seen badly but since 1914 his vision had become much worse; in 1918 he had a detachment of the retina following trauma; he had had an operation for extraction of a luxated lens. II. 5, Wilhelm J., aged 42 (1927), had seen badly since birth and had been under treatment repeatedly between the years of 1910 and 1923; he had increasing myopia; his lenses became cataractous and the left lens, with complete opacity and shrinkage, became luxated into the floor of the vitreous chamber. In 1926 the anterior chambers were very deep, there was a marked tremor of the irides, pupils reacted well; the right lens was subluxated outwards and downwards, the left lens was luxated into the vitreous and could be made to fall into the pupillary region on the patient lowering his head; R. V. = L. V. = $\frac{1}{36}$ with correction. II. 13, Frau H. D., aged 28, had always seen badly and had been under treatment many times between the ages of 11 and 22 years; she had deep anterior chambers and tremulous irides; her right pupil was excentrically placed inwards; right lens was opaque and subluxated downwards and inwards; the left lens was opaque and shrunken and was completely luxated outwards and downwards. II. 17, Paul J., aged 23, had had an operation for strabismus and had slight bilateral ptosis; his right pupil was larger than the left, the left pupil was excentrically placed upwards and inwards; the left lens was subluxated upwards and inwards and showed a slight opacity; the right lens was clear. The parents of these siblings were said to have normal eyes.

No anomaly is noted in the six siblings of the cases described nor in the seventeen members of generation III; evidently enquiries were made with regard to these members but no details concerning them are given. No consanguinity. Bibl. No. 272.

Fig. 1183. *de Caralt's Case.* Ectopia lentis in five females of two generations. I. 1 died from Raynaud's disease; I. 2 was healthy; these parents had three healthy sons and three daughters; of the latter II. 4 had congenital cataract; II. 6 had ectopia lentis and amblyopia; II. 7 had ectopia lentis, and later luxation, she also suffered from metrorrhagia. II. 4 had four daughters, of whom the first had some cerebral vascular trouble which led to mental defect. III. 2 and 3 were normal. III. 4 had bilateral ectopia lentis with later luxation; she had cataract early in life, also rickets; she was neurotic and very irritable with manifest hyperthyroidism; puberty occurred at 13 years but there was some abnormality in the development of secondary sex characters; she was liable to fainting attacks and nervous crises. II. 6 died childless. II. 7 had two healthy sons and one healthy daughter; one daughter, III. 8, had bilateral ectopia lentis, she was neurotic and had a tuberculous hip joint. III. 9 had bilateral ectopia lentis and hyperthyroidism. The condition in III. 4 and III. 8 was associated with a progressive high myopia showing resultant changes in the fundus. No consanguinity recorded. Bibl. No. 276.

Fig. 1184. *Usher's Case.* A father and daughter with both lenses dislocated. II. 4, William D., aged 41 (1909), carter, came to hospital on account of his daughter, III. 4; he stated that his father, I. 1, and mother, I. 2, had good vision and were not cousins; he was "always a little short-sighted"; II. 4 is fourth in a sibship of seven, all of his brothers and sisters had good vision; on examination his lenses were seen in the vitreous; fundi normal; R. V. with + 10 D. sph. = $\frac{6}{18}$, L. V. with + 12 D. sph. = $\frac{6}{12}$. III. 4, Sarah D., schoolgirl, aged 9 (1909), never had good sight, left eye was painful for a month two years ago, previous to this vision had been the same in each eye; a white appearance had been noticed for two or three years in her left eye; R. V. with + 15 D. sph. = $\frac{6}{43}$ not fully; pupillary part of iris blue, ciliary part green; pupil contracts feebly to light; upper edge of lens visible at extreme lower part of pupil; tension normal; fundus normal; L. V. = no perception of light; a globular bluish translucent body with dense yellowish white opacity at centre of anterior surface lies in the anterior chamber (lens dislocated); iris grey with broad pigmented pupillary band, pupil dilated, no contraction to light; it is a blind glaucomatous eye. III. 4 appears perfectly healthy and has no other deformities; respiratory, circulatory and alimentary systems normal; urine amber, acid, 1015, no sugar, no albumen; left eye was excised; III. 4 is fourth born in a sibship of five; her three sisters, III. 1, 2 and 5, have normal vision, but her brother, III. 3, does not see so well as her sisters, it is therefore just possible that he too may have dislocated lenses. The family had left the address they gave twenty-one years ago and unfortunately could not be traced. No consanguinity. Hitherto unpublished.

Fig. 1185. *Rollet and Bussy's Case.* II. 2, Leopold R., aged 28, had both lenses displaced upwards and inwards; the lower external border of the lens divided the pupils so that a third of the pupillary area was aphakic; the lenses were perfectly transparent; iridodonesis was noted; R. V. = $\frac{1}{20}$, L. V. = $\frac{1}{20}$; fundi were normal; the patient was robust; his ocular defect was noticed at the age of 5 years. III. 1, Henry R., aged 5, had lenses dislocated precisely as in his father; R. V. = L. V. = $\frac{1}{20}$. A maternal uncle of II. 2, and a son of this uncle had very bad sight which could not be corrected by glasses. No consanguinity recorded. Bibl. No. 242.

Fig. 1186. *Pinckard's Case.* II. 2, J. E., had always had bad sight; both lenses were dislocated downwards and inwards and were opaque. II. 3, Rose E., had both lenses dislocated downwards; when first seen her lenses were clear and were noted to be more convex than normal; at a later visit opacities had developed in each. II. 2 had three children, of whom III. 1, Jane E., aged 10, had both lenses dislocated upwards and inwards. III. 2, aged 6, was said to have good vision. III. 3, Rachel E., aged 5, was "mentally lacking" and had both lenses dislocated upwards and inwards. I. 2 was said to have had poor vision. No consanguinity recorded. Bibl. No. 148A.

Fig. 1187. *Breitbarth's Case.* Corectopia and ectopia lentis in two brothers; the parents, four other siblings and other relations had no similar defect. II. 2, aged 40, was a robust man, the father of many children, all of whom had normal eyes; his sclerae and corneae were normal, media were transparent; the anterior chamber in each eye was deep; irides were brown and tremulous on movement of the eyes; pupils on each side were displaced downwards and slightly outwards; they were of a long oval shape, the long axis directed obliquely from up and in to down and out; the pupils measured 2½ mm. by 1 mm., they reacted promptly to light; the lens in each eye was ectopic; extensive choroidal atrophy was noted in the region surrounding the disc; R. V. = $\frac{2}{60}$, L. V. with + 10 D. = $\frac{2}{60}$. A similar description is given of the eyes of II. 3, aged 36; his pupils however were displaced upwards and outwards and were oval in shape; the irides were tremulous on the least movement of the eyes; the lenses were ectopic; the discs were surrounded by an area of atrophic choroid; R. V. = $\frac{3 \cdot 6}{60}$, L. V. = $\frac{3}{60}$. There was no diplopia in either brother. No consanguinity recorded. Bibl. No. 116.

Fig. 1188. *Foxonet's Case.* II. 2, aged 50, complained of severe pain in her left eye; the bulb was injected, the pupil dilated, and an oval lens was in the anterior chamber, the papilla was deeply excavated; V. = perception of light; T. = + 3. At this time the right eye showed a tremulous iris and subluxated lens; fundus was normal; tension not raised; at a later date glaucoma occurred in this eye also; the patient had always had bad sight. I. 1, aged 72, also had luxation of the lens downwards in both eyes and glaucoma; cataract was noted in this case. I. 2 had good vision. II. 3, aged 35, had glaucoma with luxation of the lens in the left eye. Of the children of II. 2 two had good vision; III. 3, aged 8 years, had bilateral congenital ectopia lentis with an upward displacement. No consanguinity recorded. Bibl. No. 235.

Fig. 1189. *Tiffany's Case.* Ectopia lentis in seven children of a sibship of nine; in each case iridodonesis was present and the lens could be seen swaying slightly; none of the children complained of diplopia; the lenses all seemed slightly opaque; visual acuity varied from $\frac{20}{200}$ to as low as $\frac{3}{200}$; the direction of the displacement of the lenses in different cases was as follows: II. 1, Josephine, aged 19, both lenses outwards; II. 3, Minnie, aged 16, R. lens upwards and outwards, L. lens up and slightly outwards; II. 4, Emma, aged 15, R. lens upwards, L. lens up and inwards; II. 5, William, aged 12, R. lens outwards, L. lens upwards and outwards; II. 6, Freddie, aged 10, both lenses inwards; II. 7, Theodore, aged 8, both lenses up and outwards II. 9, Herman, aged 4, both lenses upwards and outwards. II. 2, Louisa aged 18, and II. 8, Bertha, aged 6, had V. = $\frac{2.0}{2.0}$ in each and had normally placed lenses; II. 2 had some opaque fibres of the optic nerve in the left eye. The mother, aged 40, a German, had normal eyes; the father was dead but his widow said he had something shaking in his eyes and was very near-sighted; the recorder thought he probably had the same affection as his children. The lenses in all the affected members of the family were of normal size and shape. No consanguinity. Bibl. No. 125.

PLATE LXXIV. Fig. 1190. *Usher's Case.* A pedigree with three cases of congenital dislocation of lenses in a sibship of seven; mental affection in these three cases and in a few other members on both maternal and paternal sides of the pedigree. V. 33, Annie M., aged 10 (1921), seen in Aberdeen Royal Infirmary, had been knocked down at school 11 days before admission; her right side was bruised and face cut; right eye had been swollen for some days. This child is second born in the sibship; her mother stated that she was mentally weak. On examination, there was noted R. ciliary injection, pupil widely dilated though no mydriatic had been used; anterior chamber deep; a dull red reflex. Later the upper edge of the lens was seen in the centre of the pupil, the lens being partially dislocated downwards; with focal light pale grey strands were visible, these passed upwards from the lens margin; the lower part of pupil was grey (lens) upper part is black; iridodonesis was noted; no fundus details seen. The left eye had also partial dislocation of the lens downwards, the edge of the lens is seen at junction of middle and lower thirds of pupil, upper margin was tilted slightly backwards and had grey strands passing upwards and inwards from it; anterior chamber was of uniform depth; iridodonesis was noted; fundus normal. The patient is illiterate and obviously imbecile. Urine amber, acid, 1025, no sugar, no albumen. This child died in 1928 from intestinal tuberculosis.

V. 35, Helen M., aged 10 (1924), seen in Aberdeen Royal Infirmary. The history shows that this patient has never seen well and at school requires to sit near the blackboard. No injury to eyes or head; no history of pain or redness of eyes; "she is illiterate and seems to have a simple mentality. On examination, vision was tested for both eyes but it is impossible to say what she sees, says she can see letters on the board, but will not name them; on the right, a blue-grey opaque lens lies in the anterior chamber and obscures the whole of the pupil, which contracts to light; eye movements full; T. = + 1; eye quiet; no red reflex; iris brown; on the left side the lens of a pale yellow colour lies in the anterior chamber obscuring the pupil but not completely, the upper part being quite black; pupil contracts to light; iris brown except near the pupil, above, where it has a metallic blue appearance; T. = normal; eye quiet; a brown strip of pigment is noted on upper part of lens; no red reflex; a dense white opacity is seen on the centre of anterior surface of lens; there is a dark linear area in the sclerotic at upper part of ciliary region. Heart and lungs show nothing abnormal; urine straw coloured, acid, 1018, no albumen, no sugar." A few days later the left lens was extracted by means of a spoon and still later a spoon extraction was done on the right eye. Both eyes soon healed and patient was discharged with a + 12 D. sph. for each eye. When seen seven years later (1931), she could pick up small objects such as coins quite readily; wears the + 12 D. sph.; the eyeballs appear to be of normal size; transverse diameters of cornea 11·5 mm.; fundi normal; has two decayed molars, otherwise teeth are normal.

V. 37, Peggy M., aged 12 (1931), seen at her home; mother says she is quite illiterate; is weak-minded and has learnt nothing at school. On examination, is mentally defective and has double partial dislocation of lenses; right lens is dislocated downwards, its upper edge being visible in the pupil; left lens is dislocated towards nose and its outer edge is seen at the junction of inner and middle thirds of the pupil; anterior chambers of equal depth; iris colour grey-brown; iridodonesis very marked, the whole of the iris is tremulous in each eye; refraction hypermetropia, with either eye she could distinguish a penny; eyes apparently of normal size; transverse diameter of cornea about 11·5 mm.; pupils central. Teeth were complete in lower jaw; first R. upper molar and several L. upper teeth were absent; she had had several teeth extracted.

V. 45, Annie MacC., domestic servant, aged 22, illegitimate daughter of IV. 47; her father was not the father of her half siblings V. 32—37; has good vision and is said to be clever. V. 32, Mary M., aged 21, housekeeper, has good vision, examined by school doctor. William M., the elder of V. 36, seen by Dr H. E. Smith, Jan. 1929; R. V. with − 6 D. sph. = $\frac{6}{24}$ and 1 J. = L. V.; no dislocation of lenses; media clear; fundi normal. Alex M., V. 34, and Robert M., the younger of V. 36, have, according to their parents, excellent vision. The mother, IV. 47, Jean T., aged 40, has anterior chambers of normal depth; no iridodonesis; fundi normal; reads small print, 1 J. at 10″, with either eye and V. = $\frac{6}{8}$; no mental affection; refraction hypermetropic; irides brown; pupils are equal, central, and contract to light. After the birth of her illegitimate daughter IV. 47 had the seven children V. 32—37 and no miscarriages or still-births; she and her husband were not consanguineous.

IV. 29, Arthur M., aged 52, father of the affected sibship is a crofter or small farmer in Banffshire; R. V. = L. V. = $\frac{6}{6}$; refraction emmetropic; no iridodonesis; irides blue; anterior chambers of equal depth; pupils equal, central, contract to light; is mentally sound; fundi normal. III. 32, Isabella T., though old, is robust and mentally clear; sees well; fundi normal; has had seventeen children; she herself is in a sibship of sixteen. III. 21, Alexander McC., a small farmer in Aberdeenshire, aged about 75, is working regularly; vision quite good in each eye; fundi normal; he and his family, IV. 44—63, have a bad reputation in the district of being wild people and notorious poachers; mental state appears to be satisfactory. II. 18, James T., illegitimate, lived to over 80; he was not related to his wife, II. 19, Ellen C., who was one of fourteen siblings and died aged 74. Nothing was known of ocular or mental defects in the descendants of the siblings of II. 19; no attempt has been made to follow them up. I. 4 and I. 5 were not related. I. 5 and John P., I. 6, had no children. I. 7, James C., and I. 8, Mary S., lived to old age; they were not related. II. 17, Rachael T., lived with III. 32, for 14 years; her husband II. 16, Robert L. McC., was not a cousin; he became insane in 1862 at the age of 30 and was admitted for epileptic insanity to the Aberdeen Royal Mental Hospital, where he died in 1895. Alexander McC., I. 2, father of II. 16, married twice; by his first wife he had five children, one of whom, II. 13, Jeanie McC., was admitted in 1853, at the age of 34, as an inmate of the Aberdeen Royal Mental Hospital; she had grandiose delusions, was quarrelsome and violent; she was in hospital for thirty years. III. 11, Mary E., had been hardy and sound mentally; he died from heart disease. II. 3, James E., married Annie G., II. 4, they were presumably normal. II. 1 died aged 60 of heart disease. II. 2 died old, she and her husband were unrelated.

IV. 22, William D., first cousin to IV. 29, was an epileptic imbecile, admitted in 1890 to the Aberdeen Royal Mental Hospital; his half sister, IV. 17, said that he had convulsions at the age of 2 years resulting from a fall; III. 10, father of IV. 22, had no mental defect and no such defect had been known to occur amongst his relatives. The mother, III. 9, had normal descendants from her first marriage. IV. 35, Fred C., first cousin to IV. 29, aged 34, was the youngest in a sibship of nine; he has a very large head and right hemiplegia; his sister, IV. 36, said he had a stroke in infancy after which his head became large; his fingers and wrist on the right side are markedly flexed; his head had a measure of 25″ is spherical and possibly hydrocephalic; no suggestion of tower skull or rickets; sutures are closed; left eye is divergent; pupils are equal and contract to light; no proptosis; irides blue; R. V. = finger counting at 1′, L. V. = hand movements at 1′; double optic atrophy; no nystagmus, eye movements seem to be imperfect in all directions; memory said to be good; is fond of music.

V. 57, illegitimate, is described by a medical man as peculiar though not an imbecile. The four siblings under V. 2 were reported by IV. 29 to be "all a little soft"; they are now grown up, the youngest, aged 16, in domestic service, the males at farm work; all have left home; a neighbour said that none of them is mentally affected, but that their mother was perhaps a little strange. The following went abroad, II. 5 and 7, III. 17, 18 and 23, IV. 64 (three siblings), two of IV. 39, one of IV. 34, one male and one female of IV. 80, one of V. 27, all except one male of V. 30, two males of V. 38, three males and one female (siblings) of V. 46, V. 55, one female of V. 63; VI. 3, three siblings under VI. 24, VII. 1. Those who died in infancy include III. 38, 39, two of IV. 58, one male of IV. 80, one female twin of IV. 26, three males of V. 23, one of V. 28, V. 40, one male of V. 64, one male of VI. 23. III. 35 died young, also two females of IV. 1, IV. 31, one of IV. 65, one male of V. 49, one male and one female of V. 56, one of VI. 24. V. 14 and 15 were still-born. In addition to information received from members of the pedigree help has been given by medical men in several districts. Dr Alexander Craig kindly provided the notes of II. 13 and 16 and of IV. 22. No consanguinity. Hitherto unpublished.

Fig. 1191. *Usher's Case*. Congenital dislocation of lenses in a mentally defective brother and sister; several other cases of mental defect in the pedigree. H. W., V. 6, aged 7 (1906), attends school; his right lens is dislocated into the anterior chamber, left lens partially dislocated downwards; R. V. = L. V. = finger counting at 4—5 m.; corneae are clear; optic discs are normal; tension is normal; anterior chambers are of moderate depth; on the right side slight ciliary injection is noted; the pupil is wide and circular; the left eye is quiet, the pupil, half dilated, is transversely oval and active to light; there is marked iridodonesis on the left; upper edge of lens is seen in the pupil; movement of the eyeballs is full. V. 6 was born at full time; when two years old he was 1½ hours in a "fit," said to be due to teeth; he has never been very strong, but has had none of the common children's illnesses; he is only fairly well nourished; facies is rather vacant, mouth open, shape of head brachycephalic; he is shy but not specially emotional; there is a large cicatrix on the left side of his head, parietal area; heart, lungs and abdomen are normal; no weakness is demonstrable in arms or legs; urine is straw coloured, specific gravity 1023, no albumen or sugar. This boy has always been near-sighted; three weeks before examination he came home from school at half time because his right eye was sore and red; there had been no injury to it; he was in bed for a day or two with sickness and vomiting. When in hospital the left lens of V. 6 dislocated into the anterior chamber, when escrine was used the pupils contracted but the lenses slipped back behind the irides; the child was taken home before anything was done for removal of the lenses. In 1909 the left lens was opaque and shrunken in the anterior chamber, which was deep, the eye diverged and probably had no p. l.; the right eye showed iridodonesis, pupil irregular, shallow anterior chamber. When seen in February 1931 the left eye was shrunken and of a square shape; the right eye had a blue iris with black pupil and the patient could see sufficiently, though using no glasses, to move about freely; he is very weak mentally which accounts for his inability to perform any useful work at his father's farm; he cannot read.

Plate LXXIV.   DESCRIPTIONS OF PEDIGREE PLATES   545

V. 7, N. W., aged 10 (1911), attends school; she was admitted that year to Aberdeen Royal Infirmary for dislocation of lenses with a history of sudden acute pain in the right eye a month previously and loss of vision; R. V. = hand movements at 4′; R. T. = − 1; anterior chamber was deep, pupil partially dilated; ciliary injection was noted; a purple area resembling a ruptured sclerotic was seen near the upper margin of the cornea; it may however be due to pigment in the sclerotic, nothing similar was in the other eye; iridodonesis was present; the lens was partially opaque with the upper edge visible in the pupil; the pupil was black in upper-inner part; fundus not seen, a dull red reflex up-in. L. V. = $\frac{1}{60}$; anterior chamber, generally shallow, was deeper at the periphery; iridodonesis of the whole iris; no congestion was present; tension was normal; pupil, eccentric towards the nasal side, contracted to light; disc was normal. This child had a vacant expression; was well nourished; all over her legs were small ulcerated patches varying in size from $\frac{1}{4}$ to $\frac{1}{2}$ inch in diameter; heart and lungs were normal; mental condition weak; eye movements full; no tremors of tongue; knee jerks + +, left plantar reflex showed a definite extensor response, the right was sometimes extensor, once flexor; legs held very rigid; abdominal reflexes very active on the left side, less active though present on the right side; sensation: touch, pain and muscle, good; smell: could not tell peppermint from assafoetida; taste: she would not say she could distinguish salt from sugar; she had a high arched palate and sat with mouth open; the right eye became quiet in a few days and the patient went home. Some months later there was pain in the right eye, the lens was in the anterior chamber, T. = + 3; the lens was extracted. A few weeks later the patient returned again with pain in the left eye; this lens was lying in front of the iris at the inner part and behind it at the outer; T. = + 2; lens was extracted June 1st, 1912. On Sept. 9 of that year R. V. = L. V. = $\frac{5}{60}$ with + 10 D. sph. Aug. 9th 1913, "gets on well with glasses, is at school." In January 1914, each eye, especially the left, was staphylomatous anteriorly, including the ciliary region; R. T. = + 2, L. T. = + 1; reduced by eserine to R. T. = normal, L. T. = + 1. In Feb. 1931 her father said that V. 7 had died aged 27; she became quite blind and was very difficult to manage owing to her violent temper.

The mother, III. 18, had a twin.sister; they were the last born in her sibship and, judging from accounts and photographs of them, they were probably like twins; III. 18 had only the two children V. 6 and 7, no miscarriages or still births; she was a first cousin of her husband's father; she died in 1902 at the age of 41; she had no ocular or mental defects. The father, IV. 21, a farmer, aged 69 (1931), is intelligent and has good vision and no deformities; he is an illegitimate son of III. 34 by III. 33, about whom little information could be obtained. IV. 21 wrote "my mother's name was W.,...but I can't give you much information about her family; I have heard she had a sister a little weak in mind, quite simple, but I never heard of any eye trouble or defect." No ocular or mental defect is known to have occurred in any of the seven legitimate daughters of III. 34 or their descendants, nor in any of the siblings of III. 34 or their descendants. III. 19 had an only child IV. 14 who died in infancy; IV. 21 said he was a normal child, though he died abroad and she had not seen him. IV. 21 was told that it was a good thing he had died, which meant that he thought there had been some malformation. II. 9 died when the twins, III. 18 and 19, were normal. Of those with mental defect besides V. 6 and 7, Helen M., II. 8, 4th born in a sibship of six females, was an imbecile and undersized.. Alexander H., III. 10, nominally a farmer, has stayed with his married sister, III. 15, and her husband for the last ten years; his sister regards him as peculiar, he cannot look after himself, goes away for days at a time, does not say very much; when spoken to he usually answers but sometimes just smiles and has a vacant look; his knowledge of his relatives is very limited; IV. 21 described him as "simple"; his nephew, IV. 2, shot himself for no accountable reason. I. 6, a hard-working farmer, died aged 90; latterly he became mentally affected and for a number of years had to be kept away from his work. Consanguinity. Hitherto unpublished.

Fig. 1192. *Usher's Case.* A pedigree containing one case, or probably two cases, of congenital dislocation of lenses and several individuals with mental affection. IV. 17, James T., age 6 (1924), 3rd in a sibship of six; sight had never been good; pupils, equal, contract to light; irides blue, iridodonesis; anterior chambers shallower up and in than in other parts; lenses dislocated upwards and outwards, lower edge of each lens visible in upper part of pupil; when seen again in 1931 his parents said that they had formerly believed that he was mentally affected but now regarded him as normal, and that his defective vision had accounted for their former belief. He has not been to school; fundus of each eye is normal and is focussed with a high convex glass; with + 14 D. sph. spelt words of 6 J. with his left eye; no evidence of mental derangement. His two brothers, IV. 18 and IV. 19, with blue irides, and his three sisters, IV. 15, IV. 16, IV. 20, with brown irides, have normal fundi and vision; each of them read 1 J. with each eye. Their uncle, III. 29, who died a year ago, age 35, of tubercle, possibly had dislocated lenses, because his brother, III. 20, and his sister-in-law, III. 44, who are the parents of a boy with dislocated lenses and marked iridodonesis, each independently stated that his eyes were tremulous like those of their son James, IV. 17. On the other hand his widow, III. 30, had not observed this and his notes at the Royal Mental Hospital, Aberdeen, where he had been an inmate with dementia praecox, do not mention it, though they indicate that irides were blue and pupils contracted to light and on accommodation; as a tremulous iris may readily be overlooked Usher was inclined to accept the evidence of his brother and sister-in-law who had frequently watched the tremor of the iris in their son's eyes. III. 20, father of James T., has normal fundi, blue irides, and reads 1 J. with each eye. III. 44, mother of James T., has normal fundi, brown irides, and reads 1 J. with each eye. II. 14, paternal grandmother, has normal fundi, blue irides, and shows no evidence of ectopia lentis. II. 22, maternal grandmother, refraction hypermetropic, blue irides, normal fundi. III. 24, age 45, is in a mental hospital for dementia praecox. III. 15, female, age 42, is recognised by her relatives as being insane. Her sister, III. 14, said that the mental symptoms began some years after an operation at the age of 16 for tubercular peritonitis. She does not speak civilly to anyone, not even to her mother, gets very angry and will see no strangers. II. 3, never saw well, became mentally affected and was in a home for his mental disorder. II. 16, has a large family, III. 39, in America; five of her children died in infancy, 3 in one week from diphtheria. II. 18, was mentally affected in America, was "queer" for many years, died of "sunstroke." Besides these mental cases, III. 25 with mixed astigmatism and blue irides has had a family of three children who are all very nervous. They live with their parents, the father is a farmer. The youngest, IV. 27, a boy, age 14, was with difficulty dragged, crying, into the room by his mother for examination, his pupils were equal, contracted to light, anterior chambers normal, irides blue, refraction hypermetropia, wears convex lenses, fundi normal. No examination of his brother, IV. 26, older than himself, was possible, for from nervousness he hid himself and could not be found. The mother said that likewise her married daughter is nervous, she has no children. A number of the families are abroad: IV. 4—9 in New Zealand, all see well, none mentally affected; IV. 22—24 are in Hongkong; III. 27 and his children, IV. 28—32, in Canada. The members of sibships IV. 38—44 and IV. 45—48 are all well known, none has defective vision or mental defect. IV. 45, the first born in sibship, is aged 9 years. III. 47, says she has difficulty in seeing at dusk, no opportunity to test this, but her optic discs and retinal vessels were normal and no retinal pigmentation was present to suggest retinitis pigmentosa. III. 50, irides blue with some stroma pigment, anterior chambers normal, 1 J. with each eye. III. 51, blue iris, anterior chambers normal, 1 J. with each eye. III. 52 "sees all right." III. 53, wearing glasses convex for right eye, concave for left, fundi normal, irides brown, anterior chambers normal. These four, III. 50—53, of marriageable age are all unmarried. III. 34 died, all the other members of sibship III. 33—38 see well except III. 33, the first born who requires glasses. III. 23 died in a few hours from "sunstroke" in Hongkong at age of 24, no suggestion of hereditary mental affection. We are indebted to Dr Alexander Craig, Royal Mental Hospital, Aberdeen, for notes of III. 24 and III. 29. No consanguinity. Hitherto unpublished.

Fig. 1193. *Gunn's Case.* Nineteen cases of ectopia lentis in four generations; three adults and three children were examined. The condition was bilateral in all and no further abnormality was seen; in the children, the lens could be seen floating freely in the vitreous; in one case the lens migrated into the anterior chamber and produced so great an irritation that it had to be removed. In the adults there was evidence of old iritis or irido-cyclitis, probably set up by movements of the lens. The pupils were small and fixed and the sight of all adults examined was improved by + 10 D. sph. No consanguinity recorded. Bibl. No. 195.

Plate LXXV. Fig. 1194. *Williams's Case.* Ectopia lentis in a father and in his two children. II. 1, Mary J., aged 28, had eyes slightly divergent; irides tremulous and anterior chambers deep; her pupils were central and circular, but they were small and did not dilate readily under atropine; the lenses were dislocated upwards; detachment of the retina was present; in the left eye the lens was small but transparent. II. 2, Marcus J., aged 26, had both lenses displaced upwards and on the right side slightly inwards; the lenses were a little hazy and reduced in size; he had markedly divergent eyes with the same deep anterior chambers and tremulous irides as his sister; he had small central pear-shaped pupils with sluggish reactions; this patient stuttered in his speech. The father's eyes were similarly affected; the mother and her only brother had good eyes. No consanguinity recorded. Bibl. No. 56.

Fig. 1195. *Pufahl's Case.* Corectopia in two brothers. II. 1 aged 55 had in the left eye a brown iris with a small oval pupil, 2 mm. long by $\frac{1}{2}$ mm. broad, displaced upwards and outwards; the pupil was immobile and showed no reaction to light; iris was tremulous; no lens was present in the pupillary area; T. = normal; field was much narrowed; the right eye had become completely blind and disorganised at the age of 30. II. 2, aged 53, had never seen well; both bulbs were of the normal size; the right showed a transparent cornea, normal anterior chamber, and a brown tremulous iris with a small oval pupil, $1\frac{1}{2}$ mm. by 1 mm., displaced upwards and outwards; the pupil showed no reaction to light and was without a lens; V. = finger counting at 6 inches; in the left eye conditions were similar but the pupil was less far removed from the centre of the iris and the displacement was upwards and inwards; if the patient looked down, the upper margin of the lens could be seen. Both parents and their other seven living children saw well. No consanguinity. Bibl. No. 69.

Fig. 1196. *Bryant's Case.* Congenital bilateral dislocation of the lens in five members of a sibship of seven; the parents had normal eyes. No consanguinity recorded. Bibl. No. 109.

Fig. 1197. *Wilder's Case.* I. 1 had always been healthy; at the age of 39 she had R. V. = $\frac{12}{100}$, L. V. = $\frac{6}{200}$; the R. lens was displaced, up and out, the left up and in; both lenses were clear. Of eight children of I. 1, four died in infancy; II. 2, aged 10, had R. V. = $\frac{1}{100}$, L. V. = $\frac{3}{100}$; the right lens was displaced

PLATE LXXV.   DESCRIPTIONS OF PEDIGREE PLATES   547

outwards, the left lens upwards and outwards; the lenses were clear and the child was well formed in other respects, but was mentally dull. II. 4, aged 7, and II. 7, aged 3 years, were normal. II. 5, aged 5, had normal fundi and clear lenses which were dislocated inwards. No consanguinity recorded. Bibl. No. 140.

Fig. 1198. *Hulme's Case.* Ectopia lentis in four members of a sibship of twelve; three members of the sibship died in childhood from hydrocephalus with convulsions; of these one was said to have had tremulous irides; the remaining nine were healthy and five of these had no imperfection of sight; the parents were both healthy and had excellent sight; no hereditary defect was known to have occurred previously in the family history; two of the twelve siblings were males. II. 1, E. P., aged 19, had always been near sighted; she had brown irides with circular sluggish pupils; irides were tremulous at lower and outer parts; right eye was myopic; globes were healthy and of normal shape; the right lens was displaced downwards and inwards, with commencing opacity at the edge; the disc was small and showed considerable hyperaemia; the left lens was displaced upwards and outwards, to a much greater extent and was cataractous throughout the greater part of its substance; fundus of the left eye could not be seen. II. 2, J. P., aged 18, had always been near sighted; she had brown tremulous irides; the right lens was completely cataractous and was displaced downwards and inwards; the left lens was displaced downwards and outwards but was clear; the left disc was pink and a somewhat varicose state of the vessels was noted. II. 3. F. P., aged 14, had blue irides with circular, sluggish pupils; both lenses were clear, the right was displaced downwards and inwards, the left downwards and outwards. II. 4, R. P., aged 7, saw well with the right eye in which the lens was displaced, slightly outwards and downwards, but was clear; the left lens was completely cataractous and was also displaced, slightly outwards and downwards; the left eye was blind, the right fundus showed an injected disc. No consanguinity recorded. Bibl. No. 46.

Fig. 1199. *Parker's Case.* Ectopia lentis in five cases of three generations. I. 1, aged 67 (1898), had had defective vision from her earliest childhood; the eyes of her parents were normal so far as she knew; she had six children of whom four were living; she had tremulous irides; both lenses were displaced upwards; the right lens was completely opaque, the left partly so. II. 2, aged 35, had R. V. $= \frac{15}{40}$, L. V. $= \frac{3}{300}$ without glasses; she had brown tremulous irides and bilateral upward dislocation of the lens; her three children were all similarly affected.

III. 1, Albert W., aged 15, had R. V. $= \frac{3}{210}$, L. V. $= \frac{15}{200}$ without glasses; he had brown tremulous irides and displacement of both lenses upwards and outwards. III. 2, aged 12, with brown tremulous irides had R. V. $= \frac{15}{30}$, L. V. $= \frac{15}{30}$ without glasses; he had a slight upward dislocation of both lenses. III. 3, aged 8, had R. V. $= \frac{3}{200}$, L. V. $= \frac{2}{200}$, not improved by glasses; she had brown tremulous irides and bilateral upward dislocation of the lens. All the lenses were clear except those of I. 1; the patients were intelligent; the defect was not associated with corectopia or any other anomaly. No consanguinity recorded. Bibl. No. 138.

Fig. 1200. *Eha's Case.* II. 2, aged 36 (1902), had always seen badly; he had a bilateral marked tremor of the iris; both lenses were transparent and displaced, the right downwards and the left upwards; both pupils were circular and normally situated; R. V. with $-12 \cdot 0$ D. sph. $= \frac{6}{30}$, L. V. with $-12 \cdot 0$ D. sph. $= \frac{6}{30}$; no other abnormalities or defects were present in the eyes or in the body of the patient. The parents and siblings of II. 2 had no trouble with their eyes; he had five children of whom three died shortly after birth, two had ectopia lentis.

III. 1, aged 7 years, was a cretin; he had divergent strabismus and his pupils were bilaterally displaced upwards and inwards, they reacted to light; both lenses were displaced upwards; vision could not be tested owing to the stupidity of the patient. III. 2 had normally placed pupils but both lenses were dislocated downwards and outwards; R. V. $=$ L. V. $= \frac{5}{30}$ with $-16 \cdot 0$ D. sph. or $\frac{5}{18}$ with $+12 \cdot 0$ D. sph.; no other anomalies were present. No consanguinity recorded. Bibl. No. 155.

Fig. 1201. *Eha's Case.* Ectopia lentis in a boy whose mother and uncle were similarly affected. III. 2, seen aged 6, had then R. V. with $+12 \cdot 0$ D. sph. $= \frac{3}{60}$, L. V. $=$ recognition of fingers held quite close; both lenses were opaque and were lying in the anterior chamber; the right eye had an eccentric pupil which was displaced upwards; pressure was raised in the left eye, in which acute inflammatory symptoms were present; the lenses were removed. The three siblings of the patient had normal eyes.

II. 1 had normal eyes; the house surgeon reported that II. 2 had congenital bilateral ectopia lentis; a brother of II. 2 was similarly affected; a sister of II. 2 had congenital mental defect; one member of this sibship was reported to be normal. I. 2 and I. 3 were heavy drinkers; I. 3 had two mentally defective sons who were born blind; no details of this blindness could be obtained. No consanguinity. Bibl. No. 155.

Fig. 1202. *Miles's Case.* Ectopia lentis in a mother and in six of her eight children. II. 2, Mrs L complained of pain in her left eye in 1888; the lens was found to be dislocated forwards, the edge lying on the iris and projecting a little into the anterior chamber; the right lens was dislocated into the vitreous, it was attached below and was freely moveable, coming into place when the patient bent her head forwards; none of her ancestors had trouble with their eyes; she remembered that her mother and grandmother had good sight; her husband had good vision and there was no history of eye disease in his family. III. 1, aged 27, had good health but sight had always been bad; both lenses were displaced downwards and outwards, they were freely moveable but attached at the outer side; lenses were clear. II. 2, dead, had had "very bad eyes." III. 3, aged 23, had always seen badly; lenses were dislocated into the vitreous, the right downwards, the left a little to the outer side; they were moveable and clear. III. 4, aged 20, had normal eyes. III. 5, aged 17, had both lenses slightly displaced outwards; strong concave glasses improved his vision. III. 6, aged 15, had always had good sight. III. 7, aged 10, had both lenses displaced downwards and to the left; lenses were clear; divergent strabismus was noted; this child had swollen glands in her neck, with abscess formation. III. 8, aged 3, with lenses displaced downwards and outwards, had poor vision; she had swollen glands in her neck with abscess formation. In all cases except III. 7 and 8 the irides were very tremulous; no nystagmus was present in any case. No consanguinity. Bibl. No. 128.

Fig. 1203. *Spiece's Case.* Ectopia lentis in two males and two females of two generations. III. 4, H. C., aged 7 (1918), had iridodonesis and deep anterior chambers; R. V. = L. V. = $\frac{5}{100}$; his lenses were clear, both were displaced upwards and outwards; R. V. with 10·00 D. ⊃ + 2·00 D. cyl. ax. 90° = $\frac{20}{20}$, L. V. with + 13·00 D. ⊃ +1·00 D. cyl. ax. 90° = $\frac{20}{100}$. Of the siblings of III. 4 the eldest aged 12 had R. V. = L. V. = $\frac{20}{20}$, hypermetropia 0·25 D.; III. 2, aged 10, had also R. V. = L. V. = $\frac{20}{20}$ and hypermetropia of 0·25 D. III. 3, aged 9, had a left posterior polar cataract; R. V. = $\frac{20}{30}$, L. V. = $\frac{20}{6}$. III. 5, aged 7, had R. V. = L. V. = $\frac{5}{100}$. III. 6, aged 5, had R. V. = $\frac{20}{30}$, L. V. = $\frac{20}{6}$. III. 7 was aged one year. No explanation is given of the low visual acuity of III. 5 and III. 6. The father of this sibship had good eyes; the mother II. 2, aged 38 (1918), had iridodonesis or ocular movements; R. V. = $\frac{10}{65}$, L. V. = $\frac{10}{50}$; R. V. with + 5·00 D. = $\frac{20}{6}$, L. V. with + 5·00 D. ⊃ + 0·50 D. cyl. ax. 90° = $\frac{20}{20}$ − 1; the right lens was displaced upwards and outwards, the left lens was in position; the left fundus showed disseminated choroiditis. II. 3, II. 6, and II. 9 had good eyes. II. 4 died aged 20; he had had bad sight; II. 5 died aged 4 months. II. 7, aged 27, had a divergent squint in the left eye; her anterior chambers were deep and irides tremulous; R. V. = $\frac{8}{100}$, with + 8·00 D. = $\frac{20}{6}$; L. V. = $\frac{5}{100}$, not improved by glasses; the upper outer edge of each lens could be seen on dilatation of the pupil; the right lens was transparent, the left showed early cataractous changes; this woman had a son aged 6 whose eyes were in a similar condition.

I. 1, 2 and 3 had good eyes; I. 2 died aged 52. No consanguinity recorded. Bibl. No. 227.

Fig. 1204. *Franceschetti's Case.* Ectopia lentis in three siblings whose parents were second cousins; the family were traced through six generations, a large number of members were examined and no other cases of developmental defect appear to have occurred. V. 4, aged 41 (1927), had never been seriously ill but had had defective vision since childhood and frequently suffered from an inflammatory affection of his eyes; thirty years ago he had had an operation for cataract in the left eye; both eyes showed maculae of the cornea, opacities in the vitreous, cataract of the lens, pupils centrally placed and the lens displaced outwards in the right eye and absent following operation in the left; the anterior chambers were deep; the optic nerves were a good colour; R. V. = $\frac{3}{50}$, with + 8·0 D. = $\frac{6}{24}$; at a later date the right lens had changed its position and was now displaced downwards. V. 5, aged 40, was of a delicate constitution and had always seen badly; his pupils were oval and were displaced upwards and outwards; irides were greenish yellow; anterior chambers were deep; both eyes showed traces of a persistent pupillary membrane; the right lens could not be seen, the left lens was opaque and could be seen in the vitreous. V. 5 had five children who were all free from anomalies of development. V. 14, aged 25, was robust and had never been seriously ill; her pupils were displaced upwards and outwards; irides were tremulous, lenses were opaque and displaced inwards and downwards. V. 14 was one of triplets, the two other members being free from defect. Consanguinity. Bibl. No. 273.

Fig. 1205. *Lewis's Case.* Ectopia lentis in nine males and seven females of six generations. I. 1 was reported to have been blind in both eyes; she had two sons and a daughter, of whom the daughter was believed to be normal but had two affected sons in her family of six sons and one daughter. Both the sons of I. 1 were blind in both eyes; II. 3 died aged 83 years, having had four children of whom three were affected. III. 9 was believed to have been unaffected and to have had two unaffected daughters; III. 11, aged 79 (1904), was blind in both eyes; she had an unaffected daughter; III. 12, who died aged 49, was blind in one eye only. III. 13, aged 75 (1904), had a shrunken left eye probably the result of a previous glaucomatous condition; her right lens was completely dislocated into the vitreous chamber; R. V. = $\frac{15}{200}$, with + 10·0 D. sph. = $\frac{18}{50}$. III. 13 had three children, of whom IV. 5, aged 55 (1904), had a complete dislocation of the right lens into the vitreous chamber; his left eye was shrunken to about half the normal size; he had two daughters of whom one, aged 33, was normal, the other, aged 28, was affected. Thus V. 3 had lenses displaced in a direction downwards and outwards; R. V. = $\frac{3}{200}$, L. V. = $\frac{3}{200}$ or with + 13·0 D. sph. R. V. = L. V. = $\frac{18}{50}$; eleven months later V. 3 had acute inflammation in the right eye and the dislocated lens of this eye was then seen floating in the vitreous chamber and was cataractous; seven years previously this case had been seen when there was an upward displacement of both lenses. V. 3 had three children, aged 10, 8 and 2 years respectively, who were all affected.

V I. 1 had defective vision which was first noticed at the age of 4 years; now V. = $\frac{18}{200}$ or with + 8·5 D. sph. = $\frac{18}{100}$; both lenses were displaced upwards and inwards; both lenses were clear, abnormally small and

Plate LXXV.   DESCRIPTIONS OF PEDIGREE PLATES   549

oscillated on rotation of the eyeballs; the anterior chambers were deep and irides were tremulous. VI. 2 had the right lens displaced inwards and slightly downwards, the left lens inwards and slightly upwards; R. V. = L. V. = $\frac{18}{200}$; with + 17 D. sph. R. V. = $\frac{13}{10}$, L. V. = $\frac{16}{80}$. VI. 3, aged 2 years, had a very slight dislocation of both lenses downwards and inwards. IV. 6 and IV. 8, aged 52 and 47 years respectively, were unaffected; IV. 8 had a son and two grandsons, who also were believed to be unaffected; IV. 6 had four children of whom three were affected. Thus V. 4, aged 33, had a slight upward displacement of both lenses; V. 6 and 7, aged 30 and 25 years respectively, were seen and reported upon by some other ophthalmologist. No consanguinity recorded. Bibl. No. 167.

Fig. 1206. *Dixon and Wordsworth's Case.* This case was first described by Dixon in 1857, when he saw III. 2 and her three sons, IV. 2, 3 and 5; he writes that the three younger children of III. 2 were unaffected and had excellent vision; all the affected members had tremulous irides and pupils which reacted well to light. III. 2, aged 40 (1857), with light brown irides, had her lenses displaced upwards and inwards; when her pupils were contracted the whole of the pupillary area was occupied by lens and she could see to read medium type, but could not see at any great distance. IV. 2, aged 17 (1857), with light grey irides, had both lenses displaced inwards; he also, when his pupils were contracted, saw wholly through his lenses and was able to read small type fluently. IV. 3, aged 15 (1857), with brown irides, had both lenses displaced upwards and inwards. IV. 5, aged 13 (1857), with brown irides, had both lenses displaced upwards. The displacement was considerable in IV. 3 and 5 and they could only read with difficulty.

In 1878 Wordsworth presented III. 2, two of her affected sons and three of their affected children at a meeting of the Medical Society of London; he further reports that the father of III. 2, her grandfather, and her father's youngest brother were all similarly affected. At this date III. 2, aged 59, had both lenses displaced upwards and inwards and cataract forming in the left; IV. 2, aged 37, had the right lens displaced inwards and the left lens inwards and slightly downwards; IV. 3, aged 35, had the right lens displaced upwards and inwards, the left lens inwards; V. 1, aged 10, with grey irides, had both lenses displaced inwards; V. 2, aged 5, with grey irides, had the right lens displaced upwards, the left lens upwards and inwards; V. 4, aged 7, with brown irides, had the right lens displaced upwards and outwards, the left lens upwards and inwards. No consanguinity recorded. Bibl. Nos. 39, 65.

Fig. 1207. *Macnaughton Jones's Case.* II. 4, aged 18, had congenital luxation of the right lens upwards and the left lens outwards; irides tremulous; V. = $\frac{6}{60}$. II. 3, aged 20, had corectopia, each pupil being displaced upwards and outwards; the lenses were normally placed; fundi showed a well marked crescent; V. = $\frac{1}{5}$. II. 1 and 2 had normal eyes. One of the two youngest children of this sibship had extremely near sight. The parents of II. 1—6 were healthy and had good sight; the father was addicted to drink. No consanguinity recorded. Bibl. No. 67.

Fig. 1208. *Eha's Case.* II. 1, aged 20, had in his right eye a coloboma of the iris downwards; a white lens was seen to be lying below in the vitreous; tension was not raised; in the left eye the pupil was normally placed but there was some hint of a coloboma downwards in a vertical notching of the iris; the lens was displaced downwards; R. V. with + 10·0 D. sph. = $\frac{6}{18}$, L. V. with + 8·0 sph. = $\frac{5}{12}$. The patient had two brothers and two sisters, of whom the two brothers presented the same anomaly of the eyes and had been operated on. No abnormalities of other parts were associated with the eye defect in II. 1. No consanguinity recorded. Bibl. No 155.

Fig. 1209. *Williams's Case.* Ectopia lentis in a brother and sister. I. 2, aged 35, had had a blow on her right eye from the hand of a child; vision was at once seriously impaired; vision in the left eye had always been very imperfect; now R. V. = fingers at 3 feet, lens was clear and slightly displaced downwards and outwards; the left lens, shrunken and white, was diplaced downwards; the pupil in each eye was slightly eccentric upwards. I. 3, L. B., aged 30, a well-developed labourer, had small oval pupils in a very eccentric position, upwards and outwards; they were partly covered by the upper lids; there were only a few fibres of iris between the pupil and the periphery of the cornea; the pupils responded promptly to light; in the right eye the lens was only visible under the action of atropine when the upper edge could be seen in the lower part of the pupil; in the left eye the lens was entirely outside the pupil but could be seen by looking down behind the iris; in both eyes more of the lens had been visible when examined three years previously. I. 2 had three children, all with good eyes. No consanguinity recorded. Bibl. No. 56.

Fig. 1210. *Spicer's Case.* II. 1, aged 11 (1902), had, in the right eye, a deep anterior chamber; clear cornea; the pupil was displaced upwards, nearly to the corneal margin, the sphincter was present; iris was tremulous; lens not completely opaque; the left eye was similar except that the opaque lens was lying in the anterior chamber; R. V. = $\frac{6}{36}$, L. V. = hand movements; tension normal. II. 2, aged 3, had both lenses dislocated and lying in the anterior chamber; the left lens was opaque; irides were tremulous, the pupils rather small and central. II. 3, aged 5 (1915), had tremulous irides with both pupils displaced downwards; anterior chambers were deep; in the right eye a small opaque lens was lying in the anterior chamber; the left lens was in position and not completely opaque; tension was normal; both eyes were rather small. Eight siblings were unaffected. No consanguinity recorded. Bibl. No. 217.

Fig. 1211. *Eha's Case.* Ectopia lentis in a father and in his two children. II. 1, Anna M., was seen, aged 24; she had apparently seen badly since birth but a few months before the vision of the left eye had become markedly worse; she had a marked facial asymmetry so that a line drawn through the middle of the forehead, the root of the nose and the apex of the chin was convex towards the right; in the right eye the pupil was central but the lens was displaced upwards and outwards, about half the pupil was aphakic; R. V. with + 4·0 D. sph. = $\frac{5}{10}$; in the left eye the lens was displaced upwards; opacities of the vitreous were noted; vision in this eye was reduced to an uncertain recognition of fingers; tremor of the irides was present. The patient's brother and her father were similarly affected, according to the statement of another surgeon. No consanguinity recorded. Bibl. No. 155.

Fig. 1212. *Keyser's Case.* III. 4, aged 28, had seen badly since birth; her eyes were small, the diameter of the cornea reduced; both lenses were dislocated, out and down, and were opaque; V. with + 4 D. = $\frac{15}{100}$. This patient reported that her sister and two brothers, also her mother, maternal grandfather, and three maternal uncles were similarly affected. No consanguinity recorded. Bibl. No. 57.

Fig. 1213. *Peltesohn's Case.* Ectopia lentis in four females and one male of three generations. II. 2, aged 39, the only case described, had the right lens displaced upwards, outwards and forwards, the left lens upwards, inwards and forwards; irides were tremulous. The patient reported that his mother, her sister I. 3, and a niece of the latter were similarly affected. The 6 year old daughter of II. 2 had the same anomaly, the displacement being the same in both eyes in her case. No consanguinity recorded. Bibl. No. 133.

Fig. 1214. *Bahr's Case.* Ectopia lentis in three males, coloboma lentis in two males and one female of three generations. I. 1 and 2 had ectopia lentis; the displacement was upwards, the lower margin of the lens being visible at about the middle of the pupil; the condition was bilateral in each case and the lenses were cataractous. II. 1—3 are the offspring of one or both the affected brothers of generation I.; the two daughters were examined repeatedly and had completely normal lenses; the son II. 3 was myopic and had a coloboma of the lower part of the lens. II. 4, second cousin to II. 1—3, had a coloboma of the lens; she was married and had two sons of whom III. 1 had bilateral ectopia lentis; III. 2 had coloboma lentis. No consanguinity recorded. Bibl. No. 204.

Fig. 1215. *Thompson's Case.* Ectopia lentis in two siblings and in their cousin; an aunt and a grandmother were said to have been very near, and also poor-sighted. III. 1, aged 17, had each lens displaced outwards, the inner section of the iris was tremulous; R. V. = L. V. = $\frac{20}{200}$, with − 6·00 D. sph. III. 3, aged 35, cousin to III. 1, had the left lens dislocated into the anterior chamber, the right lens was displaced outwards and was very mobile; the left lens was replaced; subsequently the right lens also became dislocated into the anterior chamber, and was replaced; severe symptoms with pain and raised tension accompanied the dislocation. III. 4, aged 24, had a tremulous lower middle portion of each iris with a tilting backwards of the corresponding part of each lens; the discs of this case were noticed to be very small. No consanguinity. Bibl. No. 96.

Plate LXXVI. Fig. 1216. *Stanford Morton's Case.* Congenital displacement of both lenses in ten members of five generations; the affected members were well developed and intelligent; all complained of "short sight," and some of having to "set" their eyes when looking at an object. The displacement was usually inwards or inwards and upwards; irides were tremulous; lenses of normal size and shape, of slightly milky appearance. III. 2, Mrs H., aged 59, used + 30 D. lenses with which she read J. 1 and sewed. IV. 2, with + 8 D. could do his work and read J. 1 at 10 inches. V. 1 was ordered + 12 D. Well marked myopic crescents were noted in IV. 2 and V. 1. No consanguinity recorded. Bibl. No. 68.

Fig. 1217. *Marlow's Case.* Ectopia lentis in three, probably in five generations. I. 1 died aged 83, having been blind for twenty-five years; of his children we are told that II. 1 lost the vision of one eye from inflammation; II. 2 was near sighted from birth; she lost the sight of one eye through inflammation and "wrong treatment" at the age of 35; II. 4 injured her eyes by "colouring," when 45 years of age, the vision gradually failed until it became very poor, finally "after grippe" she became totally blind. II. 2 had two or more children of whom III. 2, aged 55—60, had both lenses opaque and freely floating in an apparently fluid vitreous, one eye being in a state of acute glaucoma; he had had imperfect vision since childhood. III. 3 had been "near-sighted" from birth. III. 2 had a daughter, IV. 2, aged 21, who had always had defective vision and suffered from occipital headache; she had photophobia; R. V. with + 14 D. = $\frac{6}{18}$, iris tremulous, lens dislocated upwards in this eye, fundus normal; in the left eye V. with + 14 D. sph. + 1 D. cyl. ax. 140° = $\frac{6}{18}$, iris tremulous, lens dislocated inwards and upwards. IV. 2, Mrs G. W., had a son V. I who was seen to have bilateral congenital dislocation of the lens. III. 3, Mrs K. B., had three children of whom IV. 3, aged 27, had always had defective vision; his irides were tremulous below and bulged forward in the upper and inward quadrant; lenses were dislocated, up and in, leaving a third of the pupil unoccupied; R. V. with + 10 D. = $\frac{6}{24}$, L. V. with + 11 D. = $\frac{6}{24}$. IV. 4, aged 24, had the left lens displaced upwards and inwards, and the iris of this eye tremulous at the lower part; the right eye was

PLATE LXXVI.   DESCRIPTIONS OF PEDIGREE PLATES   551

apparently normal, but after dilatation of the pupil the iris of this eye also became tremulous in the lower part and there were indications of a slight displacement of the lens; fundi were normal; R. V. with − 1 D. cyl. ax. 100° = $\frac{6}{8}$, L. V. with − 0·75 D. − 1·5 D. cyl. ax. 100° = $\frac{6}{18}$; this was the only patient in the family who utilised the lens for vision. IV. 5, aged 22, had defective vision with enlargement of the right eye from birth and near-sightedness in the left; the right eye was now enormous, the cornea hazy, with a scleral staphyloma which had probably developed during the last four years; R. V. = perception of light; the patient was able to close his lids; the left eye showed a partial dislocation of the lens; L. V. = $\frac{6}{60}$, with + 6 D. + 1·5 D. cyl. ax. 80° = $\frac{6}{24}$. No consanguinity recorded. Bibl. No. 161.

Fig. 1218. *Terrien and Hubert's Case.* Bilateral congenital ectopia lentis in three, probably four, generations. IV. 2, aged 13, had a phlyctenular keralitis at the age of 4 years; her pupils were a little excentric but reacted normally; tremor of irides was noted on movements of the head; lenses were subluxated inwards and upwards; media were transparent. This patient had a brother and a sister who were unaffected, her father was alcoholic, her mother had ectopia lentis. III. 2, aged 39, had tremor of irides, pupils a little excentric; media were transparent; both lenses were displaced inwards and upwards; by her first husband, who was tuberculous, III. 2 had three still-born children. II. 1, aged 58, had always seen badly; her pupils were a little excentric but reacted normally; she had tremor of irides on movement of her head; both lenses were displaced inwards; media were transparent. Married at 18, II. 1 had five children of whom only the eldest survived infancy; she was probably the illegitimate child of her mother by a father who had had very bad sight from his infancy, and who had daughters, of whom one was said to have the same bearing of her head and the same visual troubles as II. 1. No consanguinity recorded. Bibl. No. 176.

Fig. 1219. *Starkey's Case.* The recorder had under his care a family in which the mother and her five children had double ectopia lentis. No consanguinity recorded. Bibl. No. 138.

Fig. 1220. *Franceschetti's Case.* Ectopia lentis, associated with corectopia and high myopia, in two males of a sibship of four, the offspring of a marriage between uncle and niece. IV. 4, aged 21 (1927), had always seen badly, but was healthy and had never been seriously ill; he had bilateral high myopia; his irides were greenish yellow and were tremulous; in the right eye the anterior chamber was deep; the pupil was aphakic and displaced upwards; the lens was dislocated downwards, its upper margin could be seen on dilatation of the pupil; in the left eye the pupil was of a triangular shape and was displaced downwards and slightly inwards; the lens was displaced downwards. IV. 2 had bilateral high myopia of − 30·0 D. in the right eye and − 10·0 D. in the left eye; in the right eye the pupil was oval in shape and was displaced upwards and slightly outwards; the lens was dislocated downwards, the anterior chamber deep; in the left eye the pupil was oval but was central in position and the lens was in its normal position. Consanguinity. Bibl. No. 273.

Fig. 1221. *Mules's Case.* Congenital displacement of the lens in the father I. 1 and in all his ten children by I. 2, with two doubtful exceptions in II. 1 and II. 9, who died in early infancy; seven of the ten children died under six years. Of the survivors, II. 2, aged 24, had the right lens displaced downwards and inwards, the left inwards. II. 10, aged 13, had both lenses displaced downwards. I. 2 had three normal children by her second husband. No consanguinity recorded. Bibl. No. 80.

Fig. 1222. *Eha's Case.* Ectopia lentis in a brother and sister. II. 1, aged 7 years (1902), had always seen badly; her anterior chamber was abnormally deep; pupils were in the normal position and reacted promptly; a marked tremor of the iris and of the transparent lenses was noted; the lenses were slightly displaced downwards and outwards, the inner margins of the lenses were visible after atropine; the fundi were normal except for some irregularity in the shape of the discs and in the distribution of the vessels. R. V. = finger counting at 5 m., L. V. = finger counting at 2 m.; or R. V. with − 10·0 D. sph. = $\frac{6}{30}$, L. V. with − 9·0 D. sph. = $\frac{6}{40}$. II. 2, seen aged 2, had already had several operations for epispadias; his pupils were bilaterally displaced outwards and upwards; the lenses were displaced downwards and inwards so that no lens was present in the pupillary region, but its position could be observed after atropine; fundi were normal; the patient died a few months after the examination.

No other cases of similar defect were known to have occurred in the family. No consanguinity recorded. Bibl. No. 155.

Fig. 1223. *Beauvieux's Case.* Ectopia lentis in two brothers; the father was alcoholic and died aged 45; the mother had high myopia, about 18 D. II. 1 was aged 27. II. 2 died from an accident at the age of 19; Lagrange saw him at the age of 12 years and then diagnosed congenital bilateral dislocation of the lens outwards. No consanguinity recorded. Bibl. No. 197.

Fig. 1224. *Adams's Case.* Ectopia lentis in a mother and in seven of her nine children. I. 1 considered that her defect arose as a result of her mother falling downstairs the night before she, I. 1, was born. In II. 1 the R. lens was displaced downwards leaving the upper third of the pupil clear; the L. lens was not visible in the pupil. II. 2, aged 16, had her R. lens displaced inwards, the L. lens, upwards and inwards.

II. 3, aged 14, and II. 5, aged 11, had normal eyes. II. 4, aged 12, had the R. lens displaced downwards, the L. lens down and slightly inwards; she had high myopia; R. V. with -20 D. sph. $< \frac{6}{90}$, L. V. with -20 D. sph. $< \frac{6}{35}$. II. 6, aged 10, had both lenses displaced inwards; R. V. with $+7$ D. sph. $= \frac{6}{35}$, L. V. with $+8$ D. sph. $< \frac{6}{15}$. II. 7, aged 8, had high myopia; his R. lens was displaced upwards, the L. lens up and outwards; with -20 D. sph. in each R. V. $< \frac{6}{60}$, L. V. $= \frac{6}{50}$. II. 8, aged 3, had her R. lens displaced downwards, her L. lens inwards. II. 9, aged $1\frac{1}{2}$ years, had both lenses displaced upwards. All the affected members had tremulous irides. No other congenital abnormalities were found. No consanguinity recorded. Bibl. No. 188.

Fig. 1225. *Schwarz's Case.* Corectopia in a brother and two sisters. II. 1, Peter E., aged 28, had both pupils displaced inwards and upwards to near the ciliary region; his right pupil was a little larger than the left; vision was rather better in the right eye. II. 2, aged 24, and II. 3, aged 16, had their right pupils in a position similar to those of their brother; their left pupils were displaced downwards to near the ciliary region. II. 4 and II. 5 had well developed eyes but were short-sighted. I. 1 had normal eyes. The mother I. 2, aged 58, had been blind and arthritic for 9 years; she had glaucoma and cataract; her pupils were in a normal position. No consanguinity recorded. Bibl. No. 28.

Fig. 1226. *de Haas's Case.* Ectopia lentis, with arachnodactyly, in a brother and sister; the third child in this family was healthy, also the mother; the father was dead, he was said to have had very large hands and feet and to wear spectacles of 11 D. sph. No consanguinity recorded. Bibl. No. 283.

Fig. 1227. *Weve's Case.* Ectopia lentis with arachnodactyly in four members of a family; the father, two sons and a daughter were affected. No consanguinity recorded. Bibl. No. 286.

Fig. 1228. *Zentmayer's Case.* A child, aged 7 years, had both lenses dislocated downwards and inwards; her father had a similar malformation; in the child R. V. $= \frac{3}{30}$, L. V. $= \frac{6}{36}$; her lenses were slightly cloudy but showed no localised opacity. No consanguinity recorded. Bibl. No. 271.

Fig. 1229. *Hosford's Case.* II. 1, aged 21, had normal irides, pupils and lenses, V. $= \frac{6}{6}$ and J. 1. II. 2, aged 18, had pupils displaced up and out on the R. side, upwards on the L.; her lenses were dislocated, the R. lens up and out, the L. lens upwards; R. V. $< \frac{6}{60}$, L. V. $= \frac{6}{12}$, with correction. II. 3, aged 16, had both pupils and both lenses eccentric, up and out; R. V. $= \frac{6}{18}$, L. V. $= \frac{6}{24}$ with correction. II. 4, aged 14, had both pupils and both lenses eccentric, up and out; R. V. $= \frac{6}{60}$, L. V. $= \frac{6}{18}$, with correction. II. 5, aged 12, also had both pupils and both lenses eccentric, up and out; R. V. $= \frac{6}{24}$ with correction. II. 6, aged 6, had both pupils eccentric, downwards, and both lenses dislocated inwards. The parents of this sibship were normal; no relation on either side was known to have any malformation of the eyes or other parts of the body. No consanguinity recorded. Bibl. No. 193.

Fig. 1230. *Komoto's Case.* I. 1 and 2, of whom no information is given, had three sons who all had congenital ectopia lentis; all their daughters were normal. No consanguinity recorded. Bibl. No. 190.

Fig. 1231. *Hassler's Case.* II. 2, Napoleon R., aged 22, was under examination with a view to military service; he was of a robust constitution with average intelligence, but had bad sight which had not changed since infancy; he was found to have bilateral symmetrical ectopia lentis, the displacement in each eye being inwards and slightly upwards; there was slight divergent strabismus of the left eye; no microphthalmos; R. V. $= \frac{1}{10}$, L. V. $= \frac{1}{25}$. II. 2 reported that his father, who had died at about the age of 60, had presented the same ocular lesion; one of the brothers of II. 2 had the same affection and had been declared unfit for military service; two other brothers and one sister had normal sight. No consanguinity. Bibl. No. 126.

Fig. 1232. *Kennedy's Case.* I. 1, aged 47, had bilateral ectopia lentis; his irides were tremulous, the lenses were at the bottom of the vitreous chambers; fundi were normal; R. V. $= \frac{20}{50}$, L. V. $=$ perception of light. This patient had four sons and one daughter; the eldest son and the daughter had an outward displacement of their lenses; the other three sons had normal eyes. The father and grandfather of I. 1 were reported to have had "poor eyes." No consanguinity recorded. Bibl. No. 261.

Fig. 1233. *Leoz's Case.* I. 1 was seen with secondary glaucoma following luxation of the lens in one eye and subluxation in the other. Two daughters and one son of I. 1 had bilateral subluxation of the lens outwards; one of the daughters had also a double pupil. No consanguinity recorded. Bibl. No. 248.

Fig. 1234. *Sous's Case.* Tremulous irides with subluxation of the lens downwards in a brother and sister. No consanguinity recorded. Bibl. No. 124.

Fig. 1235. *Bowman's Case.* II. 1, aged 26, whilst walking quietly along the street, found his left eye beginning to shoot and throb and water very much; symptoms of pain and inflammation became very acute and when seen a fortnight later the pupil was widely dilated and the lens was projecting into the pupil so as to fill the anterior chamber; this man said he had always had excellent vision (though short-sighted); in the right eye the iris was tremulous and flat; the lens was attached only at the upper and inner part of its circumference and would swing about according to the inclination of the head, so that on leaning towards

PLATE LXXVI.   DESCRIPTIONS OF PEDIGREE PLATES   553

the left it would disappear on the nasal side of even the dilated pupil; the lens preserved its transparency. A very full and interesting account of this case is given in the original history. The man mentioned that one of his paternal uncles, now dead, had a similar anomaly. No consanguinity recorded. Bibl. No. 33, pp. 135—138.

Fig. 1236. *Lambert's Case.* Congenital dislocation of the lenses in a brother and sister; the mother also had some dislocation of her lenses but in her the defect was of slight grade and did not interfere with her vision. II. 1 had R. V. $= \frac{4}{200}$, L. V. $= \frac{20}{200}$. II. 2 had R. V. $= \frac{20}{70}$, L. V. = finger counting only; both cases were treated by operation. Four discissions were made on each eye in both cases, with subsequent absorption of the lenses. The vision of II. 2 after operation was $\frac{20}{30}$ + in each eye with + 12·0 D. sph.; II. 1 ultimately had R. V. $= \frac{20}{50}$, L. V. $= \frac{20}{30}$ with the proper correction. No consanguinity recorded. Bibl. No. 231.

Fig. 1237. *Charles's Case.* I. 1 had ectopia lentis; nothing was known of his ancestors; of his children II. 1, a daughter, had bilateral congenital ectopia lentis; II. 2, a son, presented the same condition as II. 1 ; II. 3, a daughter, had congenital dislocation of the lens with cataract; she also had very large corneae; one or two other children of I. 1 had normal eyes. No consanguinity recorded. Bibl. No. 190.

Fig. 1238. *Wissmann's Case.* Ectopia lentis in a male who was twice married; by each wife he had two children, a boy and a girl; both the boys have ectopia lentis. The displacement in each case was inwards and upwards. No consanguinity recorded. Bibl. No. 212.

Fig. 1239. *Zirm's Case.* Bilateral ectopia lentis in a brother and sister who had eight normal siblings; the parents had normal eyes; the corneae in the four affected eyes were large and transparent, the anterior chambers deep; the irides showed very marked tremor; pupils were normal and reacted promptly to light; in the boy both lenses were dislocated up and somewhat in; the lenses were clear. The affected children, aged 14 and 8 years respectively, were the subjects of widespread rachitic changes. No consanguinity recorded. Bibl. No. 110.

Fig. 1240. *Frickhöffer's Case.* Corectopia and ectopia lentis in four siblings. I. 1 had oval pupils, the long diameter being from the inner side below to the outer side above. I. 2 had incipient cataract in the right eye, floating opacities in the vitreous, staphyloma posticum, and very defective vision. These parents had four children of whom II. 1 was not seen, her eyes were said to be the same as those of her siblings. II. 2, aged 21 (1880), had never seen well and had been unable to learn to read or write; her corneae and anterior chambers were of normal size; iridonesis was present; right pupil of normal size but elliptical shape, longest diameter from inner side below to outer side above, had a notched inner margin, and was displaced, downwards and inwards, to near the edge of the cornea; it reacted to light or to atropine; there was complete aphakia, the lens lay and moved freely in the vitreous chamber; floating vitreous opacities were noted; disc was normal but there was some atrophy of the surrounding choroid and of the pigment layer of the retina; the left pupil, of normal size and shape, had a notched margin to the outer side, its position was almost in the centre of the iris, slightly to the inner side; reaction to light and to atropine was normal; lens was partly visible in the pupil and appeared to be dislocated outwards; monocular diplopia was present; fundus normal excepting a few atrophic patches surrounding the disc. II. 3, aged 17, saw better than her siblings, she could read and write and was more intelligent than the others; she said that she saw well with the left eye but very little with the right; the cornea and anterior chamber were normal in each eye, iridodonesis was present, pupils reacted to light and to atropine; the right pupil was oval and was displaced, downwards and inwards, with its long diameter directed downwards and inwards; the lens was partly visible cutting across the pupil; fundus was normal; monocular diplopia was present; the left pupil was oval and displaced downwards with the long diameter vertical; the lens was completely in the region of the pupil and was thus ectopic in the same direction as the pupil; fundus was normal. II. 4, aged 12, had the least vision of all the siblings and could not read or write; anterior chambers and corneae were normal; iridodonesis was present in each iris; the reaction of the pupils to light and to atropine was almost absent; there was a small elliptic pupil in each eye displaced upwards and outwards with the long diameter directed downwards and inwards; the left lens was nowhere to be seen; the right lens was not in the pupillary region but could be seen lying in the vitreous chamber. No consanguinity recorded. Bibl. No. 70.

Fig. 1241. *Iwumi's Case.* Congenital ectopia lentis in two brothers; in one case the lens was in the anterior chamber. No consanguinity recorded. Bibl. No. 194.

Fig. 1242. *Baudon's Case.* Ectopia lentis in three brothers; in one case the displacement was upwards and inwards. No consanguinity recorded. Bibl. No. 74.

Fig. 1243. *Ginestous's Case.* Congenital ectopia lentis in a mother and two of her children. I. 1, aged 36, had a congenital luxation of the lens outwards; her daughter II. 1, aged 15, had a displacement upwards and inwards. II. 2, Marcel F., aged 12, had his right lens displaced downwards and outwards; the left lens showed a more accentuated ectopia and was completely outside the pupil even when this was dilated to a maximum; the lens was very mobile and could be made to occupy almost its normal position; both lenses were transparent; R. V. = $\frac{1}{10}$ or with + 9 D. = $\frac{1}{3}$, L. V. = $\frac{1}{10}$ with and without correction. No consanguinity recorded. Bibl. No. 147.

Fig. 1244. *Gehrung's Case.* Congenital bilateral ectopia lentis in a brother and sister; the mother had a coloboma lentis at the infero-internal border of each lens. II. 1 had R. V. = L. V. = $\frac{5}{200}$; both lenses were displaced upwards, about two thirds of the pupil was covered. II. 2 had R. V. = $\frac{8}{200}$, L. V. = $\frac{3}{200}$; both lenses were displaced upwards but covered about half the pupils. Both lenses of II. 1 and 2 showed a coloboma; in II. 1 it was at the upper and inner margin of the lenses on each side. The lenses in each case were clear. No consanguinity recorded. Bibl. No. 206.

Fig. 1245. *Arana's Case.* Congenital ectopia lentis in mother and son. No consanguinity recorded. Bibl. No. 237.

Fig. 1246. *Fryer's Case.* Bilateral congenital symmetrical ectopia lentis in two sisters. II. 1, Josephine V., aged 7, had R. V. = L. V. = $\frac{20}{200}$; her lenses were dislocated outwards; both lenses were slightly cloudy; the eyes were of normal size. II. 2, Willielmina V., aged 5, had both lenses dislocated in an upward and outward direction. No consanguinity recorded. Bibl. No. 83.

Fig. 1247. *Rochon-Duvigneaud's Case.* Ectopia lentis in a child aged 7 years and in its mother; during a quarrel the child's lens was luxated and fell into the anterior chamber; acute glaucoma followed and the lens was extracted. The lens was almost spherical, with the transverse diameter much less than normal. No consanguinity recorded. Bibl. No. 181.

Fig. 1248. *Morrow's Case.* Ectopia lentis in a brother and two sisters; the mother and a maternal aunt were similarly affected. In II. 1, aged 12, the lenses were displaced upwards and inwards; the condition was said to be precisely the same in II. 2. II. 3 and I. 2 were also seen. No movement of the lenses could be obtained in any of the cases. No consanguinity recorded. Bibl. No. 109.

Fig. 1249. *Kretschmer's Case.* Ectopia lentis in father and son. II. 1, aged 5 years, had tremulous irides and both lenses displaced upwards and inwards. I. 1 saw badly and had a large lens-free segment of pupil; the right lens was displaced upwards and outwards, the left lens upwards and inwards. No consanguinity recorded. Bibl. No. 210.

DESCRIPTIONS OF ILLUSTRATIVE PLATES P, Q, R, S AND T.

PLATE P. Figs. 1–15 includes examples of congenital coloboma iridis, showing the varieties which occur in shape and position of the cleft. Figs. 1 and 2 show narrow slit-shaped colobomata; von Ammon, examining about 1841, was not sure whether these clefts involved all layers of the iris or were confined to the superficial layers. Figs. 5 and 6 are examples of key-hole shaped colobomata, incomplete in Fig. 5, complete in Fig. 6. Fig 8 shows similar typical colobomata in the two eyes of an individual. Fig. 12 presents a case showing marked asymmetry in size of cornea and shape of colobomata in the two eyes of a patient. Fig. 10 is from an example of a bridge coloboma. Figs. 13, 14 and 15 show atypical colobomata directed outwards, inwards and upwards respectively. In the examples of Figs. 7 and 9 the clefts have markedly concave edges and a broad base.

Figs. 16–19 illustrate cases of Aniridia. In Fig. 16 the condition was associated with ptosis; no trace of iris was visible; a gerontoxon was noted; the patient was a female, aged 22, under the care of Gutbier. Fig. 17 shows the left eye of a man described by Henzschel (I. 1 of Ped. 1113, Plate LXX); rudiments of brownish iris were present behind the lower part of the cornea; this man had three daughters with aniridia. Fig. 18 shows the right eye of a patient of von Ammon's; a narrow barely visible rim of iris could be identified; a very dense anterior capsular cataract was present. The woman of this case was the mother of the girl whose eyes are portrayed in Fig. 19; von Ammon could detect no trace of iris in this girl; he describes the presence of an early posterior capsular cataract with the appearance of a radiating stellate structure as shown in the illustration.

The cases of this plate are taken from Plates X and XII of von Ammon's *Klinische Darstellungen der Krankheiten und Bildungsfehler des menschlichen Auges*, Th. III. (Bibl. No. 32). We are indebted to Mary Kirby for the coloured copies from the original plates.

PLATE Q. Figs. 1–9 include cases of Anophthalmia and mal-development of the eyes photographed by C. H. Usher; the cases are fully described under Plate LXVI, Ped. 982: see pp. 502–505; Figs. 1–7 represent all the living members of the sibship VI. 28–37, including the two normal members depicted in Figs. 5 and 7; Figs. 7, 8 and 9 show the normal parents of the affected children.

Plate R. Fig. 1. Portrays a little girl aged 5 years, the 14th child in a sibship of 15; the multiple anomalies exhibited by the child include bilateral supernumerary ears and colobomata of the upper eye-lids; on the right side two dermoids in the eye are shown, also macroglossia; on the left side was a coloboma of the iris and choroid. The child had a large fovea sacralis; she was unable to walk or crawl and could only say a few words. Three of her siblings, including the 15th member of the sibship, were seen to be free from developmental defect. The case was described by Bishop Harman, who kindly permits us to reproduce his illustration. (*Transactions, Ophthalmological Society of U. K.* Vol. xxiv, pp. 325–329. 1904.)

Fig. 2. This case is reproduced from von Ammon (*loc. cit.* p. 554 above) where it occurs as Fig. IV on Plate IV; it represents a case of congenital microphthalmos; the eyes were small and deeply sunken in the orbits, and showed a number of developmental anomalies including corectopia and probably choroideremia; the ocular fissure was narrow and ptosis was marked. The patient had been blind from birth; he was an imbecile and had suffered from rachitis.

Fig. 3. Shannon's cases of mal-development of the eyes in two sisters; the anomalies presented include microphthalmos with small pear-shaped cornea, and colobomata of iris and choroid. Two other siblings, their father, and other members of the family were also affected. From Vol. xv, p. 44 (1917) of the *Trans. of the American Ophthalmological Society* by kind permission. The pedigree is given on Plate LXXII, Fig. 1158: see p. 534. (Bibl. No. 223.)

Fig. 4. Enlargement of the cornea in a case of congenital buphthalmos; the right eye of this child had been destroyed in the course of the disease. The illustration is taken from Römer's *Lehrbuch der Augen-heilkunde*, Berlin and Wien, 1923, published by Herren Urban and Schwarzenberg who kindly allow this reproduction.

Fig. 5. Bilateral, symmetrical, typical coloboma iridis in a boy whose brother had a similar unilateral affection; two other siblings had normal eyes; the parents were normal and were not consanguineous. Taken from Waardenburg, P. J.: *Das menschliche Auge und seine Erbanlagen*, p. 242. Haag, 1932.

Plate S. Cases of Coloboma, Aniridia and Ectopia lentis.

Figs. 1–3 show the appearance of the fundi in Selz's cases from the pedigree, Plate LXXII, Fig. 1161; see p. 535. (Bibl. No. 150.)

Fig. 1. Coloboma of the choroid in the left eye of IV. 2 of the pedigree and in the right eye of her brother IV. 3; each case was unilateral and was associated with a normal eye on the other side; both cases had a coloboma iridis in the affected eye; in IV. 2 the affected eye was microphthalmic.

Fig. 2. Coloboma of the choroid involving the optic nerve in both eyes of IV. 1, the elder sister of the cases shown in Fig. 1; the condition was associated with bilateral coloboma iridis and microphthalmos.

Fig. 3. Coloboma of the choroid, not involving the optic nerve, in the father of the cases of Figs. 1 and 2; the condition was unilateral in his case and was not associated with coloboma iridis.

Fig. 4. Aniridia in two brothers; traces of the structure can be seen in both cases; another brother and the mother of the sibship were similarly affected. These cases were described by Mohr (Bibl. No. 123) and appear as III. 1 and III. 2 in the pedigree, Plate LXX, Fig. 1110; see p. 527.

Fig. 5. Shows anomalies in the shape and position of the pupil associated with ectopia lentis in both eyes of three siblings. The cases are described by Frickhöffer. (Bibl. No. 70.) The parents of these children had normal eyes.

Plate T. Fig. 1. Buphthalmos in a girl of 14 years of age, showing greatly enlarged corneae which occupy almost the whole of the interpalpebral areas. The original photograph is published in Lieut.-Colonel R. H. Elliot's *Treatise on Glaucoma*, London, 1922 (Bibl. No. 247), and is reproduced here by kind permission of author and publishers.

Fig. 2. Bondi's case of megalocornea in uncle and nephew, corneal diameter of uncle (Fig. 2, a) = 17 mm. and of nephew (Fig. 2, c) = 15·5 mm. on right side. Fig. 2, b is described by Bondi as the eyes of a normal individual but on the above scale as the corneae measure 10 mm. horizontally they might be described as microcorneal. Photographs given here to ½ scale. Reproduced from the *Wiener medizinische Presse* by kind permission of Herren Urban und Schwarzenberg.

CAMBRIDGE: PRINTED BY
W. LEWIS, M.A.
AT THE UNIVERSITY PRESS

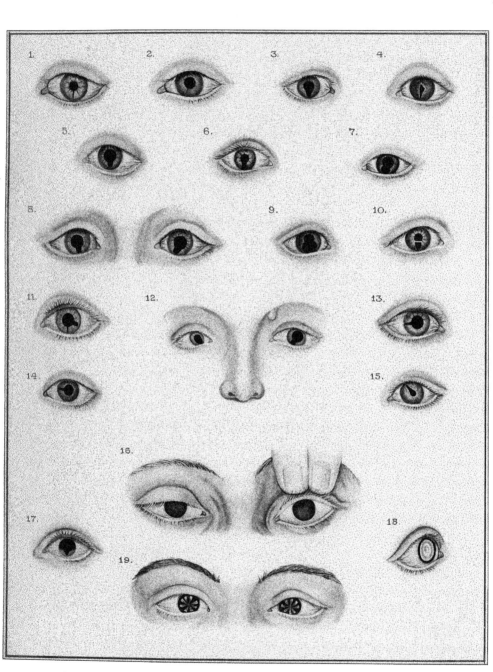

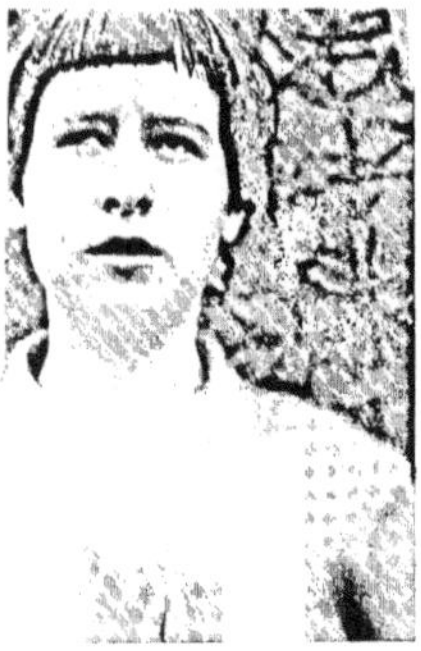

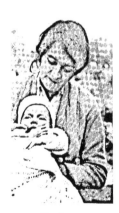

Fig. 1.

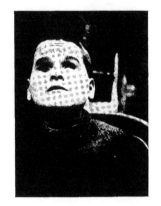

Fig. 2.

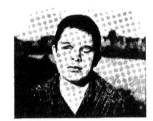

Fig. 3.

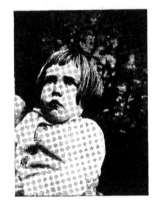

Fig. 4.

Fig. 5.

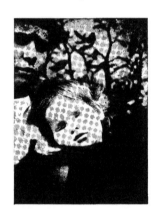

Fig. 6.

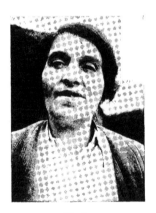

Fig. 7.

Fig. 8.

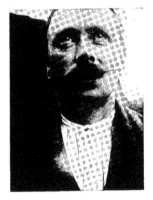

Fig. 9.

1 Parents (Figs. 7—9) and their Offspring (Figs. 1—7), five of whom show Anophthalmos or mal-development of the Eyes.

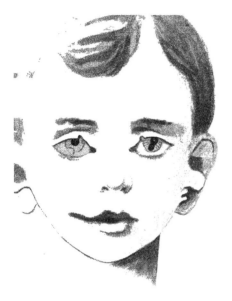

nilateral Coloboma iridis associated with other Anomalies.
By kind permission of Bishop Harman.

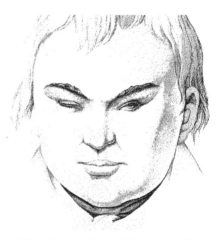

Fig. 2. Microphthalmos with other Anomalies
in an Imbecile.

After von Ammon.

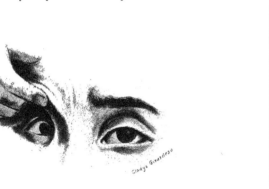

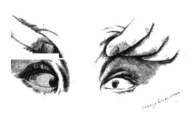

Mal-development of the Eyes in two Sisters.
After Shannon.
ermission of the American Ophthalmological Society.

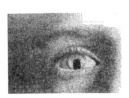

Fig. 4. Congenital Buphthalmos.
After Romer.

By kind permission of Herren Urban und
Schwarzenberg.

Fig. 5. Bilateral typical Coloboma iridis.
After Waardenburg.

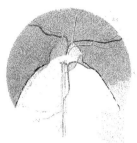

Fig. 1.

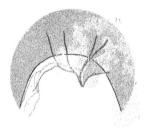

Fig. 2.

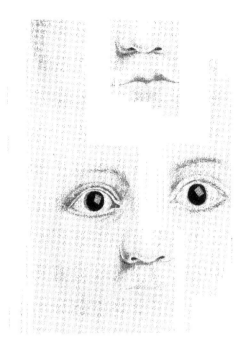

Fig. 4. Aniridia in two Siblings.
After Mohr.

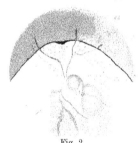

Fig. 3.
Figs. 1—3. Coloboma of the Choroid, in three members of a Family with Coloboma iridis.
After Selz.

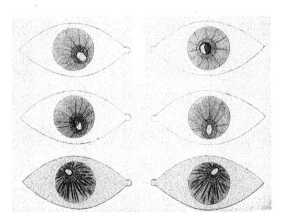

Fig. 5. Corectopia with Ectopia lentis in right and left eyes of three Siblings.
After Frickhöffer.

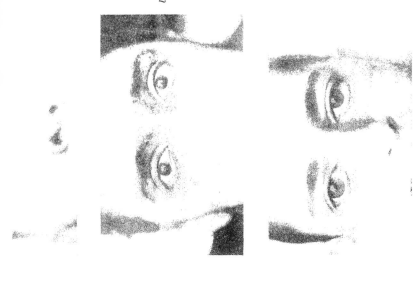
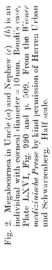

Fig. 2. Megalocornea in Uncle (*a*) and Nephew (*c*) (*b*) is an individual with corneal diameter = 10mm. Bondi's case, Plate LXVI, Fig. 990 and p. 509. From the *Wiener medizinische Presse* by kind permission of Herren Urban und Schwarzenberg. Half scale.

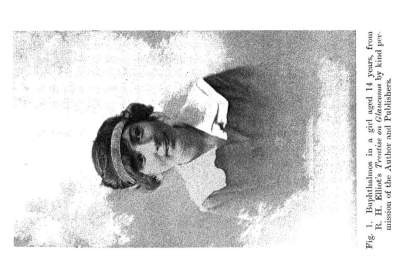

Fig. 1. Buphthalmos in a girl aged 14 years, from R. H. Elliot's *Treatise on Glaucoma* by kind permission of the Author and Publishers.

Fig. = Figure in Pedigrees, Roman capitals refer to Illustrative Plates and fig. to figures upon them.
'Associated with' = in same person but only very rarely in same pedigree.

HEREDITARY OPTIC ATROPHY.

Issued by the Francis C.

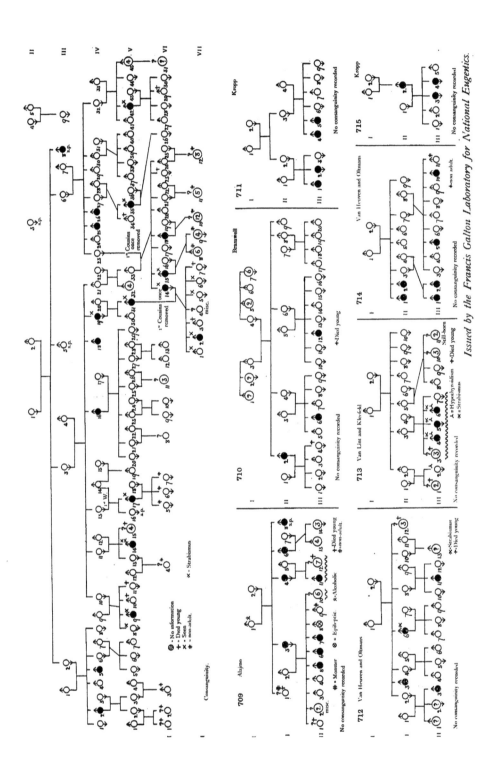

Issued by the Francis Galton Laboratory for National Eugenics.

716 Meyer Riemsloh

717

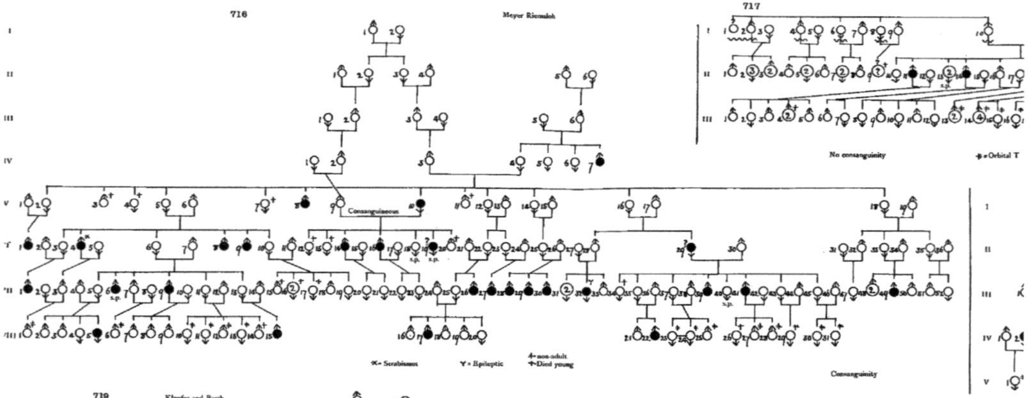

719 Klopfer and Barth

720 Render

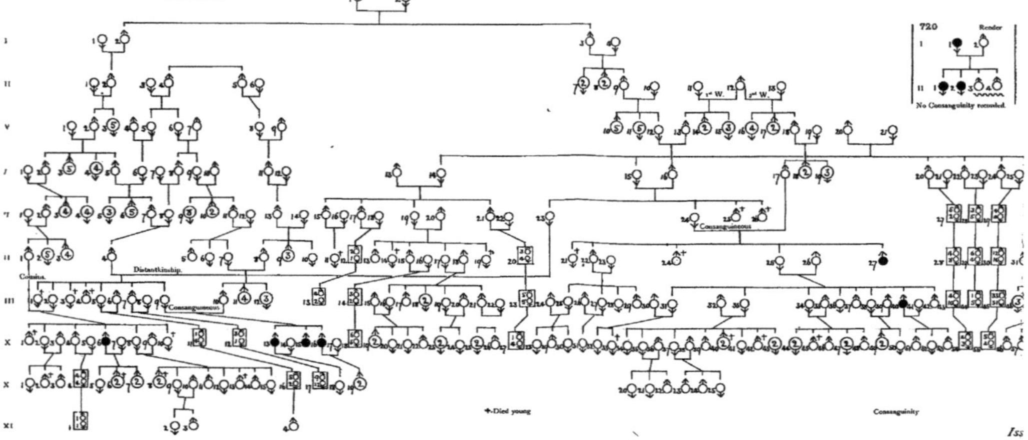

Iss

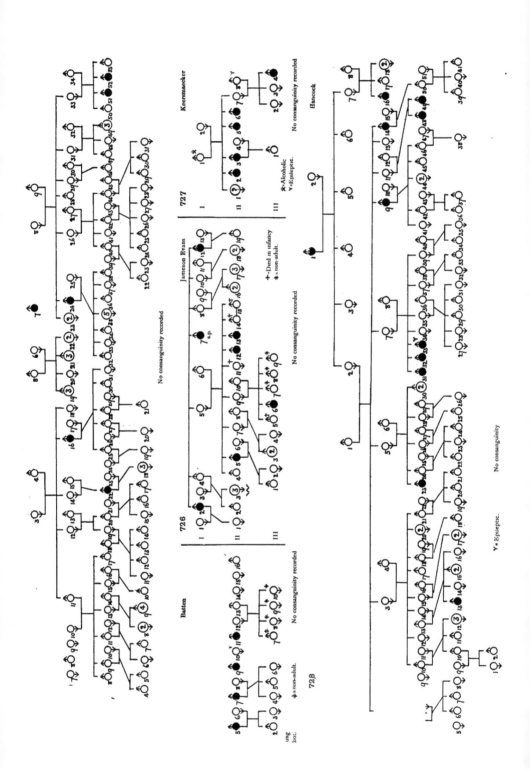

Keeremaecker

727

Jameson Evans

726

Batten

72B

Hancock

No consanguinity recorded

✗=Alcoholic
Y=Epileptic.

+ = Died in infancy
‡ = non-adult.

No consanguinity recorded

‡ = non-adult.

No consanguinity recorded

Y = Epileptic.

No consanguinity

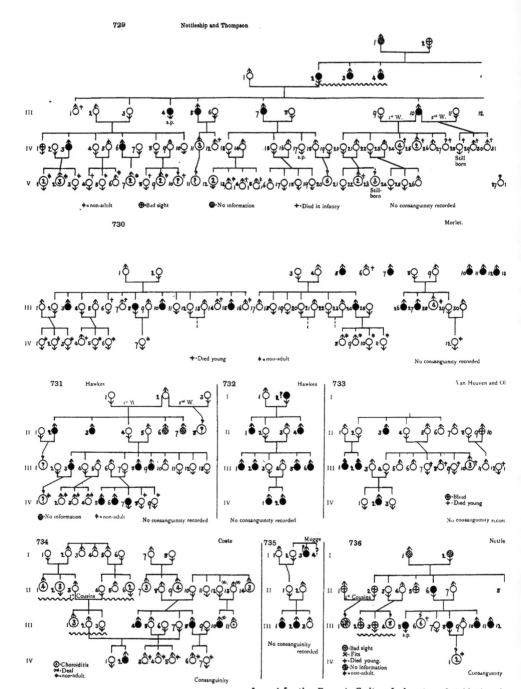

+ = non-adult   ⊕·Bad sight   ●·No information   +·Died in infancy   No consanguinity recorded

730   Morlet.

+·Died young   *·non-adult   No consanguinity recorded

731   Hawkes   732   Hawkes   733   Van Heuven and Ol

●·No information   *·non-adult   No consanguinity recorded   No consanguinity recorded

⊕·Blind
+·Died young

No consanguinity recor

734   Coste   735   Mügge   736   Nettle

⊙·Choroiditis
≈·Deaf
+·non-adult.

No consanguinity
recorded

⊕·Bad sight
✕·Fits
+·Died young.
●·No information
*·non-adult

Consanguinity   Consanguinity

Issued by the Francis Galton Laboratory for National

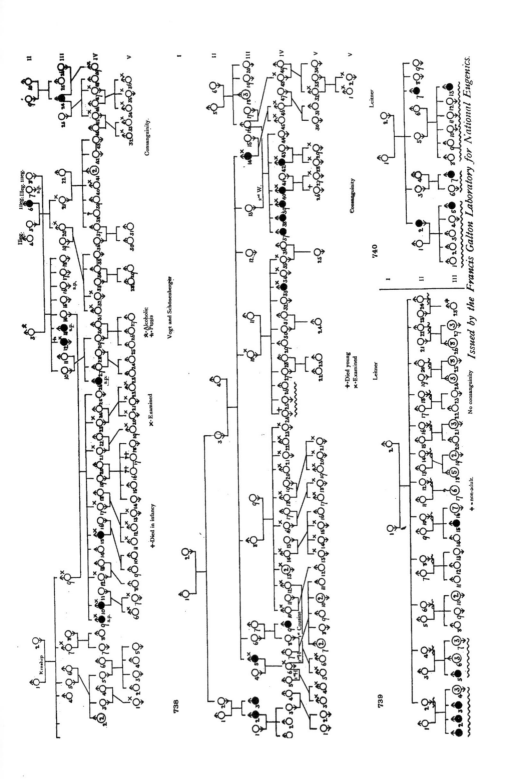

Issued by the Francis Galton Laboratory for National Eugenics.

HEREDITARY OPTIC ATROPHY.

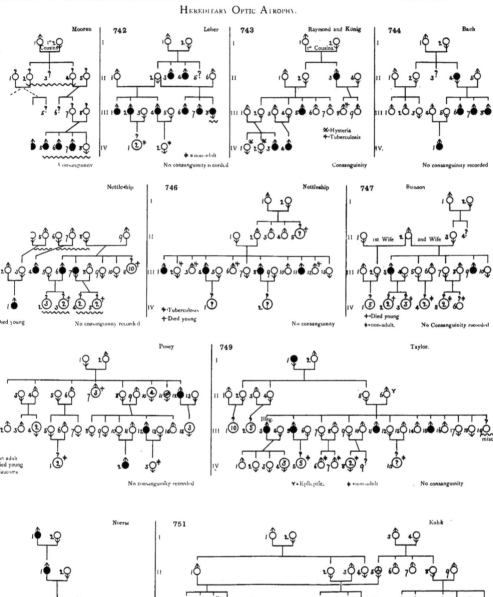

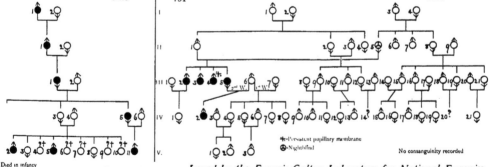

Issued by the Francis Galton Laboratory for National Eugenics.

HEREDITARY OPTIC ATROPHY.

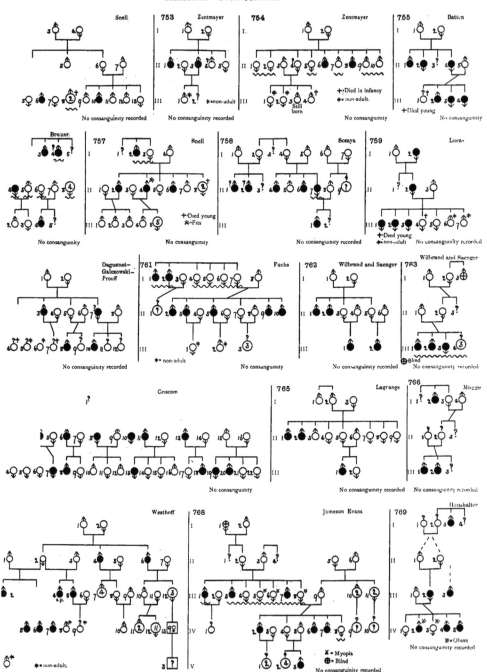

No consanguinity recorded   *= non-adult.   *+Died in infancy   *= non-adult.   +=Died young   *+=non-adult.   X = Myopia   ⊕ = Blind   ⊕=Obese

Issued by the Francis Galton Laboratory for National Eugenics.

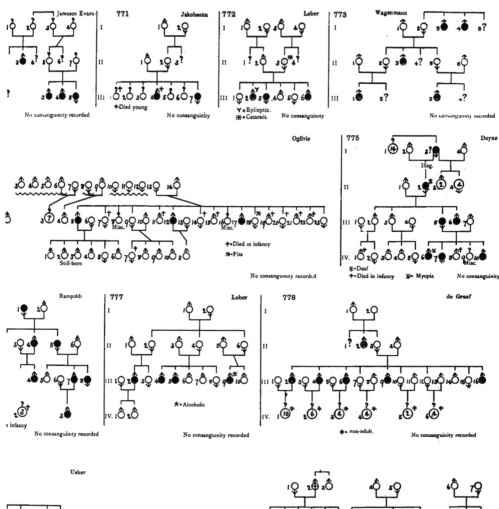

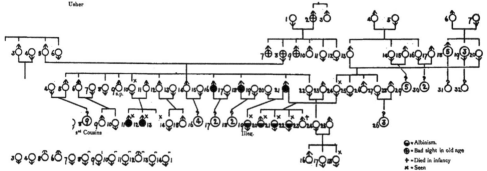

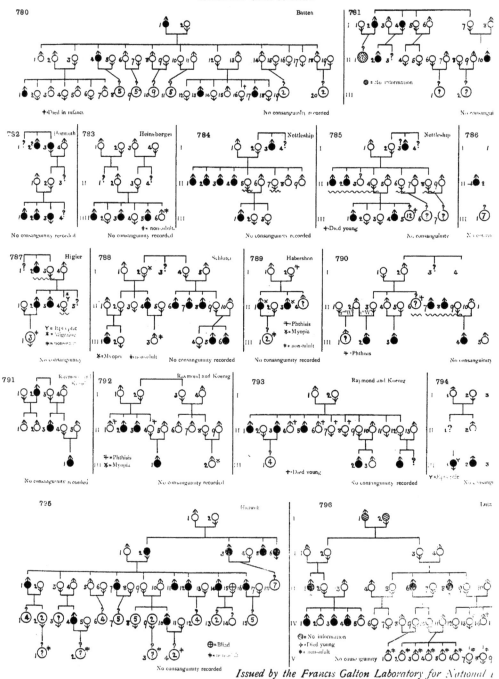

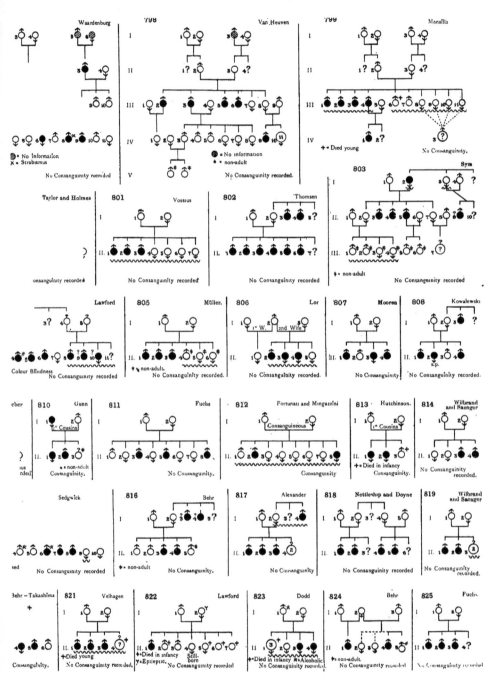

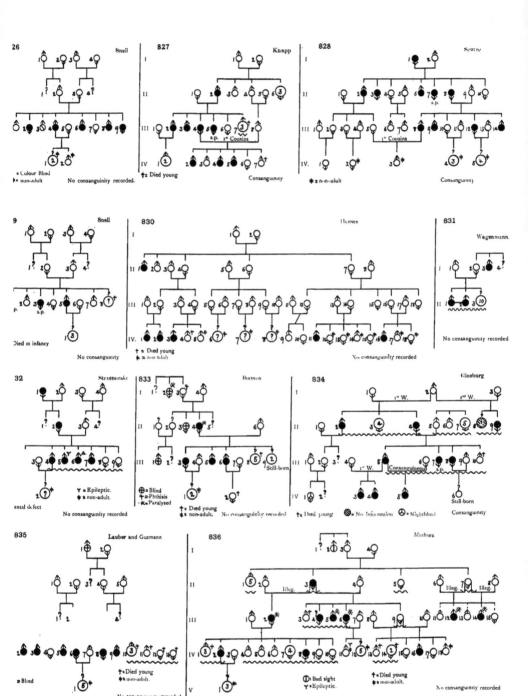

Issued by the *Francis Galton Laboratory for National Eugenics.*

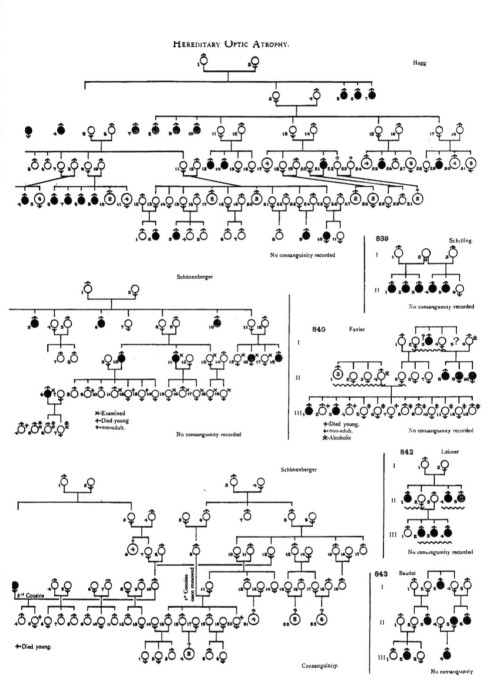

Hogg

Schilling.

839

No consanguinity recorded

Schönenberger

840   Favier

×-Examined
+-Died young
✦-non-adult.

No consanguinity recorded

+-Died young.
✦-non-adult.
×-Alcoholic

No consanguinity recorded

842   Leitner

Schönenberger

No consanguinity recorded

843   Baudot

3ʳᵈ Cousins

1ˢᵗ Cousins once removed.

✦-Died young.

Consanguinity.

No consanguinity

Issued by the Francis Galton Laboratory for National Eugenics.

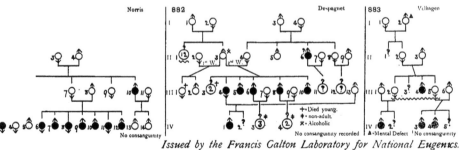

HEREDITARY OPTIC ATROPHY.

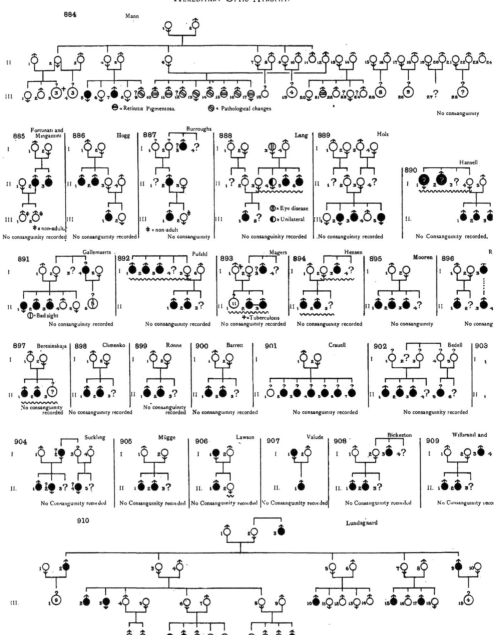

HEREDITARY OPTIC ATROPHY. (JAPANESE CASES.)

PLATE L.

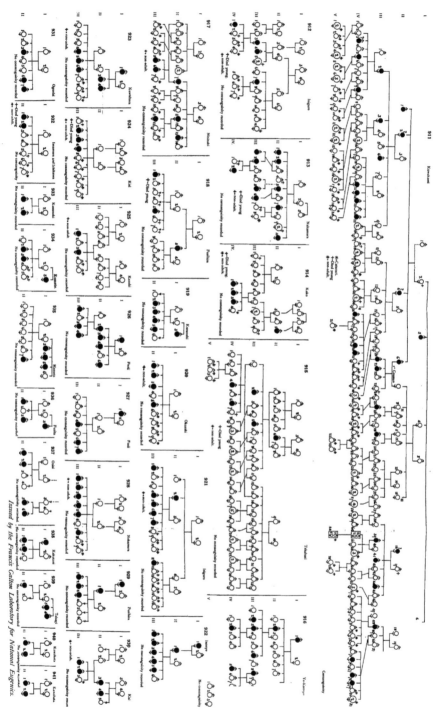

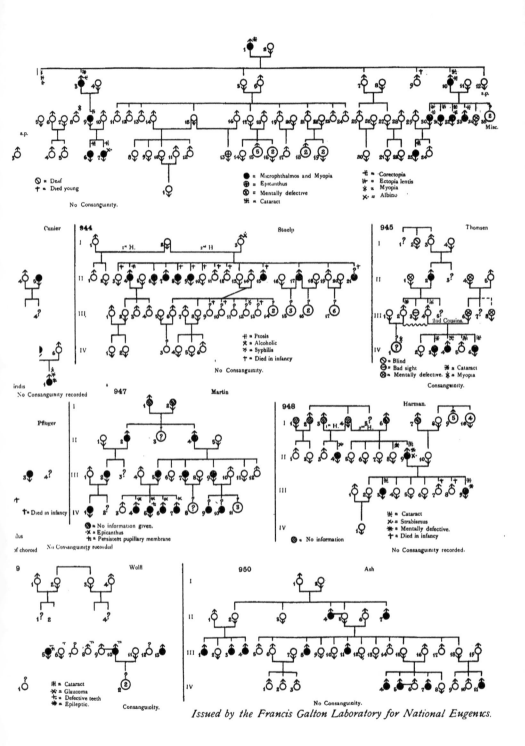

Issued by the Francis Galton Laboratory for National Eugenics.

MICROPHTHALMOS

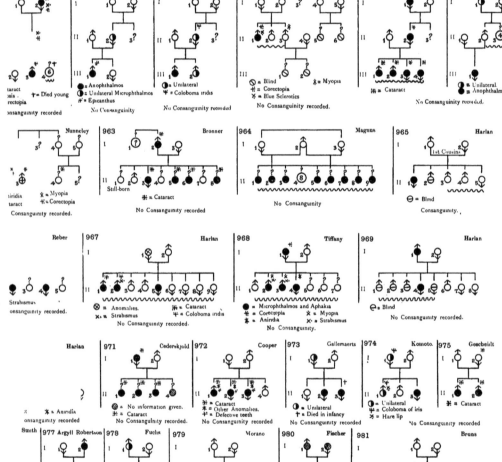

Issued by the Francis Galton Laboratory for National Eugenics.

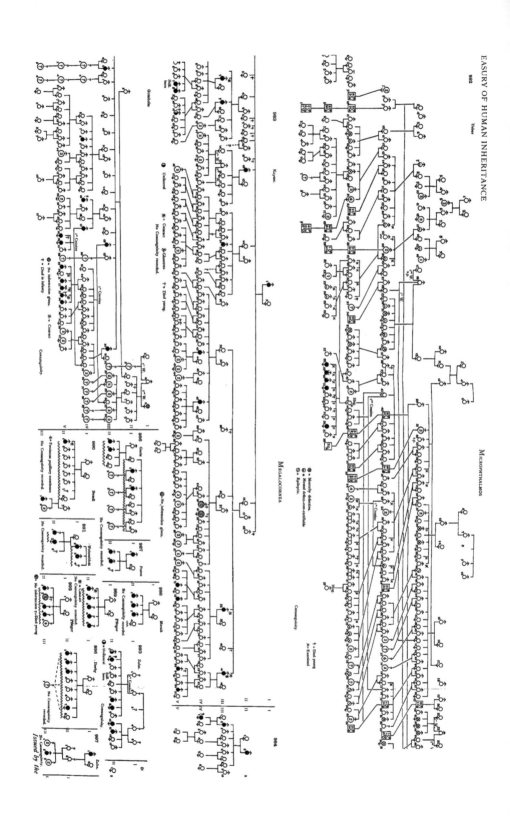

BUPHTHALMOS

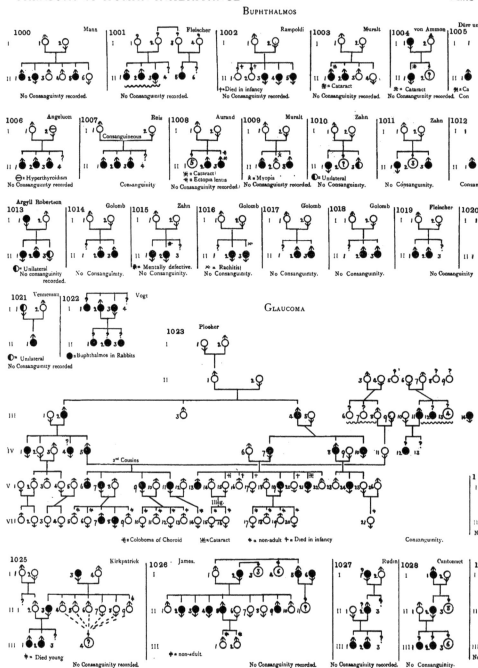

GLAUCOMA

GLAUCOMA

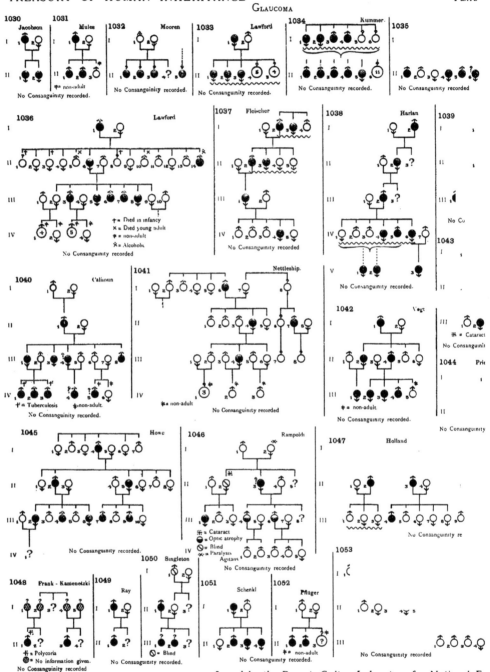

GLAUCOMA

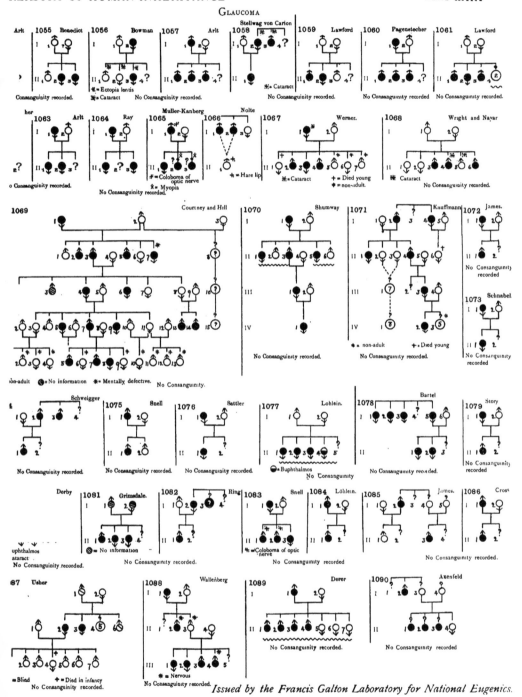

ANIRIDIA

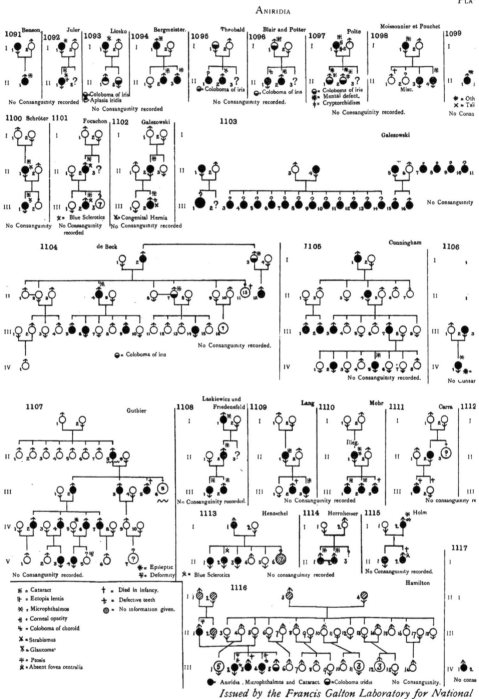

Issued by the Francis Galton Laboratory for National

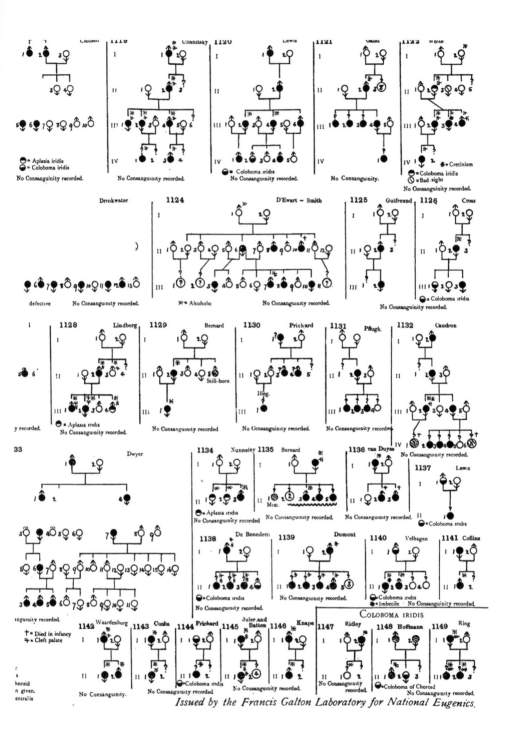

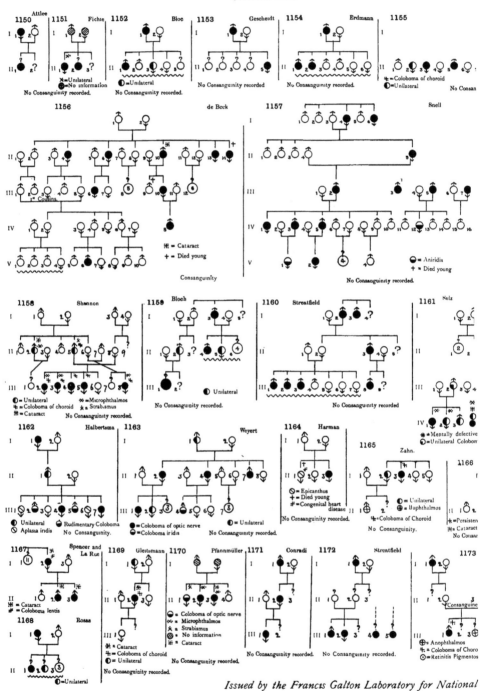

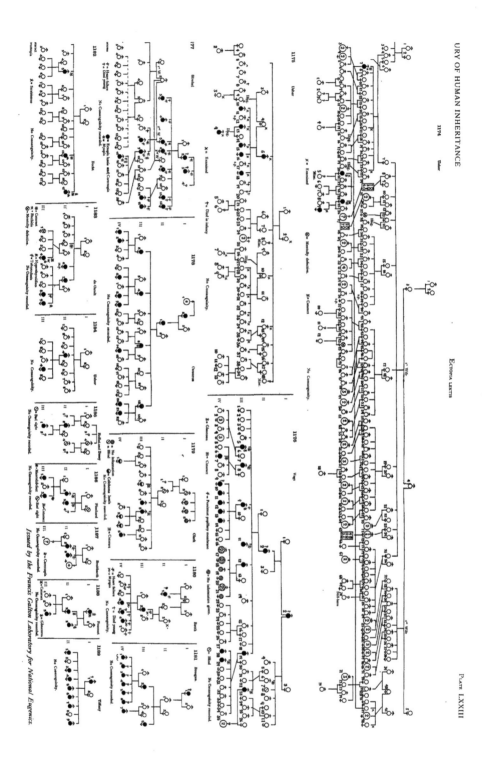

PLATE LXXIV

ECTOPIA LENTIS

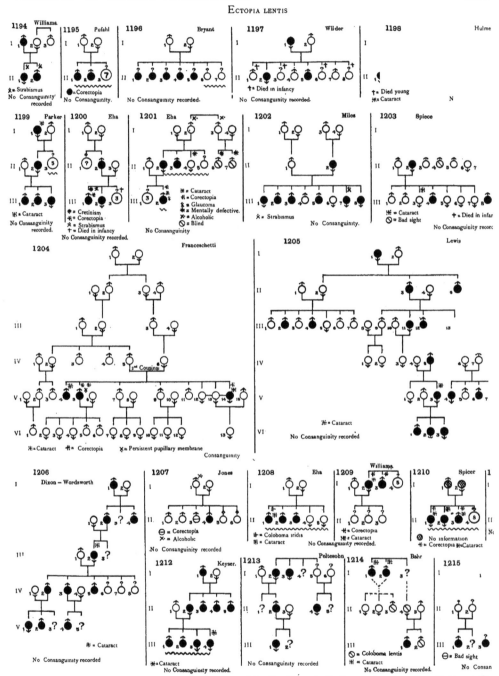

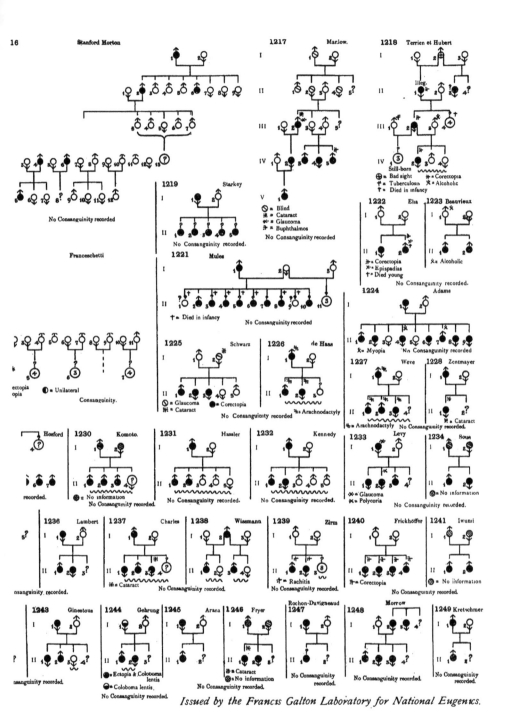

Issued by the Francis Galton Laboratory for National Eugenics.

Lightning Source UK Ltd.
Milton Keynes UK
UKHW02f0304180818
327398UK00011B/512/P